Compliments of:

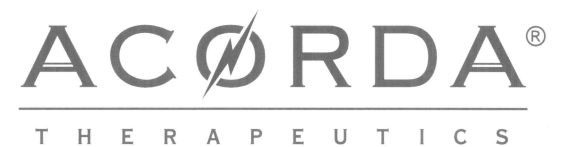

# Multiple Sclerosis

*Immunology, Pathology, and Pathophysiology*

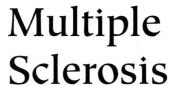

# Multiple
# Sclerosis

*Immunology, Pathology,
and Pathophysiology*

EDITOR

## ROBERT M. HERNDON, M.D.

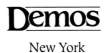

New York

Demos Medical Publishing, Inc., 386 Park Avenue South, New York, New York 10016

Library of Congress Cataloging-in-Publication Data

Multiple sclerosis : immunology, pathology, and pathophysiology / Robert M. Herndon, editor.
    p. ; cm.
Companion v. to: Multiple sclerosis: diagnosis, medical management, and rehabilitation / edited by Jack S. Burks and Kenneth P. Johnson.
Includes index.
  ISBN 1-888799-62-5 (pbk.)
  1. Multiple sclerosis. [DNLM: 1. Multiple Sclerosis—immunology.   2. Multiple Sclerosis—pathology.   3. Multiple Sclerosis—physiopathology.  WL 360 M95648 2002] I. Herndon, Robert M.   II. Multiple sclerosis.   III. Title.
  RC377 .M848 2002
  616.8'34—dc21

                                                                          2002015198

Made in the United States of America

# Dedication

This book is dedicated to the memory of three dedicated physician scientists who made important contributions to the study of MS:

Lawrence Jacobs (1938–2001) friend, colleague, and partner in the pioneering work that developed interferon beta-1a for the treatment of MS. It was his dedication to improving MS care and his drive that resulted in the early introduction of interferon beta-1a as a treatment for multiple sclerosis. He was a leader in the development of the New York State Consortium which will continue to improve the care of those with MS.

John N. Whitaker, M.D. (1940–2001) friend and fellow graduate of the University of Tennessee Medical School, a leader in neurology, who made numerous clinical and basic contributions to our understanding of MS. John was a quadruple threat. He was an outstanding administrator and clinician and a leader in both basic and clinical research. He was a true gentleman, respected by all who knew him.

John Trotter, M.D. (1943–2001) an outstanding clinician and investigator who made numerous contributions to the immunology of MS. He will be remembered as an outstanding teacher who trained a number of the outstanding immunologists currently working in the field of MS.

# Contents

# Preface

It is now more than 160 years since the first clinico-pathological descriptions of cases of multiple sclerosis (MS) by Carswell and the more extensive descriptions by Cruveilhier. It is more than 130 years since the classic clinical description and development of diagnostic criteria by Charcot yet MS remains an enigma. After decades of intense effort to find the cause, no cause has been clearly identified and the disease remains poorly understood.

Understanding the complexities of the disease requires information from a host of disciplines. As one who has been involved in the basic sciences related to MS, in clinical trials of new therapies and in the day to day care of MS patients, I have dealt with the frustration of failed attempts to discover the etiology (ies) of the disease. I have followed numerous failed and a few successful clinical trials. I have watched patients progress from normal healthy working adults to increasingly disabled wheelchair bound and bed bound states and seen patients die from complications of MS because of the inadequacy of our therapies. The situation is somewhat better since the introduction of immunomodulatory therapies and immunosuppressive regimens but it remains a devastating disease. While a great deal of progress has been made, much remains to be done. Our understanding of the disease remains limited; treatments remain inadequate and comprehensive management all too rare.

The purpose of the current work is to provide an overview of the basic sciences as they relate to MS and thus provide clinicians and investigators a better understanding of the basic aspects of the disease. While it is possible to find excellent reviews of almost any aspect of MS,

few attempts have been made to bring these very different aspects together in a single source. This volume is intended as a companion volume to *Multiple Sclerosis: Diagnosis, Medical Management, and Rehabilitation* by Jack S. Burks and Kenneth P. Johnson, Demos Medical Publishers, New York, 2000. Together, they represent an attempt to comprehensively cover the field of MS from basic research to comprehensive management and to provide a broad overview for those interested in understanding the disease better or in pursuing MS research.

Science has been compared to an expanding sphere with a core of knowledge and a surface abutting the unknown. As our volume of knowledge increases so does the interface with the unknown. However, I think the growth of knowledge is much more complex and chaotic than that, more like the growth of crystals in a eutectic medium. Spines spread out from the initial crystal and these develop as new centers of growth. The individual spines don't take up much volume but as they grow in diameter and the space between and around the spines fills in, knowledge grows rapidly. New technologies such as MRI, MR spectroscopy, polymerase chain reaction, DNA hybridization are combined with more traditional knowledge and applied to new areas, rapid increases in knowledge occur.

It is not enough to understand the immunology of experimental autoimmune encephalomyelitis (EAE). Drugs effective in EAE have rarely worked in MS but when you combine our knowledge of immunology, much of it derived from studies of EAE, with that derived from work on human disease and particularly MS, the similarities and differences provide new knowledge. When clinical studies, immunology and pathology are combined, we get new insights, which may lead to a new classification of MS. This in turn may allow new approaches to discovery of the etiology. It makes an enormous difference whether MS is one, two or several different diseases when you are searching for the etiology. If it is more than one disease, we shouldn't expect to find a single cause. In the peripheral demyelinating disease, Guillian-Barre syndrome, at least 4 causes have been identified. Insight into the various types of MS derived from recent immunopathological studies may lead to the ability to clinically distinguish the different types which would be enormously useful in identification of the causes.

Studies of remyelination in animals provided the information necessary to establish the occurrence of remyelination in MS and changed the question. It was no longer why doesn't remyelination occur or why doesn't remyelination occur in man. The question became what is the role of demyelination in recovery from attacks of MS and why is so poor later in the disease process. When information from clinical trials, basic neurobiology of demyelination and its effects on axon transport and the effects of metabolic overload on axons is combined we develop insights into the possible relationship between relapsing remitting disease and secondary progressive disease.

It is clearly not enough to understand just the pathology of MS or the neurochemistry of myelin or MRI or the physiology of demyelinated fibers. In order to conquer this disease, we need to understand all aspects of the disease process and how the various aspects relate to each other.

This volume attempts to cover the basic sciences related to MS and to integrate them so that relationships between the various disciplines are evident. Some choices have had to be made. There is undoubtedly important information in the fields of genetics and epidemiology that are inadequately covered in this volume. Readers interested in these particular areas should refer to one of the recent comprehensive reviews of these aspects of the disease.

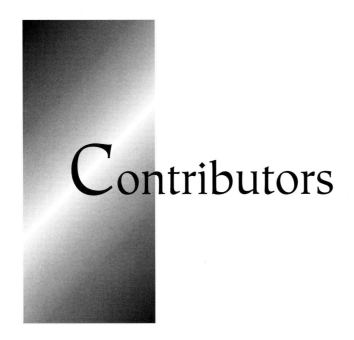

# Contributors

LaChelle R. Arredondo
Department of Neurology
University of Texas Southwestern Medical Center
Dallas, Texas

Joyce A. Benjamins, Ph.D.
Professor and Associate Chair for Research
Department of Neurology
Wayne State university School of Medicine
Detroit, Michigan

Tanuja Chitnis, M.D.
Instructor in Neurology
Harvard Medical School
    and
Associate Neurology
Department of Neurology
Brigham and Women's Hospital
Boston, Massachusetts

Suhayl Dhib-Jalbut, M.D.
Professor of Neurology
University of Maryland School of Medicine and
    Department of Veteran's Affairs
Baltimore, Maryland

Zsuzsa Fabry, Ph.D., Associate Professor
Department of Pathology
University of Wisconsin-Madison
Madison, Wisconsin

Robert S. Fujinami, Ph.D.
Department of Neurology
University of Utah School of Medicine
Salt Lake City, Utah

John E. Greenlee, M.D.
Chief of Neurology Service
VASLCHCS
    and
Professor of Neurology and Interim Chairman
University of Utah
Salt Lake City, Utah

Robert M. Herndon, M.D.
Department of Neurology
University of Mississippi Medical Center
Jackson, Mississippi

William J. Karpus, Ph.D.
Department of Pathology
Northwestern University Medical School
Chicago, Illinois

Samia J. Khoury, M.D.
Department of Neurology
Brigham and Women's Hospital
Boston, Massachusetts

Jane E. Libbey, M.S.
Department of Neurology
University of Utah School of Medicine
Salt Lake City, Utah

Amy E. Lovett-Racke
Department of Neurology
University of Texas Southwestern Medical Center
Dallas, Texas

**Harold Moses, Jr., M.D.**
Assistant Professor, Neurology
Vanderbilt University Medical Center
Nashville, Tennessee

**Michael K. Racke, M.D.**
Associate Professor of Neurology and the Center for
    Immunology
Vice Chairman of Neurology Research
University of Texas Southwestern Medical Center
Dallas, Texas

**Richard M. Ransohoff, M.D.**
The Lerner Research Institute
Cleveland Clinic Foundation
Cleveland, Ohio

**Emily K. Reinke**
Graduate Student
Neuroscience Training Program
University of Wisconsin-Madison
Madison, Wisconsin

**John W. Rose, M.D.**
Assistant Chief of Neurology
Neurovirology Research Laboratory
VASLCHCS
    and
Professor of Neurology
University of Utah
Salt Lake City, Utah

**Matyas Sandor, Ph.D.**
Associate Professor
Department of Pathology
University of Wisconsin-Madison
Madison, Wisconsin

**Fredrick J. Seil, M.D.**
Professor Emeritus of Neurology
Oregon Health and Science University
Portland, Oregon

**Diane L. Sewell, Ph.D.**
Research Associate
Department of Pathology
University of Wisconsin-Madison
Madison, Wisconsin

**Jack H. Simon, M.D., Ph.D.**
Professor of Radiology, Neurology, and Neurosurgery
University of Colorado Health Sciences Center
Denver, Colorado

**Robert P. Skoff, Ph.D.**
Professor of Anatomy and Cell Biology
Wayne State University School of Medicine
Detroit, Michigan

**Subramaniam Sriram, M.D.**
Professor of Experimental Neurology
Professor of Microbiology and Immunology
Vanderbilt University Medical Center
Nashville, Tennessee

# Multiple Sclerosis

*Immunology, Pathology, and Pathophysiology*

# 1

# Developments in Multiple Sclerosis: Research Overview

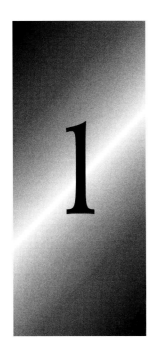

*Robert M. Herndon, M.D.*

he history of multiple sclerosis (MS) goes back at least to the early 19th century and perhaps a good deal further. In a recent review of early cases thought to be MS, Dr. T. J. Murray reviewed the early cases including the case of the blessed Lidwina of Schiedam, born April 18, 1380 (1). The daughter of a laborer with nine children, she developed an acute illness around age 15 years from which she gradually recovered. No details of this illness are recorded. In February 1396 she went skating with friends on a frozen canal and fell, and was thought to have broken some ribs on her right side. Subsequently she had difficulty walking and used furniture for support. She developed severe lancinating pains in her teeth, which suggests tic doloreux. Later she developed blindness in one eye and light sensitivity in the other. By age 19 years, walking was difficult and her right arm was paralyzed. In 1407 she began experiencing "ecstasies, and visions in which she participated in the passion of Christ, saw purgatory and heaven, and visited with the saints." A cult grew up around her. "Towns-people reported that her putrefying body gave off a fra-grant perfume." It was claimed that communion was her only sustenance during the last 17 years of her life. She slowly deteriorated, with increasing paralysis, and devel-oped pressure sores. She lived until April 1433, just short of her 54th birthday. The reports were carefully reviewed by Dr. Murray, who remarked, "I am more convinced that

the evidence suggests elements of marked religiosity, mys-ticism, histrionic behavior and even self-mutilation. Despite the possibility of some underlying neurologic dis-ease, the diagnosis must be left open."

Dr. Murray then discussed several other cases. Margaret Davis was an English housewife who died in 1701 after a prolonged illness. Her illness apparently began soon after childbirth and waxed and waned over more than 20 years, eventually leading to spastic paral-ysis of both legs and then both arms. Another is that of a Hudson Bay trader who in 1811 developed weakness in his legs at age 21 years. This was followed by visual problems and progressive weakness which caused him to give up his job and return home. Both cases are very suggestive of MS.

The most convincing early case of MS is that of Augustus d'Este, (1,2) an illegitimate grandson of George III and cousin of Queen Victoria, who kept a diary of his illness. This is a very convincing description of exacer-bations including attacks of paraparesis. The disease began with blurred vision in 1822, which gradually cleared without treatment but recurred twice during the next few years. In 1827 he again developed visual loss and diplopia. He then developed numbness in his legs. He underwent numerous therapies without benefit; the dis-ease waxed and, with continued progression of leg weak-ness, lead to his death in 1848. D'Este's diary is of par-ticular interest as it describes a very large number of treatments and remedies current at the time and gives an excellent detailed account of a disease that was undoubtedly MS.

Other early cases discussed by Dr. Murray include that of the famous German poet Heinrich Heine, the Scottish lighthouse keeper Alan Stephenson, and the Victorian writer Margaret Gatty. The absence of good descriptions of earlier cases cannot be taken as evidence that the disease was not present earlier. Rather, it likely has to do with the primitive state of medicine and the paucity of good descriptions. In reality, a disease does not exist as such until it is described and named.

The first major advance in our understanding of MS occurred with the pathologic report of cases of MS by R. Carswell, a Scottish physician working in Paris (3,4) who published in 1838 a fascicle describing the pathology of several cases. Subsequently J. Cruveilhier (5) in 1841 published a series of cases, including clinical descriptions of the course in some of those cases. Jean Martin Charcot built on that work, developing clinical criteria for the diagnosis. He made a number of important clinical and histologic observations, including the observation that demyelinated fibers are often preserved and that demyelinated fibers are capable of conduction. It was his development of clinical diagnostic criteria that established MS as a clinical disease entity (6).

The next important advance occurred with the introduction of lumbar puncture. In 1891 there were two reports of lumbar puncture. W. Essex Wynter reported the treatment of tuberculous meningitis by "paracentesis of the theca vertebralis" (7). In two cases this was done with a trocar, the other two by surgical exposure of the lumbar theca and insertion of a drain. Soon thereafter, H. Quincke reported an attempt to treat hydrocephalus by lumbar puncture and introduced the method we still use today (8). He recognized the diagnostic potential of cerebrospinal fluid (CSF). He noted the increased pressure in some of his cases and increased protein in cases of tuberculous meningitis. Within a very few years, cell count protein and sugar levels became routine tests of spinal fluid.

Application of the colloidal gold test for immunoglobulin (Ig) by Lange in 1910 (9), a test used primarily for central nervous system syphilis, to CSF in MS cases made it clear that there were Ig abnormalities in many cases of MS. The colloidal gold test was largely supplanted by a qualitative test for globulin, developed by Pande, which was used into the 1960s. This was gradually replaced by a quantitative assay for Igs initially introduced by E. A. Kabat in 1948 (10,11) although it did not become widely used until the 1960s. Further studies led to the introduction of more quantitative measures of intrathecal Ig synthesis with the development of the IgG synthesis rate (12) and the IgG index (13). Electrophoresis of CSF proteins led to the discovery of oligoclonal bands, which rapidly became a standard diagnostic test

(14). The discovery of free κ light chains and their increased specificity for MS relative to other Ig measures did not lead to a similar acceptance, most likely because of the difficulty with the assay (15). Nevertheless, the many IgG studies have contributed significantly to our diagnostic armamentarium.

The discovery of free myelin fragments in the CSF in MS (16) and the subsequent introduction of the CSF assay for myelin basic protein (MBP) (17,18) have proved considerably less useful. Although often positive in MS, the SCF assay has very limited utility, but the development of the assay for an MBP-like substance in urine by the late John Whitaker may yet prove of some value (19).

In the meantime, the discovery of experimental autoimmune encephalomyelitis (EAE) by T. M. Rivers and F. F. Schwentker (16) provided the first good animal model of a demyelinating disease. Work on this model has contributed enormously to our understanding of immunology and—even though it is clear that MS is not simply human EAE and most treatments that work in EAE have failed in MS—it has added enormously to our understanding of MS.

The demonstration that Guillian–Barre syndrome, otherwise known as acute *infectious polyneuropathy* or *postinfectious polyneuropathy*, can be caused by several agents including Epstein-Barr virus, *Campylobacter jejuni* and influenza vaccine and that it results from molecular mimicry has added much to our understanding of autoimmune disease (20). The fact that it sometimes evolves into chronic inflammatory demyelinating polyneuropathy, a relapsing disorder of peripheral myelin, has contributed to our understanding of autoimmune demyelination and to the possibility that MS could be autoimmune in origin or at least have autoimmune features.

Numerous advances in virology also have contributed to our understanding of demyelination. Several viral diseases have been used to study viral demyelination. Viruses that cause demyelination in mice and other species include JC virus, a human papova virus that causes demyelination in immunodeficient patients (21), mouse hepatitis virus (22), and Theilers' virus (23). This has contributed a great deal to our understanding of infectious demyelination and the process of remyelination.

Immunology as a field of investigation dates back to the work of Edward Jenner and the introduction of vaccination in the 1790s. The subsequent development of anthrax vaccine by Louis Pasteur in 1881 put immunology "on the map" as a science and resulted in the introduction of numerous other vaccines. This was followed by the introduction of numerous anti-sera for treatment of infections and especially for the treatment of pneumcoccal pneumonia. Use of these anti-sera disappeared with the introduction of penicillin, but their use was important to the medical armamentarium in the 1920s and 1930s.

The discovery and differentiation of T-lymphocytes and B-lymphocytes in the 1950s started a revolution in immunology. Since then, the separate roles of T and B cells in immunology and the subclassification of these cells into T-helper and T-suppressor cells, followed by further subclassification, has enormously increased our understanding of immunology. Moreover, the discovery of the role of the various cell types in different inflammatory diseases, the special character of immune reactions in the brain (as discussed in Chapter 5) and the discovery of cytokines, chemokines, and interferons (discussed in section III), have added to our understanding of the complex immune reactions in MS.

The independent discovery of interferons by two different groups (24,25) in the late 1950s led to the development of means to manufacture them. One of the major hypotheses regarding the etiology of MS was that it was a viral disease, so interferons were soon tried in MS. The early trials of interferons were unsuccessful, probably largely as a result of inadequate sensitivity in trial design and too low a dosage (26). In 1986 L. Jacobs and colleagues reported the first successful trial of B interferon with the intrathecal route (26). Subsequently, trials of subcutaneous interferon B-1b (27,28), followed by the intramuscular and later subcutaneous interferon B-1a, led to their introduction into our therapeutic armamentarium (29,30).

During that period, glatiramer acetate (Copaxone® formerly copolymer-1) underwent several clinical trials that eventually led to its introduction into our therapeutic armamentarium (31).

The study of remyelination began in the late 1950s when M. B. Bunge and colleagues reported remyelination in the cat after demyelination by barbotage (32). Subsequent work by R. M. Herndon, S. K. Ludwin, L. Arenella and O. R. Hommes (33–36) demonstrated that mature oligodendrocytes were capable of dividing, that new oligodendrocytes could be regenerated from undifferentiated precursor cells, and that remyelination was a regular event in every species tested. Subsequently, J. W. Prineas and E. Connell demonstrated that remyelination can be seen regularly in early MS in humans (37).

The introduction of polymerase chain reaction (PCR) in the 1980s and the subsequent development of representational difference analysis led to the identification of herpes type VI in MS tissue and in oligodendroglia in one case of MS (38). Further investigation associated activated herpes VI and VII with MS (38–40), but not with other neurologic diseases. This approach carries considerable promise for identifying infectious agents in MS patients.

Knowledge has been described as being like an expanding sphere, with the volume of knowledge contacting a surface on the unknown. The more knowledge expands, the more the surface area contacts with the unknown. I prefer the analogy of an enlarging crystal in a eutectic environment. Numerous spines stick out from the core of the crystal, and their tips serve as new centers of growth while the core expands and spines steadily expand at their base. The spines represent new discoveries in a narrow field, such as the introduction of polymerase chain reaction, immunocytochemistry, or the development of monoclonal antibodies. These add only a small increment to the volume of knowledge, but as they develop, the spines expand, their tips serve as new centers of growth, and their new applications spread the base. They then are used in combination with other techniques and applied to various problems, filling in the space between the spines, and resulting in a marked increase in the volume of knowledge.

I have touched only on a few of the many fields that have affected our understanding of MS. The fields of neurophysiology, neurochemistry, genetics, epidemiology, and many others have made important contributions. In doing research on MS, it is not enough to know clinical neurology, neurochemistry, neuroanatomy, or pathology. If you are working in one of these areas, it is not enough to know only that area; you also need to understand the areas that relate to what you are doing and to have some notion of how ideas from these areas relate to and affect your work. It is also useful to know how your work is likely to affect other areas. Only by combining techniques can we add to the knowledge base in major ways and begin to understand the complexities of the disease. This volume is intended to provide an overview of MS-related research. Inevitably, some areas will be left out, but it is my hope that the general overview presented in this volume will prove useful to many investigators in the field and help to advance our efforts to cure this thus far intractable disease.

# References

1. Murray J. The saint, the king's grandson, the poet, and the victorian writer: Instances of MS when the disease did not have a name. *Int J Mult Scler Care* [serial online]. June 2001; 3(2): 1.
2. Firth D. *The Case of Augustus d'Este.* Cambridge: Cambridge University Press; 1948.
3. Carswell R. *Pathological Anatomy: Illustrations of the Elementary Forms of Disease.* London: Longmans, Green and Co., 1838.
4. Compston A. The 150th anniversary of the first depiction of the lesions of multiple sclerosis. *J Neurol Neurosurg Psychiatry* 1988; 51:1249–1252.
5. Cruveilhier J. *Anatomie Pathologique du Corps Humain.* Paris: Bailliere, 1835–1842.
6. Charcot, JM. *Lectures on Diseases of the Nervous System* London: The New Sydenham Society, 1877.
7. Wynter WE. Four cases of tubercular meningitis in which paracentesis of the theca vertebralis was performed for relief of the fluid pressure. *Lancet* 1893; 12:172–175.
8. Quincke H. Die Lumbalpunktion des Hydrocephalus. *Klin Wochenschr* 1891; 32:861–862, 929–933.
9. Lange KC. Ueber die ausflockung von Goldsol durch Liquor cerebrospinalis. *Klin Wochenschr.* 1912; 49:897–901.
10. Kabat EA, Glusman M, Knaub V. Quantitative estimation of the albumin and gamma globulin in normal and pathologic cere-

brospinal fluid by immunochemical methods. *Am J Med* 1948; 4:653–662.

11. Kabat EA, Freedman DA, Murray J, Knaub V. A study of the crystalline albumin, gamma globulin and total protein in the cerebrospinal fluid of one hundred cases of multiple sclerosis and in other diseases. *Am J Med Sci* 1950; 219:55–64.

12. Tourtellotte WW, Potvin AR, Fleming JO, et al. Multiple sclerosis: Measurement and validation of central nervous system IgG synthesis rate. *Neurology* 1980; 30:240–244.

13. Link, H, Tibbling G. Principles of albumin and IgG analyses in neurological disorders. II. Evaluation of IgG synthesis within the central nervous system in multiple sclerosis. *Scand J Clin Lab Invest* 1977; 37:397-401.

14. Lowenthal A, van Sande M, Karcher D. The differential diagnosis of neurological disease by fractionating electrophoretically the CSF G-globulins. *J. Neurochem* 1960; 6:51–56.

15. Rudick RA, Pallant A, Bidlack JM, Herndon RM. Free kappa light chains in MS spinal fluid: A sensitive test with enhanced MS specificity. *Ann Neurol* 1986; 20:63–69.

16. Rivers TM, Schwentker FF. Encephalomyelitis accompanied by myelin destruction experimentally produced in monkeys. *J Exp Med* 1935; 61:689–702.

17. Cohen S, Herndon RM, McKhann G. Radioimmunoassay of myelin basic protein in spinal fluid: An index of active demyelination. *New Engl J Med* 1976; 295:1455–1457.

18. Bashir RM, Whitaker JN. Molecular features of immunoreactive myelin basic protein in cerebrospinal fluid of persons with multiple slcerosis. *Ann Neurol* 1980; 7(1):50–57.

19. Whitaker JN, Wolinsky JS, Narayana PA, et al. Relationship of urinary myelin basic protein-like material with cranial magnetic resonance imaging in advanced multiple sclerosis. *Arch Neurol* 2001; 58:49–54.

20. Ho TW, McKhann GM, Griffin JW. Human autoimmune neuropathies. *Ann Rev Neurosci* 1998; 21:187–226.

21. Padgett BL, ZuRhein GM, Walker DL, Eckroade RJ. Cultivation of a papova-like virus from human brain with progressive multifocal leukoencephalopathy. *Lancet* 1971; 1:1257–1260.

22. Weiner LP. Pathogenesis of demyelination induced by a mouse hepatitis virus (JHM virus). *Arch Neurol* 1973; 28:298–303.

23. Lipton HL. Theiler's virus infection in mice: An unusual biphasic disease process leading to demyelination. *Infect Immun* 1975; 11:1147–1155.

24. Isaacs A, Lindenmann J. Virus interference I: the interferon. *Proc Royal Soc Lond* 1957; 147:258–267.

25. Nagano Y, Kojima Y. Inhibition de l'infection vaccinale par un facteur liquide dans le tissu infect par le virus homologue. *C R Soc Bio* 1958; 152:1627–1629.

26. Jacobs L, Salazar AM, Herndon R, et al. Multicenter, double-blind study of effect of intrathecally administered natural human fibroblast interferon on exacerbations of multiple sclerosis. *Lancet* 1986; 2:1411–1413.

27. Camenga D, Johnson KP, Alter M, et al. Systemic recombinant alpha-1 interferon therapy in relapsing multiple sclerosis. *Arch Neurol* 1986; 43:1239–1246.

28. IFNβ Multiple Sclerosis Study Group and the University of British Columbia MRI Analysis Group. Interferon beta-1b in the treatment of multiple sclerosis. *Neurology* 1995; 45:1277–1285.

29. Jacobs LD, Cookfair DL, Rudick RA, et al., and the MS Collaborative Study Group. Intramuscular interferon beta-1a for disease progression in relapsing multiple sclerosis. *Ann Neurol* 1996; 39:285–294.

30. PRISMS Study Group. Randomized double-blind placebo-controlled study of interferon β-1a in relapsing/remitting multiple sclerosis. *Lancet* 1998; 352:1498–1504.

31. Johnson KP, Brooks BR, Cohen JA, et al. Copolymer 1 reduces relapse rate and improves disability in relapsing-remitting multiple sclerosis: Results of a phase III multicenter, double-blind, placebo-controlled trial. *Neurology* 1995; 45:1268–1276.

32. Bunge MB, Bunge RP, Ris H. Ultrastructural study of remyelination in an experimental lesion in adult cat spinal cord. *J Biophys Biochem Cytol* 1961; 10:67–94.

33. Herndon RM, Price DL, Weiner LP. Regeneration of oligodendroglia during recovery from demyelinating disease. *Science* 1977; 195:693–694.

34. Ludwin SK. An autoradiographic study of cellular proliferation in remyelination of the central nervous system. *Am J Pathol* 1979; 95:683–696.

35. Arenella L, Herndon RM. Mature oligodendrocytes: Division following demyelination in the adult central nervous system. *Arch Neurol* 1984; 41:1162–1165.

36. Hommes OR. Remyelination in human CNS lesions. *Prog Brain Res* 1980; 53:39–63.

37. Prineas JW, Connell F. Remyelination in multiple sclerosis. *Ann Neurol* 1979; 5:22–31

38. Challoner PB, Smith KT, Parker JD, MacLeod DL, et al. Plaque-associated expression of human herpesvirus 6 in multiple sclerosis. *Proc Natl Acad Sci USA* 1995; 92:7440–7444.

39. Alvarez-Lafuente R, Martin-Estefania C, de Las Heras V, et al. Prevalence of herpesvirus DNA in MS patients and healthy blood donors. *Acta Neurol Scand* 2002; 105:95–99.

40. Tomsone V, Logina I, Millers A, Chapenko S, et al. Association of human herpesvirus 6 and human herpesvirus 7 with demyelinating diseases of the nervous system. *J Neurovirol* 2001; 7:564–569.

# I

# MORPHOLOGIC SUBSTRATES OF DEMYELINATION

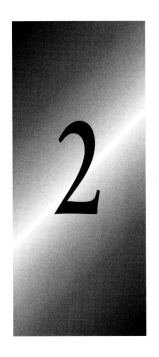

# 2 Morphology of Oligodendrocytes and Myelin

*Robert Skoff, Ph.D.*

Macroglia are composed of oligodendrocytes and astrocytes. They account for 95 percent of the glia in the parenchyma of the central nervous system (CNS); microglia make up the remainder. The major function of oligodendrocytes is to form and maintain myelin for the purpose of saltatory conduction. According to Penfield (1), these cells were first described by Robertson in 1899 and 1900 who called these cells *mesoglia*. Oligodendrocytes and microglia were described in detail by Ramon y Cajal in 1911 (2) but lumped together into the category of the "third element." The first accurate description of oligodendroglia as a distinct cell type is generally credited to del Rio-Hortega who, in 1921, (3) modified the silver carbonate method to distinguish oligodendrocytes from microglia. The prefix *oligo* is somewhat of a misnomer because, although they display fewer processes than astrocytes in silver preparations, we now know from a variety of techniques that they have an elaborate network of fine processes. Oligodendrocytes, believed to be most numerous in white matter tracts of the CNS, are classically referred to as *interfascicular oligodendrocytes* (Figure 2.1), because they are often aligned in rows between the myelinated fibers. However, oligodendrocytes are surprisingly numerous in many regions of the gray matter, where their cell bodies, or perikarya, are often opposed to the perikarya of neu-

rons. Because of this location, they are referred to as *satellite* or *perineuronal oligodendrocytes* (Figure 2.2A). It is still unclear whether satellite oligodendrocytes myelinate a few axons or have metabolic functions not directly related to myelin. Certainly, many myelinated fibers enter and leave the gray matter (Figure 2.2B), and oligodendrocytes that form myelin in gray matter contribute greatly to their total cell number. The spinal cord illustrates this point well (Figure 2.2B) but cortical gray matter presents a similar picture. Electron microscopic cell counts of oligodendrocytes in spinal cord gray matter greatly outnumber those of astrocytes (4), although one might think the converse is true. The density of oligodendrocytes in gray matter can be appreciated with immunocytochemistry or in situ hybridization with the use of oligodendrocyte markers that stain the cell body but leave myelin sheaths unstained (Figure 2.2C). The carbonic anhydrase II isoform, selective for oligodendrocytes (5), is particularly revealing in this regard because it stains up only the perikarya of oligodendrocytes. Because their perikarya are small, approximately 8 to 15 μm in diameter, they are very difficult to identify at the light microscopic level in paraffin or frozen sections stained with classic dyes, including hematoxylin and eosin. Certain classic metallic stains, developed by Ramon y Cajal and del Rio-Hortega, specifically impregnate oligodendrocytes and their processes. However, they stain a fraction of their

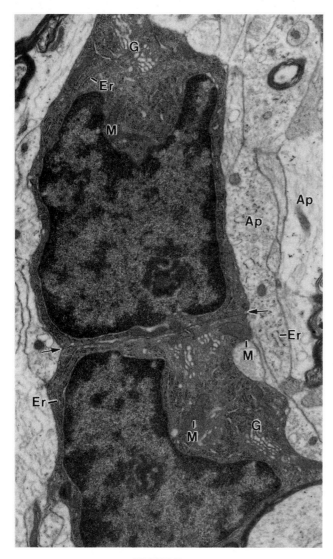

**FIGURE 2.1**

Electron micrograph of oligodendrocytes in white matter of a 47-day-old-rat. The electron density of the two oligodendrocytes contrasts with the electron lucency of adjacent astrocytic processes (Ap). Oligodendrocytes are often aligned in rows parallel to myelinated fibers. The plasma membrane (arrows) between adjacent oligodendrocytes is often obscure, probably due to their electron density. The cytoplasm and processes of oligodendrocytes in ultrathin sections are commonly aligned at one pole of the cell. However, thick sections that reveal the whole cell body connected to its processes show these processes extending in multiple directions (Figure 2.7). The inherent electron density of the cytoplasmic matrix masks organelles that occupy most of the cytoplasm. Golgi apparatus (G), rough endoplasmic reticulum (Er), mitochondria (M), and free ribosomes are much more abundant in oligodendrocytes than in astrocytes and microglia. The endoplasmic reticulum (Er) forms narrow, long strands in oligodendrocytes compared with the thick, short strands in astrocytes. The chromatin in mature oligodendrocytes forms distinct clumps beneath the nuclear membrane and the nucleoplasm. 13000X

total number. Even in 1-μm semithin plastic sections, which provide much better preservation and resolution of tissue, identification of oligodendrocytes is not always possible (Figure 2.2A).

Our understanding of the complex morphology of oligodendrocytes and their intimate relation to other glia and neurons has been achieved, not just from one technique but by the blending of many different techniques. In the 1990s, intracellular injections of horseradish peroxidase or fluorescent dyes into individual cells showed additional details about the 3-dimensional morphology of oligodendrocytes and astrocytes. The combination of horseradish peroxidase labeling, which fills the finest processes, and the resolution of electron microscopy has provided information about the relation between structure and function of oligodendrocytes with regard to astrocytes and neurons (6–8).

## SUBTYPES OF OLIGODENDROCYTES

Del Rio-Hortega and others (9,10) described subtypes of oligodendrocytes based on the size of the oligodendrocyte cell body, the number of internodes formed by an individual oligodendrocyte, and the thickness and length of the internode. Del Rio-Hortega distinguished oligodendrocytes with small cell bodies and fine processes (types I and II) from those with larger cell bodies and fewer processes (types III and IV). Types I and II are much more numerous than types III and IV, myelinate numerous axons, and are found throughout the CNS. Types III and IV are involved with myelination of the largest diameter fibers such as those located in the spinal cord and brainstem. Although oligodendrocytes differ morphologically, a commonly held perception is that all oligodendrocytes are created equal in terms of their lineage and biochemical composition. However, recent studies of glial lineages and application of antibody double-labeling methods have led to a re-examination of whether different morphologic subtypes of oligodendrocytes correlate with different biochemical compositions. More recently, Butt et al. (11) found oligodendrocytes that myelinated numerous; small-diameter myelin sheaths were positive for RIP (an oligodendrocyte marker) and carbonic anhydrase II but oligodendrocytes that myelinated a few large-diameter axons were positive for RIP and negative for carbonic anhydrase II. These cells correspond to del Rio-Hortegas types I and II and types III and IV, respectively. Whether these "biochemically" distinct oligodendrocytes have separate lineages has not been investigated. In the chicken, molecular heterogeneity was demonstrated with an antibody that stains oligodendrocytes and myelin surrounding large- but not small-diameter fibers (12). The question of whether different subtypes of oligodendrocytes are intrinsically pro-

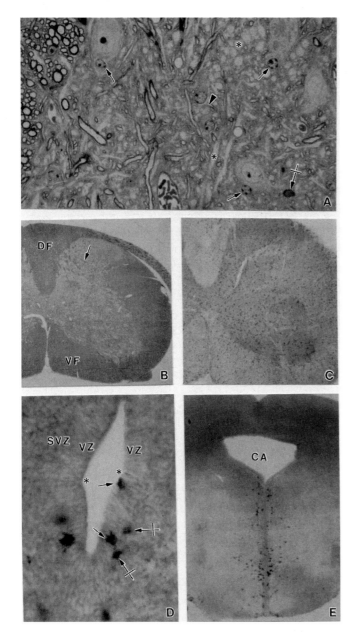

FIGURE 2.2

Light micrographs show the morphology and distribution of oligodendrocytes in white and gray matter (A–C) and the location of oligodendrocyte progenitors during embryonic development (D–E). **A.** A 1-μm plastic embedded section of cervical spinal cord shows the transition between white and gray matter. Myelin sheaths are visualized as dark rings surrounding axons. Dendrites (asterisks) are unmyelinated and of large caliber. At this magnification, the nuclei of glial cells are distinct but their cytoplasm is small and difficult to visualize. Nuclei of oligodendrocytes (arrows) have a thin rim of chromatin around the nuclear membrane and dense clumps of chromatin scattered throughout the nucleus. Nuclei of astrocytes are weakly stained (arrowhead) and oval, and the contrast between chromatin and nucleoplasm is not as pronounced as in oligodendrocytes. A possible microglial cell (crossed arrow) with a bean-shaped nucleus and dense staining is present. **B.** Low magnification plastic-embedded section of cervical spinal cord shows myelinated fibers (arrow) entering gray matter from dorsal funiculi (DF) and leaving through ventral funiculi (VF). **C.** A 50-μm-thick section of a 1-year-old mouse cervical spinal cord immunostained with an antibody against carbonic anhydrase II. The antigen recognized by this antibody is restricted to the cell bodies of oligodendrocytes and allows comparison of their numbers throughout the white and gray matter. In spinal cord, oligodendrocytes are as abundant in gray as in white matter. They tend to be evenly dispersed throughout white and gray matter, and with this antibody they appear larger and more intensely stained in gray than in white matter. **D.** A 100-μm Vibratome section from embryonic day 14 mouse spinal cord. The section was probed for MBP message by using the procedure described by Bessert and Skoff (47). This method provides high resolution and it is possible to distinguish ventricular (VZ) from subventricular (SVZ) layers. Two cells (arrows) are in the ventricular layer, and other cells (crossed arrows) have already begun to migrate away from the proliferative zone toward the basal floorplate. The sulcus limitans (asterisk) delineates ventral and dorsal ventricular halves. **E.** A 100-μm Vibratome section from embryonic day 18 mouse mesencephalon. Cells expressing MBP message are streaming from the cerebral aqueduct (CA) ventrally toward the base of the brainstem. They are also migrating laterally into surrounding neurophil from the cerebral aqueduct. MBP, myelin basic protein.

grammed to myelinate small- or large-diameter axons was addressed by transplantating oligodendrocytes from the optic nerve, where they normally myelinate small-diameter axons, into the spinal cord, where oligodendrocytes myelinate small- and large-diameter axons. Fanarraga et al. (13) found that optic nerve oligodendrocytes could myelinate the larger-diameter axons in the spinal cord of myelin-deficient rats. Other morphologic classifications of oligodendrocytes have been based mostly around the developmental appearance of oligodendrocyte-specific antigens.

The principal function of oligodendrocytes is to facilitate rapid conduction of axon potentials along axons, but other functions associated with specific subtypes of oligodendrocytes are being discovered. One of the most interesting and unsuspected is the finding of glutamatergic synapses on a subset of oligodendrocytes in the hippocampus. Investigators have identified a stage in the differentiation of oligodendrocytes that is characterized by extensive branching of radial processes resembling a snowflake. With the use of an antibody to a proteoglycan to detect these oligodendrocytes or by microinjecting biocytin into cells, these snowflakelike cells in the hippocampus were shown with electron microscopy to possess synapses on their processes. Bergles et al. (14) found that the axonal presynaptic elements contain aggregates of synaptic vesicles congregated near a presynaptic membrane and form a close apposition with a postsynaptic oligodendrocyte membrane. By combining morphology with electrophysiologic techniques, the investigators were able to show that the presynaptic component is derived from pyramidal neurons and that excitatory inward currents are elicited in the oligodendrocytes. These low-affinity α-amino-3-hydroxy-5-methyl-4-isoxazole-propionate (AMPA) receptors on oligodendrocytes are mediated by glutamate. The effect of these synapses on oligodendrocyte precursors is unknown, but they may modulate interactions between neurons and oligodendrocytes via calcium and other ions. They also might downregulate oligodendrocyte proliferation because these cells seemingly do not proliferate in the adult nervous system after experimental injury. Interestingly, these oligodendrocytes are postsynaptic to hippocampal neurons, and these synapses possess the morphologic features of typical asymmetrical synapses. The oligodendrocytes respond to non-N-methyl-D-aspartic acid (non-NMDA) receptors and possess electrophysiologic properties of propagating action potentials. With tissue culture, other investigators have found non-NMDA receptors on oligodendrocytes (15).

Age-related changes in the number of oligodendrocytes have been difficult to quantify, but several studies have indicated that they slowly increase with age (16). In the macaque striate cortex, they increased dramatically in postnatal development but continued to increase in 4- to 8-year-old animals (17). As oligodendrocytes age, they acquire nuclear filaments and other organelles, but the biochemical significance of these observations is unclear (18–20). Although little information is available about the aging of oligodendrocytes, this is an area that needs additional investigation because biochemical changes involving turnover of glial messages and proteins may be factors in the initiation or progression of demyelinating diseases and Alzheimer disease.

## ULTRASTRUCTURE OF OLIGODENDROCYTES

Viewed through the electron microscope, each of the three types of adult glia has unique features that permit their definitive identification. It is presumptuous, however, to assume that all glia in the adult nervous system are mature and that all glia have features sufficient to be categorized even in very thin sections. Proliferation and maturation of glial precursors, although modest, occur in the subventricular zone and throughout the white matter in adults (18,21), and identification of these cells at the electron microscopic level as multi-, bi-, or unipotential glial pre-

cursors is open to additional studies. The difficulty in identifying glial cells in the embryonic and early postnatal rodent nervous systems is even more taxing because many immature glia lack diagnostic features of mature glia.

It is usually the combination of several different features that permit identification of a specific glial cell type as an astrocyte, oligodendrocyte, or microglia. Researchers select for publication pictures that exhibit stereotyped features of macroglia, but when viewed through the electron microscope many glia are cut near their edge and have only a few diagnostic features. In semi- and ultrathin sections, the electron density of mature oligodendrocytes stands out as an overall distinguishing feature (Figures 2.1 and 2.2A). Their electron densities contrast sharply with the electron-lucent nature of astrocytes and the more moderate density of microglia. The nuclei and cytoplasm of oligodendrocytes are electron dense. Their nuclear membranes are rimmed by electron-dense clumps of chromatin that extend into the more lightly stained nucleoplasm. In gray matter, the contrast between chromatin and nucleoplasm is not as pronounced in white matter oligodendrocytes, leading to possible misidentification of oligodendrocytes as astrocytes or microglia. The nuclear membrane of the oligodendrocyte is conspicuously more dilated than that of the astrocyte and microglia and abundantly studded with ribosomes.

With regard to the oligodendrocyte's general shape, the plasma membrane of the oligodendrocyte is often irregular, and has angled borders that abut myelinated fibers and astrocytic and microglial processes. This morphologic profile is helpful for oligodendrocyte identification because the plane of section in electron micrographs often fails to show much of the cytoplasm. When cytoplasm is abundant, it tends to be eccentrically located at one pole of the cell body, with the nucleus at the other pole (Figure 2.1). Rough endoplasmic reticulum of oligodendrocytes is much more abundant than in astrocytes and microglia and consists of cisternae of endoplasmic reticulum stacked layer upon layer. The lumen of the endoplasmic reticulum is narrower than that of astrocytes but less so than that of microglia, and the membrane is abundantly studded with ribosomes. The abundance of endoplasmic reticulum is a reflection of the cell's massive protein synthesis machinery. Free ribosomes are also abundant in oligodendrocytes and extend into the cell's distalmost processes, even as far as the node of Ranvier. The occurrence of free ribosomes in the oligodendrocyte's processes is a property distinguishing it from small-diameter unmyelinated axons that lack ribosomes. Messenger RNA for myelin basic protein (MBP), one of the two major proteins of myelin, and messages for several other minor components of myelin, including oligodendrocyte MBP, are transported on free ribosomes into the processes (22–24). This finding suggests that all the translational machinery, including transfer RNA, are likewise transported down the processes. The signal to initiate translation at the tips of the processes is unknown. The Golgi apparatus is also prominent in oligodendrocytes, situated near the nucleus, and consists of four to five cisternae that have a beaded appearance. Mitochondria and microtubules are relatively more abundant in oligodendrocytes than in astrocytes and microglia. Microtubules are randomly oriented in the perikarya but become fasciculated as they enter the oligodendrocytic processes. They undoubtedly play a role in the transport of free ribosomes and other molecules into the distal processes. Mature oligodendrocytes lack intermediate filaments and glycogen, which are abundant in astrocytes.

Freeze-fracture analyses of oligodendrocytic membranes show features not easily interpretable with the electron microscope. The most important of these structural membrane components are aggregates of particles characteristic of gap junctions. With the use of combinations of antibodies and electrophysiologic studies, investigators identified connexin 32 (25–26) as the major gap junctional protein and connexin 45 as a minor gap junctional protein in oligodendrocytes (27). Gap junctions sandwiched between adjacent oligodendrocyte cell bodies, their processes, and myelin at paranodal regions are most common, but they also exist between astrocytes and oligodendrocytes. Interestingly, gap junctional proteins between different types of cells need not be composed of the same protein (homologous) but are often composed of two different proteins (heterologous). In the case of oligodendrocytes and astrocytes, connexin 32 in oligodendrocytes is coupled to connexin 43, the major connexin in astrocytes (28). Gap junctions are channels between adjacent cells that permit the flow of ions, second messengers, and small molecules directly from one cell's cytoplasm to another's. It has been proposed that the coupling of oligodendrocytes and astrocytes functions as a K+ buffer, but other functions cannot be ruled out given the diverse functions of these structures (29). After electrical stimulation, K+ may flow by means of gap junctions through the paranodal loops and then into astrocytes through heterologous channels. Interestingly, connexin 32 immunostaining appears to be restricted to subpopulations of oligodendrocytes that correspond to types I and II of del Rio-Hortega, whereas other subtypes do not express connexin 32 (26).

In electron micrographs, oligodendrocytes in postnatal brain often lack features distinctive of mature oligodendrocytes yet most still have properties sufficient to distinguish them from astrocytes and microglia (Figure 2.3). With 1-h pulses of tritiated thymidine to label cells in the S phase of the cell cycle, Skoff et al. (30) found that, during the second and third postnatal weeks, most labeled cells in the optic nerve are immature oligodendrocytes. The cytoplasm and nucleus were not as electron dense as in mature oligodendrocytes, but they exhibited stacks of

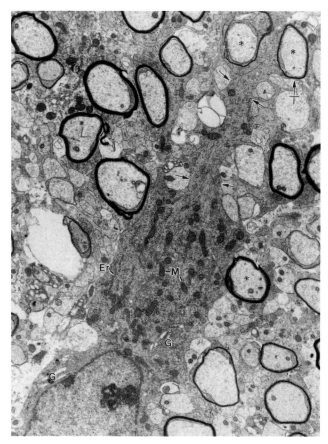

**FIGURE 2.3**

Low magnification electron micrograph of an actively myelinating oligodendrocyte in spinal cord white matter of a 5-day-old mouse. Actively myelinating oligodendrocytes have larger nuclei and more abundant cytoplasm than do mature oligodendrocytes. They are less electron dense than mature oligodendrocytes and, hence, may be confused with astrocytes. Their cytoplasm contains numerous mitochondria (M), Golgi apparatus (G), and rough endoplasmic reticulum (Er). This oligodendrocyte is in direct contact with several myelinated fibers (asterisks) that it is probably myelinating. However, direct connections between the process of an oliogdendrocyte and a myelin sheath are difficult to demonstrate except for the distal tip of this oligodendrocyte's process (arrows), which is directly connected to a nascent myelin sheath (crossed arrow). 10600X

rough endoplasmic reticulum and Golgi apparatus characteristic of mature oligodendrocytes. Although these cells often have several processes, most do not appear to be myelinating axons. Mori and Leblond (18) also used the electron density of oligodendrocytes to distinguish recently generated from mature oligodendrocytes. After examining the electron densities of thymidine-labeled cells at longer and longer intervals after tritiated thymidine injections, they found that immature oligodendrocytes show a weak stain as opposed to mature cells that show stronger stains. These findings agree with light and electron microscopic observations showing that proliferating oligodendrocytes are more weakly stained than mature oligodendrocytes. More detailed ultrastructural descriptions about oligodendrocytes and the history surrounding their identification can be found elsewhere (31).

## ORIGINS AND LINEAGES OF OLIGODENDROCYTES

All macroglia and neurons arise from precursor cells in the ventricular layer of the embryonic nervous system. The ventricular layer is a pseudostratified layer of cells that surrounds the ventricles and extends from the rostral tips of the lateral ventricles to the caudal end of the spinal canal. The subventricular layer immediately adjacent to the ventricular layer is also, especially in adults, a source of glial precursor cells. In adults, the subventricular layer is absent or thinned except at the dorsolateral boundary of the lateral ventricles, where it remains a highly proliferative zone. The *origin* of glia may be defined as the location or region along the neuraxis wherein glial precursors are generated. It is well established that glial precursor cells proliferate in the ventricular layer, migrate laterally from the ventricular layer into the surrounding neuropil, and continue to proliferate and/or differentiate (see reviews in 32–33). However, only recently has it been appreciated that glial precursors also migrate rostrocaudally along the neuraxis for considerable distances (34–36). Therefore, the origin of a glial cell in adult white or gray matter is not necessarily the ventricular layer closest to a particular oligodendrocyte. Of particular relevance to glial migration and glial lineage studies, oligodendrocyte precursors have been found to be present in embryonic development much sooner than previously suspected. By using a combination of different techniques including immunocytochemistry, in situ hybridization, and oligodendrocyte-specific transgenes linked to reporter genes, investigators have examined the origin of oligodendrocyte precursors in the ventricular and subventricular layers. Results from these studies indicated that oligodendrocyte precursors are located only at certain regions along the neuraxis (37–40). Oligodendrocyte precursors in the spinal cord, although present from the cervical to the lumbar levels, are restricted to the ventral half of the spinal cord (Figure 2.2D) (41–44). In the brainstem, they are found principally in restricted areas of the diencephalon and rhombencephalon. In the diencephalon, cells expressing proteolipid protein message are present as soon as embryonic day 9.5 in the mouse (37). The ventricular origins of oligodendrocytes destined for telencephalic structures including the cerebral cortex, striatum, and corpus callosum are still unclear. They may arise exclusively from the diencephalon or from still undetermined locations in the telencephalon (45). During postnatal development we found scattered proteolipid protein and MBP message-positive cells along the lateral and dorsal ventricular layers of the lateral ventricles (46). This observation suggests that the lateral ventricles can generate oligodendrocyte precursors throughout postnatal life. In the spinal cord, cells labeled for myelin-specific genes or with oligodendrocyte-specific markers have been found exclusively in the ventral half of the embryonic spinal cord, but the spatial resolution obtained with radioactive probes and use of frozen sections usually do not provide sufficient resolution to determine whether labeled cells are in the ventricular layer or the adjacent neuropil. This is problematic because cells could migrate longitudinally along the ventricular neuraxis from one area to another, leading to the impression that labeled cells are generated in the adjacent ventricular zone. With in situ hybridization techniques that provide very high cellular resolution, we examined the location of cells expressing MBP and proteolipid protein (PLP) messages. Embryos are perfused intracardially to obtain excellent fixation and complementary DNAs are coupled to digoxigenin to provide high spatial resolution (47). In agreement with previous studies, MBP and PLP transcripts are located only in cells in the ventral half of the central canal between embryonic days 12 and 16 (Figure 2.2D). In the cerebral aqueduct, cells stream ventrally from ventricular layer along the midline to the ventral brainstem and then spread laterally (Figure 2.2E). Not previously reported, the labeled cells in spinal cord always formed a single pair in the ventricular zone opposite each other in the central canal at 14 days of gestation. They also were located stereotypically 4 to 6 cells from the bottom of the basal plate. In the horizontal plane, the pair of cells did not form a continuous band but appeared approximately every 6 cells. Occasionally, an unpaired cell was immediately below the sulcus limitans (Figure 2.2D). The stereotypic location of these oligodendrocytic precursors indicates that adjacent cells interact closely with cells expressing the myelin gene. Whether these signals from surrounding cells are excitatory or inhibitory are unclear. Sonic hedgehog, a morphogenetic protein localized to the notochord and basal floorplate is required for oligodendrocytic development (48–51). By 16 days of gestation, MBP- and PLP-expressing cells in the spinal cord are not found in the ventricular layer but in the subventricular zone and are in the process of migrating ventrally to spread into the mantle and marginal zones. Here, they quickly acquire the phenotypic properties—i.e., several processes and small round nuclei—of immature oligodendrocytes. Our studies showed that the time of origin of oligodendrocyte precursors in the ventricular zone of the spinal cord is limited to just a few days, an important finding. The fact that these cells expressed oligodendrocyte- and myelin-specific transcripts in the ventricular zone strongly suggests that they are committed to becoming oligodendrocytes. Mice that express the PLP/DM20 transgene linked to a reporter molecule during early embryonic development do not yet express the classic myelin glycolipids and proteins; however, during late embryonic and postnatal development, the reporter molecule colocalizes with these myelin glycolipids and proteins in vivo and in vitro (36). This indicates that the embryonic PLP-expressing cells turn into oligodendrocytes. However, it is unclear whether myelin protein gene expression identifies all oligodendrocyte precursors because another set of oligodendrocyte precursors that expresses platelet-derived growth factor α receptor was identified during embryonic development (52). Although cells positive for the platelet-derived growth factor α receptor were in the same vicinity of the cells expressing myelin gene transcripts, they did not precisely colocalize in their position with cells expressing myelin protein genes. Furthermore, they did not seem to be double labeled during embryonic development or postnatal development (53), suggesting that oligodendrocytes may derive from separate lineages.

*Lineage* is used by scientists in many different ways to identify precursors cells of the mature, specialized cells of the body. Lineage can be viewed as tracing one's family tree and, in the case of an astrocyte or oligodendrocyte, its origin from a given cell in the ventricular layer. Ultimately, a particular cell in the ventricular layer can be traced all the way back to the ovum. The *lineage* of a cell should not be confused with the *plasticity* of a cell, which is the potential of a cell to change from its normal in vivo fate to that of another type of cell. Many "lineage" studies are performed with cultured cells and involve experimental manipulation of cells. Cell transformation may depend on the introduction of different growth factors not normally present in its environment, the introduction of transgenes, and altering the type of cells that the cell is not normally in contact with in vivo. The use of the word *lineage* preferably should be limited to in vivo studies to define a cell's normal developmental history or ancestry without regard to what its fate might become in the dish. The lineage of a particular cell type can be determined without knowledge of how cell-to-cell interactions and environmental factors influence a cell's fate. The rediscovery of the stem cell in embryonic and adult animals and their potential to generate many different types of cells in the dish illustrate the plasticity of brain cells (see below).

Lineages of glial cells in vivo have been traced with two different approaches. In the first, described as an anterograde approach, glial lineages are traced forward in time from their proliferation in the ventricular layer as progenitor cells to a mature macroglial cell in adult animals. The strategy in this approach involves randomly labeling ventricular precursors, usually with a retroviral reporter gene, and then determining the types of cells in

a clone. In the second approach, lineages are traced backward in a retrograde method by identifying morphologic and molecular properties of mature cells in less mature cells. With regard to the study of glial lineages, the first approach is more direct than the second, but comparison of the results of both approaches have led to the same basic conclusions.

To trace the lineage of a precursor cell in the ventricle and subventricle, noncompetent retroviruses are injected into the ventricle of embryonic or neonatal rodents. These noncompetent retroviruses transmit the viruses to the cells' progeny but cannot infect adjacent cells. They are further engineered to contain a reporter gene, usually the lacZ gene, which codes for the protein β-galactosidase. Colorimetric development of β-galactosidase permits visualization of the progenitors' progeny. By integrating data from numerous studies (34,54–55; and see reviews in 32–33), the retroviral studies showed that divergence of progenitor cells begins on embryonic day 13 in the cerebellum and embryonic day 15 in the forebrain. At these times and in these structures, more than 85% of the clones consist of astrocytes, oligodendrocytes, or neurons. Interestingly, astrocyte clones were generally restricted to white or gray matter, with little intermixing between the two. All the in situ retroviral studies found mixed clones but fewer than 5% of all clones were bi- or multipotential. These mixed clones consisted of different combinations of neurons and oligodendrocytes, neurons and astrocytes, and astrocytic and oligodendrocytic clones. Radial glial cells, which give rise to astrocytes, have recently been shown to generate in vivo not only astrocytes but also neurons in the neocortex (56). These neurons migrate along the radial glia and then contribute to the radially or vertically organized columns of the neocortex. With the use of time-lapse videomicroscopy, Noctor et al. (56) showed that the neurons migrating along the radial glial processes are derived by asymmetric cell division of the radial glia precursors, one of which remained a glial cell and the other a neuron. The generation of neurons and glia from the same progenitor may depend on the embryonic age of the rodent because clones isolated during embryonic days 14 to 16 generated mostly neurons, whereas more mixed clones were found at later time points (57). Interestingly, clones containing microglial cells have not been described, suggesting that they have a separate, non-neural lineage from macroglial cells. Our current knowledge about neuroglial lineages during in vivo development is shown in Figure 2.4.

The retroviral studies indicating divergence of neuroglial lineages in midembryonic development dovetail with in situ hybridization studies (see above) that found cells in the ventricular and subventricular zones express oligodendrocyte- and myelin-specific genes. Classic electron microscopic autoradiographic studies of postnatal rat optic nerve showed most glia in the S phase

**E15-P0
VENTRICULAR/SUBVENTRICULAR
ZONE**

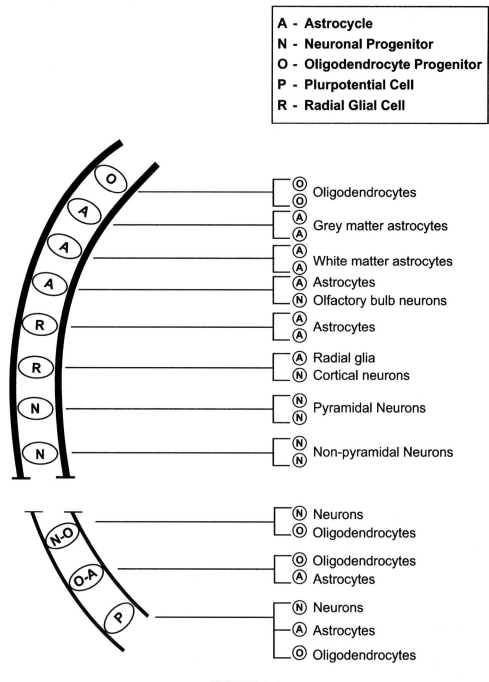

**FIGURE 2.4**

The ventricular and subventricular zones of the brain from mid to late embryonic development are composed of a mosaic of progenitor cells that have the potential to generate adult brain neurons and glia. Based on in vivo retroviral labeling paradigms, this diagram shows the fate of different progenitor cells in the cerebrum. The lineages capped by bold lines show progenitor lines that are likely to form the vast majority of glia and neurons in the cerebrum. The lineages capped by narrow lines represent lineages that have been shown to occur in vivo but probably generate fewer total brain cells. Each lineage may be dominant at different times during development, and it is still unclear which lineage generates the most oligodendrocytes and astrocytes in the adult brain. EI5, embryonic day 15; PO, postnatal day 0.

of the cell cycle expressing the morphologic features of astrocytes and oligodendrocytes (30). A small percentage of microglial cells also was labeled with radioactive thymidine 1h after injection, indicating that they proliferate in situ during postnatal CNS development. Although these studies of the postnatal CNS did not directly identify the lineage of macroglial cells, they indicated that immature astrocytes and oligodendrocytes proliferate and generate mature macroglia. With regard to proliferating oligodendrocytes, these oligodendroblasts are morphologically similar to the cell shown in Figure 2.3 but are somewhat smaller. The oligodendroblasts appear, in most cases, to be premyelinating cells because connections of mitotic or S-phase cells to myelin sheaths are seldom found (58–60). Numerous classic studies have shown that proliferation and mitosis of macroglial cells is not limited to the ventricular and subventricular zones during development but also occurs in white and gray matter tracts (61). Because oligodendroglial proliferation occurs simultaneously around the ventricle and in adjacent white matter tracts during postnatal development, it is difficult to determine the percentage contributions from these different sources. The same conclusion can be drawn for adult animals, where ventricular and white matter proliferation occurs. Tritiated thymidine recently was combined with oligodendrocyte-specific markers to determine which myelin-specific markers are expressed by dividing oligodendroblasts. Those studies found that oligodendroblasts express myelin-specific glycolipids, particularly sulfatide but sometimes galactocerebroside (62). These oligodendroblasts were distributed abundantly throughout the white matter in the postnatal brain, suggesting that local proliferation is the major source of mature oligodendrocytes (62). Occasionally, a few proliferating cells were MBP+ but none were PLP+, suggesting that myelin-specific proteins are not abundantly expressed by proliferating cells. However, the failure to detect myelin proteins in proliferating cells may be due in part to the insensitivity of immunocytochemistry to detect very low levels of myelin proteins. This cautionary statement is based on the observations of many laboratories of the strong expression of myelin gene messages during embryonic and early postnatal development. Whether myelin proteins are immediately degraded or very low levels of proteins are generated in these oligodendrocyte progenitors is still unclear.

In the 1980s and 1990s, tissue culture studies focused on characterization of a bipotential cell named the O-2A cell because this progenitor cell in tissue culture gives rise to oligodendrocytes and a subtype of astrocyte, with certain properties similar to those of the fibrous astrocyte (63–64). These cells in culture, depending on which growth factors are added to the medium and the method of culture, could generate oligodendrocytes or an astrocyte that had long, thin processes, called the type II astrocyte. The type II astrocyte was thought to have arisen after oligodendrocytes were generated and to have a specific function that involved ensheathment of the node of Ranvier (65). However, re-evaluation of the time of origin of astrocytes in the optic nerve showed no major astroglial proliferation after the bulk of oligodendrocyte proliferation (66). Transplantation of all O-2A progenitors harvested from tissue culture and transplanted into the brain developed into oligodendrocytes rather than into astrocytes (67). The counterpart of the type II astrocyte in vivo is unknown. In addition to the bipotential O-2A glial precursor cell, a tripotential glial cell was found in tissue culture that could generate oligodendrocytes and the two subtypes of astrocytes (68).

The pluripotentiality of glial precursors, as first shown in tissue culture, has been extended to neurons. The classic doctrine that no new neurons are generated in the adult brain has been shattered by numerous studies showing modest renewal of neurons in certain regions of brain, especially the hippocampus and olfactory cortex (69–70). Other studies have harvested brain tissue and shown that in the dish neurons, astrocytes, and oligodendrocytes can be generated from a single pluripotent stem cell. The discovery of multipotent stem cells harvested from bone marrow, brain, and other tissues in rodents and humans is relevant to multiple sclerosis because these cells might provide unlimited sources of progenitor cells that can be expanded with growth factors to become oligodendrocytes (71–72). One group identified stem cells in the ventricular and subventricular zones that can be cultured to generate neurons and macroglia (73). In culture, astrocytic monolayers generated neurons and astrocytes, but in this system generation of oligodendrocytes was not reported (73). Other researchers found stem cells in the adult spinal cord that could be clonally expanded to generate neurons, astrocytes, and oligodendrocytes (74). Transplantation of these clonally expanded cells into spinal cord and hippocampus produced neurons, oligodendrocytes, or astrocytes, depending on the local microenvironment. Whether these cells confer the ability to perform normal functions when amplified and transplanted into diseased brains remains to be tested. Relevant to oligodendrocytes is the finding that rodent neocortex contains small numbers of cycling progenitor cells that express NG2, a marker of immature oligodendroglia.

## MYELIN

This section focuses on the structural organization of the myelin sheath (Figure 2.5); the molecular composition of myelin is presented in Chapter 4. The first description of myelin harkens back to the grinding of lenses for light microscopes and Leeuwenhoek who, in 1717, described

A

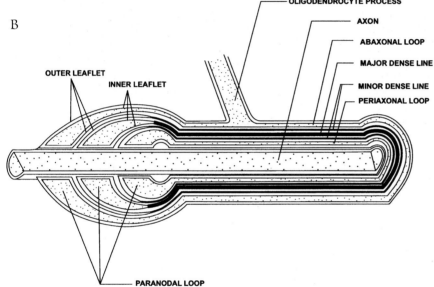

B

C

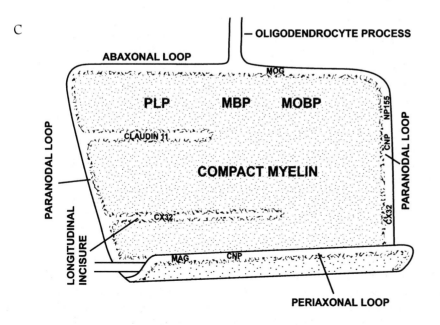

**FIGURE 2.5**

Illustration of the structure of the myelin sheath at different levels of resolution. **A.** Two oligodendrocytes in the white matter extend processes to axons. The node of Ranvier is the unmyelinated segment of the axon. Details of one myelin sheath (boxed area) are drawn at higher magnification in B. **B.** Three-dimensional drawing of a myelin sheath shows the process of an oligodendrocyte continuous with the abaxonal loop (outer loop) of myelin. The outer loop is continuous with the paranodal loops, which in turn is ultimately continuous with the periaxonal (inner) loop. Hence, cytoplasmic continuity between the oligodendrocyte process and the periaxonal loop is always present. In compact myelin, the single inner leaflets of the plasma membrane come together to form the major dense line, and the two outer leaflets fuse to form the minor dense line. **C.** An unfurled myelin sheath illustrates the continuity between longitudinal incisures, which contain cytoplasmic and paranodal loops. The compartmental distribution of the major proteins in myelin are shown.

nervules exiting from the spinal cord and surrounded by fatty tunics; for an engaging history of myelin see Rosenbluth (75). The next major advance in the description of myelin was Ehrenberg's teasing out of a single nerve fiber in the 1830s, not only in the peripheral nervous system (PNS) but also in the CNS; a sobering reflection for myelin biologists in the twenty-first century who pride themselves on their teased fiber preparations. However, general confusion reigned over whether the fatty substance was a sheath surrounding the nerve fiber or somehow deposited within the fiber, like marrow inside bone. The Greek word *myelin*, or *marrow*, was used by Virchow in 1858 to refer to the medullary substance between the axon and its external membrane. In 1871 Ranvier wrote that myelin is not a continuous structure along the axon cylinder but interrupted periodically along its length. Schmidt in 1874 and Lanterman in 1877 described slits running obliquely through the myelin sheath. The birefringence of myelin made it a favorite for X-ray diffraction studies in the 1930s and 1940s. Electron microscopes, although developed at the same time, were primitive in terms of the resolution they offered and did not offer novel insights into myelin structure. Not until the 1970s, with the increased resolution of electron microscopy, were accurate descriptions of the complex structure of the myelin sheath provided. Not to downplay the resolution of electron microscopy, but the development of new fixatives, intracardiac perfusion, and hard resins in the 1970s contributed as much new technology as the electron microscope toward understanding the fine structure of myelin. Also in the 1970s, freeze-fracture analyses of myelinated fibers revealed additional structural features of myelinated fibers such as gap junctions. After much debate, the ultrastructure of the myelin sheath was agreed to in the 1970s, and ultrastructural studies in the 1980s and early 1990s added only modest refinements to our understanding of myelin structure. Myelin studies were revived in the late 1990s by the identification of novel myelin proteins and the use of immunocytochemical methods showing that these myelin proteins have unique distributions in the myelin sheath. And, most importantly, some of the mechanisms involved in the formation of the myelin sheath have been revealed by studying animals which lack or overexpress these myelin proteins; see review by Baumann and Pham-Dinh (76).

Myelin consists of the spiral wrapping of plasma membrane by the oligodendrocyte or Schwann cell around the axon. A segment of myelin is called an *internode*, and, at the distal ends of each internodal myelin segment, the axon is unmyelinated and referred to as the *node of Ranvier* (Figure 2.5A). The schematic is quite misleading with regard to the comparison of internodal length with the size of the oligodendrocyte cell body. Internodes longer than 1 mm (1000 μm) have been found in spinal cord (77), but the average diameter of an oligo-dendrocyte perikaryon is 5 to 15 μm, for a 100-fold difference between maximum lengths of the two structures. Obviously, axons in long tracts of the body are myelinated by many different oligodendrocytes. Because some pyramidal fibers in humans extending from the cortex to the lumbar cord are approximately 1 m long, and an internode is approximately 1 mm, roughly 1000 different oligodendrocytes have contributed to the ensheathment of a single pyramidal axon.

Numerous classic and contemporary studies have examined the relation of the length and thickness of the internode to the axon. Correlation of myelin thickness and internodal length to axon diameter are more easily established in the PNS than in the CNS because individual fibers in the PNS can be teased out and axonal and myelin parameters can be measured more easily than in CNS. The classic literature has extensively documented a positive linear correlation between axonal diameter, myelin sheath thickness, and internodal length for the PNS and CNS (e.g., 78–79). In the PNS, myelin sheath thickness generally correlates with the diameter of the axon (80–82). In the CNS, this same general relation exists, but recent studies have shown the interrelation between the two is not as tightly correlated as in the PNS (83). The anterior medullary velum, or roof of the fourth ventricle, was used to study axon–myelin relation because this structure is very thin and myelin sheaths are scattered throughout the neuropil, permitting examination of single fibers. Predictably, smaller-diameter fibers have shorter internodes than do larger-diameter fibers, but the internodal length of these small-diameter fibers was significantly less than plotted by linear regression analyses (83).

Although considerable evidence exists that axons modulate oligodendrocytic differentiation and regulate myelin sheath thickness (84), less research has focused on the role of oligodendrocytes and myelin in regulating axonal properties. Oligodendrocytes and their processes, even when they do not form myelin sheaths, appear capable of modulating the diameter of axons and the spacing of neurofilaments (85). The evidence partly derives from examination of mutant mice whose oligodendrocytes do not form compact myelin but whose processes loosely enwrap axons. Two proteins in the PNS, peripheral myelin protein 22 kD and myelin-associated glycoprotein, also play roles in modulating the caliber of axons because trembler mice deficient in peripheral myelin protein 22kD (86) and in myelin-associated glycoprotein deficient mice (87) have smaller axonal diameters and decreased neurofilament spacing.

In the CNS, the node of Ranvier was reported to be surrounded by fine astrocytic processes that encircle the bare axolemma (8,88). Three-dimensional reconstructions of these "astrocytic" cells that form the node have shown processes extending to the pia limitans or blood

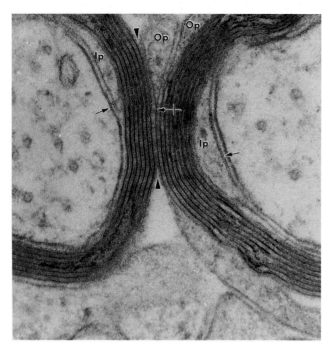

**FIGURE 2.6**

High magnification electron micrograph from the spinal cord of a 57-day-old postnatal mouse. Several outer (Op) and inner (Ip) tongues of myelin sheaths are present. The trilaminar composition of the plasma membrane can be visualized in several areas (arrows). The inner leaflet of the plasma membrane fuses together to form the major dense line (crossed arrow). The two outer leaflets of the plasma membrane fuse together to form the minor dense line (arrowhead). Interestingly, and difficult to explain, the outer loop may be connected to two different myelin sheaths, as is the case here. 175000X

## MATURATION OF OLIGODENDROCYTES AND FORMATION OF THE MYELIN SHEATH

The maturation of oligodendrocyte precursors into myelinating oligodendrocytes occurs at different times in different fiber tracts during development. A general principle is that myelination of fiber tracts begins with the phylogenetically oldest fiber tracts. Hence, myelination of motor and sensory fiber roots and cerebellar peduncles precedes association with cortical areas. This pattern is dramatically illustrated in the human, wherein motor and sensory roots in the PNS begin myelination as early as the fourth fetal month and is completed within several months after birth, whereas association areas are still being myelinated into the third decade (90). Another rule of thumb is that myelination proceeds rostrocaudally in the spinal cord but caudorostrally in the brainstem. In the mouse, myelination begins in the ventral funiculi at birth, in the optic nerve 5 days postnatally (Figure 2.6), and in the corpus callosum approximately 14 days postnatally. Although gradients of myelination can be ascribed to different regions of the brain and spinal cord, the gradient is not precisely tuned and can differ from one species to another. In optic nerves of rats, myelination proceeds from the optic nerve head at the retina toward the chiasm (91–92). In optic nerves of rabbits, the pattern of myelination is more homogeneous than in the rat (92). In both species, myelination is retarded near the optic canal, indicating that local factors modulate myelination along axons. Interestingly, the first myelinated fibers were found adjacent to blood vessels, suggesting factors from the vascular system accelerate oligodendrocyte differentiation (92).

After migration from the ventricular and subventricular zones into the presumptive white and gray matter, the oligodendrocytic precursors undergo a dramatic change in their morphology from bipolar cells to snowflake-shaped cells with multiple radial processes (Figure 2.7A). These snowflake-shaped cells completely blanket the neuropil, such that their processes are likely to be in direct contact with all axons contained within their sphere. The premyelinating cells already express most myelin proteins including MBP (Figure 2.7A) and glycolipids including galactocerebroside and sulfatide (93). These observations indicate that an intrinsic genetic program in oligodendrocytes activates myelin gene expression. The axons "selected" for myelination by an oligodendrocyte are not necessarily the axons closest to the cell body, and all axons touched by oligodendrocyte processes are not ensheathed. The oligodendrocyte shown in Figure 2.7B extends processes to two bundles of fibers on opposite sides of the cell body. This static picture may at first glance give the impression that specific trophic stimuli from axons have persuaded the oligodendrocyte to send processes to these bundles. However, it is likely that the radial processes of the oligo-

vessels, in keeping with traditional theory that all astrocytes contribute processes to form the "blood–brain barrier." The concept that a specialized type of astrocyte, the type II astrocyte, is generated after oligodendrocytes and specialized to form nodal processes (65) has not been proved by extensive light and electron microscopic autoradiographic and immunocytochemical microscopic studies (66). More recently, in addition to classic astrocytes, oligodendrocyte progenitors identified with the NG2 antibody were shown to form processes at the nodes of Ranvier (89). They did not appear to be positive for carbonic anhydrase or glial fibrillary acidic protein (markers for oligodendrocytes and astrocytes, respectively), in keeping with the hypothesis that these cells are likely to be immature glial precursors. It remains unclear whether nodal cells identified as astrocytes in previous studies are all immature oligodendrocyte progenitors or a combination of astrocytes and immature oligodendrocytes.

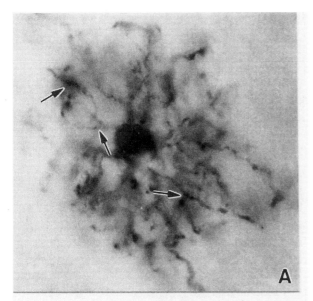
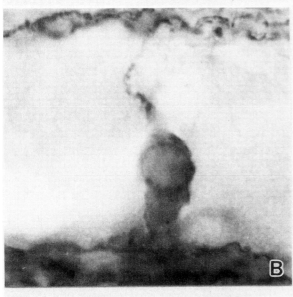
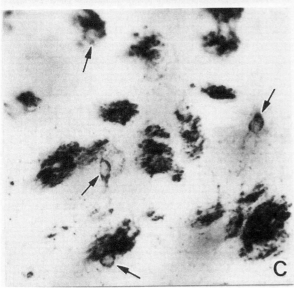

**FIGURE 2.7**

Oligodendrocytes in different stages of differentiation. **A.** A pre-myelinating oligodendrocyte in the cerebrum of a neonatal mouse. The section, immunostained for myelin basic protein, shows an oligodendrocyte with multiple, thin processes that radiate in all directions from the cell body. The processes often branch and interdigitate with each other (arrows) to create a snowflake appearance. 700X. **B.** A myelinating oligodendrocyte in cerebrum of a 5-day-old mouse is visualized with myelin basic protein immunocytochemistry. Immunoreaction product surrounds the spherical nucleus and fills two processes that emerge from opposite sides of the perikaryon. The processes contact several axons that are being myelinated. 1000X. **C.** Striatum of a 14-day-old mouse brain immunostained with an antibody (A007) that recognizes different glycolipids (93). Cell bodies of oligodendrocytes (arrows) in gray matter send their processes into bundles of fibers; other oligodendrocytes are immediately adjacent to fiber bundles; still others, difficult to visualize, are present in the center of white matter fibers. Most antibodies to myelin proteins and glycolipids in late postnatal and adult tissue stain myelin and cell bodies, making it difficult to identify and quantify oligodendrocyte cell numbers in adult tissue. 300X dendrocyte are already in contact with these axons and that axon–oligodendrocytic contacts trigger myelination (94–95). Interestingly, one side of an oligodendrocyte may retain the snowflake appearance, whereas the other side has only long processes that have begun to ensheath some axons. Using confocal microscopy, Hardy and Friedrich (94) found that the first stage of myelin investment consists of the elaboration of a long thin process parallel to the longitudinal axis of the axon. The second stage consisted of the spiral ensheathment and longitudinal enlargement of the oligodendrocyte process around the axon. As the oligodendrocyte begins to form more myelin sheaths, it loses a number of radial processes. Morphologically, axons generally attain a certain diameter for myelination to begin, but this diameter-dependent effect is most likely contingent upon biochemical changes in the axon. Those axons that are myelinated in the anterior medullary velum overlying the fourth ventricles express neurofilament as 200 kD subunits (95). The appropriate diameter might be accompanied by electrical activity because tetrodotoxin blocked myelination in an in vitro system (96). Conversely, α-scorpion toxin facilitates myelination by causing repetitive electrical activity (97–98). Based on electron microscopic studies (99–101), investigators extrapolated that a single oligodendrocyte can form as many as 40 different internodes around axons. However, when using antibodies to label the oligodendrocyte and its connecting processes to myelin internodes, 15 to 20 internodes were the maximum number counted (94,102). In adult CNS, the density of white matter myelin makes it difficult to demonstrate connections of a single oligodendrocyte to all its sheaths (Figure 2.7C).

## STRUCTURE OF THE MYELIN SHEATH

The 3-dimensional structure of the myelin sheath is best appreciated from reconstructions (Figures 2.5B and 2.5C), and in comparison with the high magnification electron micrograph (Figure 2.6). Adjacent to the node of Ranvier, the compacted layers of myelin membrane become unraveled, the inner leaflets of the fused plasma membranes split, and the intervening space is filled with cytoplasm (Figure 2.5B). This region of myelin is called the *paranode* and is enriched in many proteins not normally found in the compacted myelin sheath (Figure 2.5C). A low magnification electron micrograph of internodal, compact myelin cut transversely shows alternating layers of light and dark lines (Figure 2.5B). The dark line, termed the *major dense line*, represents the apposition of the inner leaflets of two plasma membranes in which the cytoplasm between the two adjacent plasma membranes has been extruded during myelin formation. The terms *extruded* and *squeezed out* are often used to describe the

apposition of the two inner leaflets but are undoubtedly misnomers because the mechanism by which the two inner leaflets become opposed is unknown. The formation of the dark line is best visualized at the outermost or innermost lamella, where the two plasma membranes separate and are filled with cytoplasm (Figure 2.6). Usually, a thin rim or tongue of cytoplasm lies adjacent to the outermost and innermost layers of myelin and are termed the *outer* (abaxonnal) and *inner* (periaxonal) *mesaxons*, respectively. The light line represents the fusion of the two outer leaflets of the plasma membrane, and their formation can be visualized in favorable sections at the outer and inner mesaxons (Figures 2.5B and 2.6). The major dense lines are continuous with one another and can be traced as one spiral extending from the outer surface of the myelin sheath to the inner surface adjacent to the axolemma. The layers, or lamellae, are counted from 1 major dense line to another and the larger the number, the thicker the myelin sheath. As one might surmise, very high magnification shows a still more elaborate morphology of the major and minor dark lines. The two outer leaflets do not fuse completely, leaving an intervening gap of 2 nm. Interestingly, this gap has been shown to be penetrable to small molecules including lathanum but not to larger molecules such as ruthenium red or ferritin. Penetration of lathanum occurs despite the tangential rings of tight junctions at the paranodes, at the inner mesaxon, and between cytoplasmic gaps. Similarly, at magnifications greater than 200000X, the major dense line is composed of two lines representing the fusion of the two inner leaflets of the plasma membrane.

The morphologic complexity of myelin is matched by an asymmetric distribution of myelin proteins and lipids. Compact myelin is composed mainly of PLP and MBP; the inner and outer loops are enriched with myelin-associated glyco protein 2',3'-cyclic nucleotide 3'-phosphodiesterase, and myelin oligodendrocyte glycoprotein, and the paranodal loops are enriched with connexin 32 and myelin-associated oligodendrocytic basic protein. Tight junctions between compact myelin and noncompact myelin are enriched with claudin 11 (103–105) and paranodal/axonal membranes are enriched with neurofascin 155 (106). How different myelin proteins and glycolipids are sorted into nodal, paranodal, inner, and outer loops is a matter of intensive investigation (107–108). In addition to segregation of myelin proteins at paranodes and tight junctions, the axon at the nodal and paranodal regions expresses many specific ion channels and proteins. These proteins are discussed further in Chapter 4 and are the subject of a special issue of the *Journal of Neurocytology* (1999;28) devoted to myelin. The recent discovery of many different myelin proteins and their unique distributions in myelin has re-energized the field of myelin research, with the task at hand being to decipher their function in the membrane.

## Acknowledgments

The data in this chapter were supported by grants from the NIH and NMSS. I thank Denise Bessert and Mirela Cerghet for assistance in preparing the manuscript and for performing the immunocytochemistry and in situ hybridization.

# References

1. Penfield W. Neuroglia: normal and pathological In: Penfield W, (ed.) *Cytology and Cellular Pathology of the Nervous System.* Vol II. New York: Hafner Publishing Co, 1965; 423–479.

2. Ramon y Cajal S. *Histologie du système nerveux de l'Homme et des vertébrés.* Vol I and II. Paris: Maloine; Reprinted Madrid, Consejo Superior de Investigaciones Cientificas, 1952.

3. del Rio-Hortega P. Estudios sobre la neuroglia. La glia de escasas radiciones (oligogendroglia). *Bol Real Soc Esp Hist Nat,* 1921; 63–92.

4. Kerns JM, Frank MJ. Non-neuronal cells in the spinal cord of nude and heterozygous mice. I. Ventral horn neuroglia. *J Neurocytol* 1981; 10:805–818.

5. Ghandour MS, Langley OK, Vincendon KG, Gombos G. Double labeling immunohistochemical technique provides evidence of the specificity of glial cell markers. *J Histochem Cytochem* 1979; 27:1634–1637.

6. Butt AM, Ransom BR. Visualization of oligodendrocytes and astrocytes in the intact rat optic nerve by intracellular injection of lucifer yellow and horseradish peroxidase. *Glia* 1989; 2:470–475.

7. Butt AM, Ransom BR. Morphology of astrocytes and oligodendrocytes during development in the intact rat optic nerve. *J Comp Neurol* 1993; 338:141–158.

8. Butt AM, Duncan A, Berry M. Astrocyte associations with nodes of Ranvier: Ultrastructural analysis of HRP-filled astrocytes in the mouse optic nerve. *J Neurocytol* 1994; 23:486–499.

9. Ramón-Moliner E. A study on neuroglia. The problem of transitional forms. *J Comp Neurol* 1958; 110:157–171.

10. Stensaas LJ, Stensaas SS. Astrocytic neuroglial cells, oligodendrocytes and microgliacytes in the spinal cord of the toad. I. light microscopy. *Z Zellforsch Mikrosko Anat* 1968; 84:473–489.

11. Butt AM, Ibrahim M, Ruge FM, Berry M. Biochemical subtypes of oligodendrocyte in the anterior medullary velum of the rat as revealed by the monoclonal antibody rip. *Glia* 1995; 14:185–197.

12. Anderson ES, Bjartma C, Westermark G, Hildebrand C. Molecular heterogeneity of oligodendrocytes in chicken white matter. *Glia* 1999; 27:15–21.

13. Fanarraga ML, Griffiths IR, Zhao M, Duncan ID. Oligodendrocytes are not inherently programmed to myelinate a specific size of axon. *J Comp Neurol* 1998; 399:94–100.

14. Bergles DE, Roberts DB, Somogyi P, Jahr CE. Glutamatergic synapses on oligodendrocyte precursor cells in the hippocampus. *Nature* 2000; 405:187–191.

15. Fern R, Moller T. Rapid ischemic cell death in immature oligodendrocytes: A fatal glutamate release feedback loop. *J Neurosci* 2000; 20:34–42.

16. Ling EA, Leblond CP. Investigation of glial cells in semithin sections II. Variation with age in the numbers of the various glial cell types in rat cortex and corpus callosum. *J Comp Neurol* 1973; 149;73–82.

17. O'Kusky J, Colonnier M. Postnatal changes in the number of astrocytes, oligodendrocytes, and microglia in the visual cortex (area 17) of the macaque monkey: A stereological analysis in normal and monocularly deprived animals. *J Comp Neurol* 1982; 210:307–315.

18. Mori S, Leblond CP. Electron microscopic indentification of three classes of oligodendrocytes and a preliminary study of their proliferation activity in the corpus callosum of young rats. *J Comp Neurol* 1970; 139:1–30.

19. Vaughan DW, Peters A. Neuroglial cells in the cerebral cortex of rats from young adulthood to old age: An electron microscope study. *J Neurocytol* 1974; 3:405–429.

20. Monteiro RAF, Conceição LEC, Rocha E, Marini-Abreu MM. Age changes in cerebellar oligodendrocytes: The appearance of nuclear filaments and increase in the volume density of the nucleus and in the number of dark cell forms. *Arch Histol Cytol* 1995; 58:417–425.

21. Paterson JA, Privat A, Ling EA, Leblond CP. Investigation of glial cells in semithin sections III. Transformation of subependymal cells into glial cells, as shown by radioautography after 3H-thymidine indjection into the lateral ventricle of the brain of young rats. *J Comp Neurol* 1973; 149:83–102.

22. Barbarese E, Brumwell C, Kwon S, Cui H, Carson JH. RNA on the road to myelin. *J Neurocytol* 1999; 28:263–270.

23. Gould RM, Freund CM, Barbarese E. Myelin-associated oligodendrocytic basic protein mRNAs reside at different subcellular locations. *J Neurochem* 1999; 73:1913–1924.

24. Gould RM, Freund CM, Palmer F, Feinstein DL. Messenger RNAs located in myelin sheath assembly sites. *J Neurochem* 2000; 75:1834–1844.

25. Dermietzel R, Spray DC. Gap junctions in the brain: Where, what type, how many and why? *Trends Neurosci* 1993; 16:186–192.

26. Li J, Hertzberg EI, Nagy JI. Connexin-32 in oligodendrocytes and association with myelinated fibers in mouse and rat brain. *J Comp Neurol* 1997; 379:571–591.

27. Kunzelmann P, Blümcke I, Traub O, Dermietzel R, Willecke K. Coexpression of connexin-45 and -32 in oligodendrocytes of rat brain. *J Neurocytol* 1997; 26:17–22.

28. Ochalski PA, Frankenstein UN, Hertzberg EL, Nagy JI. Connexin-43 in rat spinal cord: Localization in astrocytes and identification of heterotypic astro-oligodendrocytic gap junctions. *Neuroscience* 1997; 76:931–945.

29. Chiu SY. Functions and distribution of voltage-gated sodium and potassium channels in mammalian Schwann cells. *Glia* 1991; 4:541–558.

30. Skoff RP, Price DL, Stocks A. Electron microscopic autoradiographic studies of gliogenesis in rat optic nerve. *J Comp Neurol* 1976; 169:291–312.

31. Wood P, Bunge RP. The biology of the oligodendrocyte In: Norton WT (ed.), *Oligodendroglia.* New York: Plenum Press; 1984, 1–45.

32. Skoff RP, Knapp PE. The origins and lineages of macroglial cells. In: Kettenmann H, Ranson BR (eds.), *Neuroglia.* New York: Oxford Press; 1995; 135–148.

33. Skoff RP. The lineages of neuroglial cells. *Neuroscientist* 1996; 2:335–344.

34. Price J, Thurlow L. Cell lineage in the rat cerebral cortex: A study using retroviral-mediated gene transfer. *Develop* 1988; 104:473–482.

35. Walsh C, Cepko CL. Widespread dispersion of neuronal clones across functional regions of the cerebral cortex. *Science* 1992; 255:4334–4440.

36. Spassky N, Goujet-Zalc C, Parmantier E, et al. Multiple restricted origin of oligodendrocytes. *J Neurosci* 1998; 18:8331–8343.

37. Timsit SG, Bally-Cuit L, Colman D, Zalc B. DM20 messenger RNA is expressed during the embryonic development of the nervous system of the mouse. *J Neurochem* 1992; 58:1172–1175.

38. Pringle NP, Nudhar HS, Collarini EJ, Richardson WD. PDGF receptors in the rat CNS: During late neurogenesis, PDGF alpha-receptor expression appears to be restricted to glial cells of the oligodendrocyte lineage. *Development* 1992; 115:535–551.

39. Yu WP, Collarini EJ, Pringle NP, Richardson WD. Embryonic expression of myelin genes: Evidence for a focal source of oligodendrocyte precursors in the ventricular zone of the neural tube. *Neuron* 1994; 12:1353–1362.

40. Dickinson PJ, Fanarraga ML, Griffiths IR, Barrie JM, Kyriakides E, Montague P. Oligodendrocyte progenitors in the embryonic spinal cord express DM-20. *Neuropathol Appl Neurobiol* 1996; 22:188–198.

41. Warf BC, Fok-Seang J, Miller RH. Evidence for the ventral origin of oligodendrocyte precursors in the rat spinal cord. *J Neurosci* 1991; 11:2477–2488.

42. Noll E, Miller RH. Oligodendrocyte precursors originate at the ventral ventricular zone dorsal to the ventral midline region in the embryonic rat spinal cord. *Development* 1993; 118:563–573.

43. Ono K, Yasui Y, Rutishauser U, Miller RH. Focal ventricular origin and migration of oligodendrocyte precursors into the chick optic nerve. *Neuron* 1997; 19:283–292.

44. Pringle NP, Guthrie S, Lumsden A, Richardson WD. Dorsal spinal cord neuroepithelium generates astrocytes but not oligodendrocytes. *Neuron* 1998; 20:883–893.

45. Price J. Glial cell lineage and development. *Curr Opin Neurobiol* 1994; 4:680–686.

46. Skoff RP, Bessert DA, Barks JDE, Song D, Cerghet M, Silverstein FS. Hypoxic-ischemic injury results in acute disruption of myelin gene expression and death of oligodendroglial precursors in neonatal mice. *Int J Dev Neurosci* 2001; 19:197–208.

47. Bessert DA, Skoff RP. High resolution in situ hybridization and Tunel staining with free-floating brain sections. *J Histochem Cytochem* 1999; 47:693–701.

48. Miller RH. Oligodendrocyte origins. *Trends Neurosci* 1996; 19:92–96.

49. Orentas DM, Miller RH. The origin of spinal cord oligodendrocytes is dependent on local influences from the notochord. *Dev Biol* 1996; 177:43–53.

50. Poncet C, Soula C, Trousse F, et al. Induction of oligodendrocyte progenitors in the trunk neural tube by ventralizing signals; effects of notochord and floor plate grafts, and of sonic hedgehog. *Mech Dev* 1996; 60:13–32.

51. Pringle NP, Yu WP, Guthrie S, et al. Determination of neuroepithelial fate: Induction of the oligodendrocyte lineage by ventral midline cells and sonic hedgehog. *Dev Biol* 1996; 177:30–42.

52. Pringle NP, Richardson WD. A singularity of PDGF alpha-receptor expression in the dorso-ventral axis of the neural tube may define the origin of the oligodendrocyte lineage. *Development* 1993; 117:525–533.

53. Butt AM, Hornby MF, Ibrahim M, Kirvell S, Graham A, Berry M. PDGF-alpha receptor and myelin basic protein mRNAs are not coexpressed by oligodendrocytes in vivo: A double in situ hybridization study in the anterior medullary velum of the neonatal rat. *Mol Cell Neurosci* 1997; 8:311–322.

54. Vaysse PJ, Goldman JE. A clonal analysis of glial lineages in neonatal forebrain development in vitro. *Neuron* 1990; 5:227–235.

55. Luskin MB, Parnavelas JG, Barfield JA. Neurons, astrocytes, and oligodendrocytes of the rat cerebral cortex originate from separate progenitor cells; an ultrastructural analysis of clonally related cells. *J Neurosci* 1993; 13:1730–1750.

56. Noctor SC, Flint AC, Weissman TA, Dammerman RS, Kriegstein AR. Neurons derived from radial glial cells establish radial units in neocortex. *Nature* 2001; 409:714–720.

57. Malestata P, Hartfuss E, Gotz M. Isolation of radial glial cells by fluorescent-activated cell sorting reveals a neuronal lineage. *Development* 2000; 127:5253–5263.

58. Sturrock RR. Electron microscopic evidence for mitotic division of oligodendrocytes. *J Anat* 1981; 132:429–432.

59. Sturrock RR, McRae DA. Mitotic division of oligodendrocytes which have begun myelination. *J Anat* 1980; 131:577–582.

60. Meinecke DL, Webster HdeF. Fine structure of dividing astroglia and oligodendroglia during myelin formation in the developing mouse spinal cord. *J Comp Neurol* 1984; 222:47–55.

61. Privat A, Leblond CP. The subependymal layer and neighboring region in the brain of the young rat. *J Comp Neurol* 1972; 146:277–302.

62. Skoff RP, Ghandour MS, Knapp PE. Postmitotic oligodendrocytes generated during postnatal cerebral development are derived from proliferation of immature oligodendrocytes. *Glia* 1994; 12:12–23.

63. Raff MC, Miller RH, Noble M. A glial progenitor cell that develops in vitro into an astrocyte or an oligodendrocyte depending on culture medium. *Nature* 1983; 303:390–396.

64. Raff MC, Abney ER, Cohen J, Lindsay R, Noble M. Two types of astrocytes in culture of developing rat white matter: Differences in morphology, surface gangliosides, and growth characteristics. *J Neurosci* 1983; 3:1289–1300.

65. Miller RH, David S, Patel R, Abney ER, Raff MC. A quantitative immunnohistochemical study of macroglial cell development in the rat optic nerve: In vivo evidence for two distinct astrocyte lineages. *Dev Biol* 1985; 111:35–41.

66. Skoff RP. Gliogenesis in rat optic nerve: Astrocytes are generated in a single wave before oligodendrocytes. *Dev Biol* 1990; 139:149–168.

67. Espinosa A, Monteros deL, Zhang M, de Vellis J. O2A progenitor cells transplanted into the neonatal rat brain develop into oligodendrocytes but not astrocytes. *Proc Natl Acad Sci USA* 1993; 90:50–54.

68. Rao MS, Noble M, Mayer-Pröschel M. A tripotential glial precursor cell is present in the developing spinal cord. *Neurobiology* 1998; 95:3996–4001.

69. Kuhn HG, Winkler J, Kempermann G, Thal LJ, Gage FH. Epidermal growth factor and fibroblast growth factor-2 have different effects on neural progenitors in the adult rat brain. *J Neurosci* 1997; 17(15):5820–5829.

70. Isacson O. The neurobiology and neurogenetics of stem cells. *Brain Pathol* 1999; 9:495–498.

71. Svendsen CN Smith AG. New prospects for human stem-cell therapy in the nervous system. *Trends Neurosci* 1999; 22:357-364.

72. Galli R, Borella U, Gritti A, et al. Skeletal myogenic potential of human and mouse neural stem cells. *Nat Neurosci* 2000; 3:986–991.

73. Laywell ED, Rakic P, Kukekov VG, Holland EC, Steindler DA. Identification of a multipotent astrocytic stem cell in the immature and adult mouse brain. *Proc Natl Acad Sci USA* 2000; 97:13883–13888.

74. Shihabuddin LS, Horner PJ, Ray J, Gage FH. Adult spinal cord stem cells generate neurons after transplantation in the adult dentate gyrus. *J Neurosci* 2000; 20:8727–8735.

75. Rosenbluth J. A brief history of myelinated nerve fibers: One hundred and fifty years of controversy. *J Neurocytol* 1999; 28:251–262.

76. Baumann N, Pham-Dinh D. Biology of oligodendrocyte and myelin in the mammalian central nervous system. *Physiol Rev* 2001; 81:871–927.

77. Murray JA, Blakemore WF. The relationship between internodal length and fibre diameter in the spinal cord of the cat. *J Neurol Sci* 1980; 45:29–41.

78. Friede RL, Bischhausen R. The precise geometry of large internodes. *J Neurol Sci* 1980; 48:367–381.

79. Smith KJ, Blakemore WF, Murray JA, Patterson RC. Internodal myelin volume and axon surface area. A relationship determining myelin thickness? *J Neurol Sci* 1982; 55:231–246.

80. Friede RL, Samorajski T. Relation between the number of myelin lamellae and axon circumference in fibers of vagus and sciatic nerves of mice. *J Comp Neurol* 1967; 130:223–231.

81. Williams PL, Wendell-Smith CP. Some additional parametric variations between peripheral nerve fibre populations. *J Anat* 1971; 109:502–526.

82. Fraher JP. A quantitative study of anterior root fibers during early myelination. II. longitudinal variation in sheath thickness and axon circumference. *J Anat* 1973; 115:421–444.

83. Ibrahim M, Butt AM, Berry M. Relationship between myelin sheath diameter and internodal length in axons of the medullary velum of the adult rat. *J Neurol Sci* 1995; 133:119–127.

84. Kidd GJ, Hauer PE, Trapp BD. Axons modulate myelin protein messenger RNA levels during central nervous system myelination in vivo. *J Neurosci Res* 1990; 26:409–418.

85. Sánchez I, Hassinger L, Paskevich PA, Shine HD, Nixon RA. Oligodendroglia regulate the regional expansion of axon caliber and local accumulation of neurofilaments during development independently of myelin formation. *J Neurosci* 1996; 16:5095–5105.

86. Suter U, Welcher AA, Ozcelik T, et al. Trembler mouse carries a point mutation in a myelin gene. *Nature* 1992; 356:241–244.

87. Yin X, Crawford TO, Griffin JW, et al. Myelin-associated glycoprotein is a myelin signal that modulates the caliber of myelinated axons. *J Neurosci* 1998; 18:1953–1962.

88. ffrench-Constant C, Miller RH, Kruse J, Schachner M, Raff MC. Molecular specialization of astrocyte processes at nodes of Ranvier in rat optic nerve. *J Cell Biol* 1986; 102:844–852.

89. Butt AM, Duncan A, Hornby MF, et al. Cells expressing the NG2 antigen contact nodes of Ranvier in adult CNS white matter. *Glia* 1999; 26:84–91.

90. Yakovlev PI, Lecours AR. The myelinogenic cycles of regional maturation of the brain. In: Minkovski A (ed.), *Regional Development of the Brain in Early Life*. Oxford, UK: Blackwell, 1966; 3–70.

91. Skoff RP. The pattern of myelination along the developing rat optic nerve. *Neurosci Lett* 1978; 7:191–196.

92. Skoff RP, Toland D, Nast E. Pattern of myelination and distribution of neuroglial cells along the developing optic system of the rat and rabbit. *J Comp Neurol* 1980; 191:237–253.

93. Bansal R, Stefansson K, Pfeiffer SE. Proligodendroblast antigen (POA), a developmental antigen expressed by A007/O4-positive oligodendrocyte progenitors prior to the appearance of sulfatide and galactocerebroside. *J Neurochem* 1992; 58:2221–2229.

94. Hardy RJ, Friedrich VL. Progressive remodeling of the oligodendrocyte process arbor during myelinogenesis. *Dev Neurosci* 1996; 18:243–254.

95. Butt AM, Ibrahim M, Berry M. The relationship between developing oligodendrocytes units and maturing axons during myelinogenesis in the anterior medullary velum of neonatal rats. *J Neurocytol* 1997; 26:327–338.

96. Kaplan MR, Meyer-Franke A, Lambert S, et al. Induction of sodium channel clustering by oligodendrocytes. *Nature* 1997; 386:724–728.

97. Demerens C, Stankof B, Logak M, et al. Induction of myelination in the central nervous system by electrical activity. *Proc Natl Acad Sci USA* 1996; 93:9887–9892.

98. Colello RJ, Devey LR, Imperato E, Pott U. The chronology of oligodendrocyte differentiation in the rat optic nerve: Evidence for a signaling step initiating myelination in the CNS. *J Neurosci* 1995; 15:7665–7672.

99. Peters A, Proskauer CC. The ratio between myelin segments and oligodendrocytes in the optic nerve of the adult rat [abstract]. *Anat Rec* 1969; 163:243.

100. Peters A, Vaughn JE. Morphology and development of the myelin sheath. In: Davison AN, Peters A, (eds.), *Myelination*. Springfield Ill.: Charles C. Thomas, 1970; 3–79.

101. Matthews MA, Duncan D. A quantitative study of the morphological changes accompanying the initiation and progress of myelin production in the dorsal funiculus of the rat spinal cord. *J Comp Neurol* 1971; 142:1–22.

102. Sternberger NH, Itoyama Y, Kies MW, Webster HdeF. Immunocytochemical method to identify basic protein in myelin-forming oligodendrocytes of newborn rat CNS. *J Neurocytol* 1978; 7:251–263.

103. Gow A, Southwood CM, Li JS, et al. CNS myelin and sertoli cell tight junction strands are absent in Osp/claudin-ll null mice. *Cell* 1999; 99:649–659.

104. Morita K, Sasaki H, Fujimoto K, Furuse M, Tsukita S. Claudin-11/OSP-based tight junctions of myelin sheaths in brain and Sertoli cells in testes. *J Cell Biol* 1999; 145:579–588.

105. Bronstein JM, Tiwari-Woodruff S, Buznikov AG, Stevens DB. Involvement of OSP/claudin-11 in oligodendrocyte membrane interactions: Role in biology and disease. *J Neurosci Res* 2000; 59:706–711.

106. Tait S, Gunn-Moore F, Collinson JM, et al. An oligodendrocyte cell adhesion molecule at the site of assembly of the paranodal axo-glial junction. *J Cell Biol* 2000; 150:657–666.

107. Kim T, Pfeiffer SE. Myelin glycosphingolipid/cholesterol-enriched microdomains selectively sequester the non-compact myelin proteins CNP and MOG. *J Neurocytol* 1999; 28:281–293.

108. Krämer E-M, Schardt A, Nave K-A. Membrane traffic in myelinating oligodendrocytes. *Microsc Res Tech* 2001; 52:656–671.

# 3 Astrocytes: Structure and Function

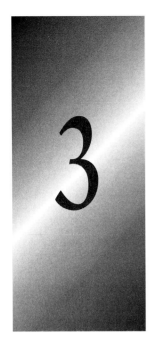

*Robert M. Herndon, M.D.*

Astrocytes play a far more important role in multiple sclerosis (MS) than has been generally recognized. Not only do they form the dense firm scars in areas of demyelination, which led to the term plaque in MS, but they also have important functions in the development and control of the immune response in the nervous system. They are typically stellate, or star shaped cells, although some have highly specialized shapes. They are derived from the neuroectoderm and phylogenetically are closely related to ependymal cells. Their developmental origin and relationship to precursor cells and oligodendrocytes is discussed in Chapter 2. Historically, they were regarded primarily as supporting cells that provide structural support for other cells in the central nervous system and react to injury by forming scars.

Their main role relative to MS was seen as scar formation. Beginning in the 1960s, it became clear that astrocytes are far more complex than previously suspected. They perform a large number of essential functions in the developing and the mature central nervous system (1–3). Many of these functions have been elucidated only in the past two decades, and additional information continues to be added. Functions for which there is substantial evidence include: 1) guidance of cell migration during development, 2) removal of cell debris, 3) structural support, 4) active uptake and metabolism of neurotransmitters, 5) control of the extracellular ionic environment, 6) induction of the blood–brain barrier, 7) elaboration of extracellular matrix constituents, 8) scar formation after injury, 9) regulation of synaptic density, and 10) maintenance of postsynaptic specialization after denervation.

## STRUCTURE AND CLASSIFICATION

There are two basic types of astrocytes: *protoplasmic* astrocytes found primarily in gray matter and *fibrillary* astrocytes found primarily in white matter (Figure 3.1) (4). In addition, a number of highly specialized astrocytes found in particular locations within the central nervous system including tanycytes, Müller cells of the retina, and the Golgi epithelial cells of the cerebellum (Figure 3.2). Intermediate filaments containing glial fibrillary acidic protein (GFAP) are characteristic of astrocytes and rarely, if ever, found in other cell types. These intermediate filaments are much more abundant in fibrillary than in protoplasmic astrocytes and increase dramatically in reactive astrocytes. Astrocytes have few cytoplasmic organelles (Figure 3.1) and an electron lucent cytoplasm. They typically are seen to contain a few mitochondria, a sparse Golgi apparatus, occasional lysosomes and multivesicular bodies, and a very sparse granular endoplasmic reticulum. GFAP-containing intermediate filaments are relatively abundant in fibrillary astrocytes and reactive astrocytes but are sparse in protoplasmic astrocytes.

Astrocytes contain virtually all of what little glycogen there is in the brain and have unique, membrane-associated, orthogonal particle complexes consisting of 5-nm particles arranged in a square on the P face of astrocytic membranes in freeze-fracture preparations (5). The basic unit is a group of four particles arranged in a square, but these aggregate to form rectangular aggregates and parallel arrays of varying length. Although they occur in other cell types outside the nervous system, within the nervous system they are seen only on astrocytes.

Astrocytes in the form of radial glia develop quite early in embryogenesis and play a critical role in development (6). Adult astrocytes remain capable of proliferation, but new astrocytes can develop in the adult from stem cells in the adult brain and spinal cord (7). These glial precursor cells have been shown in culture to be capable of differentiation into astrocytes or oligodendrocytes under the appropriate influences (8). Highly specialized astrocytes include the unipolar Golgi epithelial cells (Bergmann glia) (9) of the Purkinje cell layer of the cerebellum, specialized glia in the inferior hypothalamus called *tanycytes* (10) that extend from the ventricular surface to the pial surface, and the Müller cells of the retina (9).

Astrocytes have a number of important relationships to other structures. Many of their processes have end feet that attach to neurons or capillaries. They form the *glia limitans* at the surface of the brain and spinal cord. End feet closely surround capillaries and venules, and astrocytic processes surround and isolate synapses and synaptic complexes from adjacent brain structures. These close relationships are extremely important to their many functions.

## ROLE OF ASTROCYTES IN GUIDANCE OF CELL MIGRATION DURING DEVELOPMENT

In the development of the cerebral cortex, astrocytes in the form of radial glia extend from the ventricle to the external surface of the developing hemispheres. These serve as guides for neuroblasts that develop in the germinal zone and migrate along the glial processes to reach their final position in the cortex. These radial glia undergo asymmetric division, with one daughter cell remaining as a radial glial cell and the other migrating along the radial process to become a neuron, an oligodendrocyte, or a more peripherally located astrocyte. Successive waves of migrating neuroblasts form the various layers of the cortex.

In the cerebellum, the radial glia serve as guides for the inward migration of the external germinal cells that migrate in, past the Purkinje cell layer, and develop into granule cells. These radial glia lose their ventricular attachment and translocate to the Purkinje cell layer where they become Golgi epithelial cells (Bergmann glia) (11). The role of the radial glia in embryogenesis has been studied in considerable detail by Rakic (6).

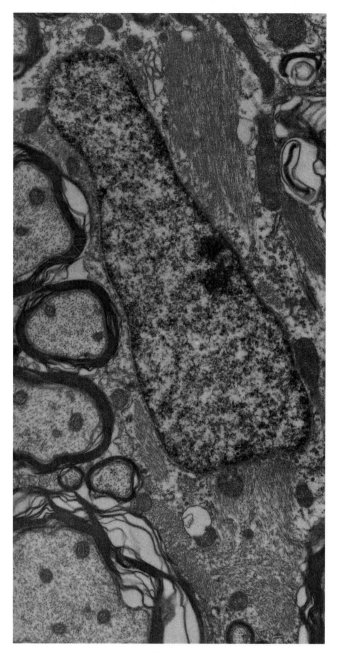

**FIGURE 3.1**

Fibrillary astrocyte in the white matter of normal mouse brain. Note the numerous glial filaments and sparse organelles. A bit of Golgi apparatus can be seen at the top. Original magnification, X 19000 X.

## PHAGOCYTIC ROLE OF ASTROCYTES

Astrocytes are capable of phagocytosis. They appear to play an important role in removing the debris left by programmed cell death. It has been estimated that up to 50% of the neurons formed during embryogenesis die by apoptotic mechanisms as part of development. Removal of the debris left by these apoptotic cells is a substantial task and appears to be carried out largely by astrocytes without any evidence of an inflammatory response. They are not as effective or efficient as microglia or macrophages in clearing cell debris but clearly play an important role in cleaning up cell debris during developmental apoptotic cell death, remodeling of neural processes, and during recovery from injury (12,13). They probably play a role in removing debris when cell death occurs during normal aging and in pathologic processes.

## STRUCTURAL SUPPORT

The structural support function of astrocytes is apparent in the term *glia*, or glue. Clearly, early anatomists recognized a structural function, an idea that has been reinforced by the discovery of glial cell adhesion molecules and by their demonstrated ability to synthesize the matrix materials fibronectin and laminin. In addition to providing the structural framework for neural development, as development proceeds, their terminal processes develop end feet and form the glia limitans over the surface of the brain and spinal cord (1). During that period, they form a network closely investing all of the small blood vessels. Thus, with the blood vessels, they form a framework that supports, nourishes, and protects the neurons and oligodendroglia.

Astrocytes react very actively to injury. They proliferate and hypertrophy, their cytoplasm expands, and they develop more cytoplasmic organelles including large numbers of ribosomes, which are involved in the production of GFAP-containing intermediate filaments and other structural products needed by the reacting cell. The result is a dense fibrous scar. In MS, these scars form in areas of demyelination, forming the plaques typical of this disease. Tenascin-R and tenascin-C, which form a portion of the extracellular matrix, inhibit glial reaction but are destroyed by macrophages in MS plaques (14). These macrophages also appear to produce an astrocyte attractant or attractants (astrokines) such as osteopontin (15).

### Role in Axonal Transmission

There is very good evidence that astrocytes regulate the extracellular ionic milieu. In the white matter, astrocytic processes are regularly found adjacent to central nodes (16). They contain sodium channels, potassium channels, and Na,K-ATPase–mediated potassium uptake (17). At central nodes, where the ionic milieu is critically important for transmission of nerve impulses, astrocytes appear to regulate extracellular sodium and potassium during transmission. Without rapid removal of excess potassium from the perinodal area, accumulation of extracellular potassium would reduce the membrane potential, thereby interfering with impulse conduction.

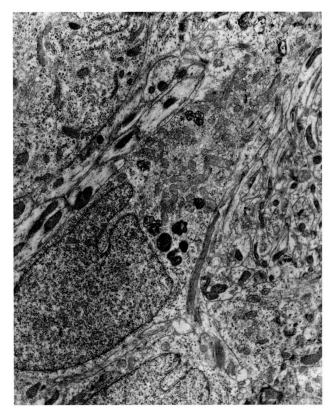

**FIGURE 3.2**

Golgi epithelial cell (Bergmann astrocyte) in normal mouse brain. This specialized protoplasmic astrocyte has considerably more organelles than most protoplasmic astrocytes with numerous mitochondria and a number of lysosomes. The granular endoplasmic reticulum and Golgi apparatus are sparse. The edge of a Purkinje cell can be seen at top left.

In remyelinated nerve fibers, in which there is usually a very short distance between nodes, it is likely that rapid removal of potassium is even more important. The amount of potassium that passes through the nodal membrane at each node is probably about the same as in a normal fiber, but the close proximity of adjacent nodes means that the total potassium efflux per unit length of axon with each impulse is much larger. Thus removal of excess potassium becomes even more critical in areas of remyelination.

### Role in Formation of the Blood–Brain Barrier

Astrocytes appear not to play a direct structural role in the blood–brain barrier. Rather, the barrier is formed by the capillary endothelial cells. In the brain, the capillary endothelial cells, have astrocytes covering about 90% of their surface. The astrocytes appear to induce changes in the endothelial cells causing them to develop the changes that constitute the blood–brain barrier (18). Endothelial cells in the brain, excluding those few areas such as the area postrema and subfornical organ in which the blood–brain barrier is absent, differ from endothelial cells elsewhere. They are thinner, they have more mitochondria, they are not fenestrated, and they have much tighter junctional complexes between adjacent endothelial cells than their peripheral counterpart (19).

To establish the effect of brain tissue on the capillary endothelium, Stewart and Wiley transplanted embryonic quail brain into the coelomic cavity of chick hosts (20). The chick capillaries that grew into the embryonic quail brain developed the morphologic characteristics typical of cerebral vessels. The distinctive morphology of the quail cells allowed identification of the vessels as being of chick origin. When bits of unvascularized quail somite were transplanted into chick brain, the chick vessels growing into the somite did not develop barrier characteristics.

Goldstein isolated and cultured endothelial cells and astrocytes separately (21). When the two were cultured together, the endothelial cells developed tight junctions similar to those seen in vivo. Further evidence that astrocytic secretion plays a critical role in induction of the blood–brain barrier was provided by Hurwitz and coworkers who cultured endothelial cells and astrocytes on opposite sides of a synthetic permeable membrane (22). They demonstrated the induction of blood–brain barrier–specific proteins in the endothelial cells under these culture conditions (22).

Another blood–brain barrier–related function of astrocytes appears to be at least partial control of glucose transporter expression. When endothelial cells were incubated in medium conditioned with glucose deprived astrocytes, an increase in the GLUT1 isoform of the glucose transporter was seen, whereas no effect was seen with media conditioned by astrocytes that were not glucose deprived (23).

## ELABORATION OF EXTRACELLULAR MATRIX CONSTITUENTS

The extracellular matrix (ECM) in the central nervous system is far more complex and far more important in development and in immunologic and pathologic processes than was earlier suspected. It is highly complex and contains more than two dozen different matrix molecules and their receptors (24). They have a substantial number of highly specific functions. The ECM and its relationship to MS has been reviewed by Sobel (24). Some of the matrix molecules aggregate into visible structures such as the basal lamina, whereas others bind to specific membrane components. The ECM provides functional signals to glial cells and neurons that influence a wide variety of behaviors including growth, proliferation, migration, differentiation, and apoptosis.

The ECM is composed of aggregates and polymers, the majority of which are proteoglycans. Other matrix components include laminin, type IV collagen, fibronectin, proteases, and protease inhibitors (25). Proteoglycans are 80- to 400-kD proteins with one or more glycosaminoglycan side chains (24). There are more than 25 species of proteoglycan core proteins (25). If we consider the variation in amount and location of the side chains on the core proteins, it can be seen that there is a broad diversity of structure and likely a corresponding diversity in function. A family of proteoglycans designated *lecticans* is abundant in central nervous system white matter. These are large chondroitin sulfate proteoglycans and include versican, aggrecan, neurocan, and brevican. Of these, neurocan and brevican appear restricted to the central nervous system (26). Aggrecan, neurocan, decorin, and biglycan have been designated as "antiadhesive" proteoglycans (24). They inhibit attachment and spreading on surfaces that normally permit attachment.

Other antiadhesive proteoglycans include tenascin-C, thrombospondin-1, and secreted protein, acidic and rich in cysteine, or "SPARC." Tenascin-C can exhibit adhesive or antiadhesive properties depending on in vitro conditions (24).

## Role in Synaptic Regulation, Function, and Maintenance of Postsynaptic Specializations

Astrocytes play a variety of roles related to synaptic transmission. They surround and isolate synaptic complexes such as the cerebellar glomeruli. They take up and inactivate neurotransmitters, play an important role in regulating synaptic density in a number of regions, and in some areas of the brain play an important role in maintaining postsynaptic specialization after denervation.

In cerebellar cultures made deficient in astrocytes by treatment with cytosine arabinoside, the Purkinje cell somata become hyperinnervated by Purkinje cell recurrent collaterals. When astrocytes from optic nerve are added to the cultures, they invade the culture, surround the Purkinje cell somata, and displace many of the synapses, thereby reducing the synaptic density to near normal levels (27). Physiologically, the hyperinnervated Purkinje cells show marked inhibition. After the introduction of astrocytes, inhibition returns to near normal (28). Purkinje cell spines in cultures deficient in astrocytes and granule cells do not show postsynaptic specializations; however, they do show these specializations when competent astrocytes are present in adequate numbers. When cerebellar cultures deficient in granule cells are treated with the matrix molecule laminin, the number of Purkinje cell dendritic spines increases and they develop a postsynaptic web (29).

In the cerebellum in vivo, when granule cell axons are destroyed, astrocytic processes envelop the vacated

Purkinje cell spines and are able to maintain not only the spine itself but also the postsynaptic apparatus and synaptic cleft material (30,31) (Figure 3.2). The maintenance of the postsynaptic web and cleft material does not occur without functionally competent astrocytes (27).

In the hypothalamus, the glial process covering the magnocellular oxytocin neurons is significantly reduced after stimulation, allowing for more extensive contact with synaptic terminals. This process is accompanied by synaptic remodeling, resulting in an increased number of GABAergic, glutamatergic, and noradrenergic contacts. At the same time, remodeling of astrocytes in the neurohypophysis results in enhanced neurohemal contact with the cell processes (32).

After axotomy, neurons typically undergo a reactive change called central chromatolysis. The granular endoplasmic reticulum is largely replaced with free ribosomes. When this process occurs in anterior horn cells, astrocytic processes insinuate themselves between the cell soma and the terminal boutons, removing them from the reacting motor neuron (33). When the axon reconnects with its target, the process is reversed, astrocytic processes withdraw, and new synapses are formed.

The role of astrocytes in synaptic transmission is still being elucidated. Astrocytes have high affinity uptake systems for most neurotransmitters and have been shown to take up and metabolize a number of transmitters including glutamate, γ-aminobutyric acid, glycine, taurine, alanine, (34) catecholamines, and serotonin (35). They also appear to serve as ion sources and sinks, thus playing a critical role in the maintenance of appropriate ion concentrations in the extracellular fluid in synaptic regions, as they do at central nodes.

### Role in Immune Response

Astrocytes appear to play an important role in immune reactions in the central nervous system. They do not normally express class I and class II histocompatability antigens or express them at extremely low levels, (36) even though they are normally present on most nucleated cells. These antigens are critical for immune interactions and specifically for antigen presentation. Interferon-γ induces class I and II antigens on astrocytes in vivo. (37). Astrocytes also have been shown to be capable of secreting interleukin-1. The combination of interleukin-1 and histocompatibility antigens allows astrocytes to function as antigen presenting cells (38). This appears extremely relevant to MS because there is clear evidence that interferon-γ, unlike type 1 interferons, induce acute attacks of MS (39).

Astrocytes have been shown to secrete the chemokines IP-10/CXCL10, MCP-1/CCL2, and CX3CL1/fractalkine in response to treatment with tumor necrosis factor-α and interferon-γ. These appear to be secreted when T-cells invade the central nervous system and appear to be involved in the elaboration of the local inflammatory response (see Chapter 11).

### SUMMARY

Astrocytes are far more complex and have far more functions in the nervous system than anyone would have suspected a few decades ago. They serve as guides to cell migration during development, induce formation of the blood–brain barrier, play an active role in immune function in the nervous system, serve as ion sources and sinks, isolate synapses and remove neurotransmitter from the extracellular fluid, and play a role in controlling synaptic number in a variety of settings. Additional functions are likely to appear as research continues. Many of their functions in disease states and particularly in MS remain to be elucidated. As these functions are further defined, some may become targets for therapeutic intervention in a number of diseases including MS.

## References

1. Federoff S, Vernadakis A. *Astrocytes: Development, Morphology and Regional Specialization of Astrocytes.* London: Academic Press; 1986.
2. Federoff S, Vernadakis A. *Astrocytes: Biochemistry, Physiology and Pharmacology of Astrocytes.* London: Academic Press; 1986.
3. Federoff S, Vernadakis A. *Astrocytes: Cell Biology and Pathology of Astrocytes.* London: Academic Press; 1986.
4. Privat A, Rataboul P. Fibrous and protoplasmic astrocytes. In: Federoff S, Vernadakis A. (eds.), *Astrocytes: Development, Morphology and Regional Specialization of Astrocytes.* London: Academic Press, 1986; 105–129.
5. Landis DMD, Reese TS. Membrane structure in mammalian astrocytes: A review of freeze-fracture studies on adult, developing, reactive and altered astrocytes. *J Exp Biol* 1982; 95:35–48.
6. Rakic P. Neuronal migration and contact guidance in the primate telencephalon. *Postgrad Med* 1978l :54 (suppl 1):S25–S40.
7. Shihabuddin LS, Horner PJ, Ray J, Gage FH. Adult spinal cord stem cells generate neurons after transplantation in the adult dentate gyrus. *J Neurosci* 2000; 20:8727–8735.
8. Raff MC, Miller RH, Noble M. A glial progenitor cell that develops in vitro into an astrocyte or an oligodendrocyte depending on culture medium. *Nature* 1983; 303:390–396.
9. Roots BI. Phylogenetic development of astrocytes. In: Federoff S, Vernadakis A. (eds.), *Astrocytes: Development, Morphology and Regional Specialization of Astrocytes.* London: Academic Press, 1986; 1–34.
10. Rafols JA. Ependymal tanycytes of the ventricular system in vertebrates. In: Federoff S, Vernadakis A, (eds.), *Astrocytes: Development, Morphology and Regional Specialization of Astrocytes.* London: Academic Press, 1986; 131–148.
11. Shiga T, Ichikawa M, Hirata Y. A Golgi study of Bergmann glial cells in developing rat cerebellum. *Anat Embryol (Berl)* 1983; 167(2):191–201.
12. Ronnevi LO. Origin of the glial processes responsible for the spontaneous postnatal phagocytosis of boutons on cat spinal motoneurons. *Cell Tissue Res* 1978; 189:203–217.
13. Egensperger R, Maslim J, Bisti S, Hollander H, Stone J. Fat of DNA from retinal cells dying during development: uptake by microglia and macroglia (Muller cells). *Brain Res Dev Brain Res* 1996; 97:1–8.

14. Gutowski NJ, Newcombe J, Cuzner ML. Tenascin–R and C in multiple sclerosis lesions: relevance to extracellular matrix remodelling. *Neuropathol Appl Neurobiol* 1999; 25:207–214.

15. Ellison JA, Barone FC, Feuerstein GZ. Matrix remodeling after stroke. De novo expression of matrix proteins and integrin receptors. *Ann NY Acad Sci* 1999; 890:204–222.

16. Black JA, Friedman B, Waxman SG, Elmer LW, Angelides KJ. Immuno–ultrastructural localization of sodium channels at nodes of Ranvier and perinodal astrocytes in rat optic nerve. *Proc R Soc Lond B Biol Sci* 1989; 238:39–51.

17. Thio CL, Waxman SG, Sontheimer H. Ion channels in spinal cord astrocytes in vitro. III Modulation of channel expression by coculture with neurons and neuron–conditioned medium. *J. Neurophysiol* 1993; 69:819–831.

18. Janzer RC, Raff MC. Astrocytes induce blood–brain barrier propertien in endothelial cells. *Nature* 1987; 325:253–257.

19. Stewart PA, Coomber BL. Astrocytes and the blood–brain barrier. In: Federoff S, Vernadakis A (eds.), *Astrocytes: Development, Morphology and Regional Specialization of Astrocytes.* London: Academic Press, 1986; 311–328.

20. Stewart PA, Wiley MJ. Developing nervous tissue induces formation of blood brain barrier characteristics in invading endothelial cells: A study using quail–chick transplantation. *Dev Biol* 1981; 84:183–192.

21. Goldstein GW. Endothelial cell–astrocyte interactions. A cellular model of the blood–brain barrier. *Ann NY Acad Sci* 1988; 529:311–339.

22. Hurwitz AA, Berman JW, Rashbaum WK, Lyman WD. Human fetal astrocytes induce the expression of blood–brain barrier specific proteins by autologous endothelial cells. *Brain Res* 1993; 625:238–243.

23. Morchoisne RA, Borson S, McCall AL, Drewes LR, Roux F. Factor(s) released by glucose–deprived astrocytes enhance glucose transporter expression and activity in rat brain endothelial cells. *Biochim Biophys Acta* 2001; 1540:233–242.

24. Sobel RA. The extracellular matrix in multiple sclerosis. *J Neuropathol Exp Neurol* 1998; 57:205–217.

25. Lander AD. Proteoglycans in the nervous system. *Curr Opin Neurobiol* 1993; 3:716–723.

26. Gary SC, Zerillo CA, Chiang VL, et al. cDNA cloning, chromosomal localization, and expression analysis of human BEHAB/brevican, a brain specific proteoglycan regulated during cortical development and in glioma. *Gene* 2000; 256:139–147.

27. Meshul CK, Seil FJ, Herndon RM. Astrocytes play a role in regulation of synaptic density. *Brain Res* 1987; 402:139–145.

28. Drake-Baumann R, Seil FJ. Influence of functional glia on the electrophysiology of Purkinje cells in organotypic cerebellar cultures. *Neuroscience* 1999; 88:507–519.

29. Herndon RM. Thiophen–induced granule cell necrosis in the rat cerebellum. An electron microscopic study. *Exp Brain Res* 1968; 6:49–68.

30. Seil FJ. The extracellular matrix molecule, laminin, induces Purkinje cell dendritic spine proliferation in granule cell depleted cerebellar cultures. *Brain Res* 1998; 795:112–120.

31. Herndon RM, Margolis G, Kilham L. The synaptic organization of the malformed cerebellum induced by perinatal infection with the feline panleukopenia virus. II. The Purkinje cell and its afferents. *J Neuropathol Exp Neurol* 1971; 30:557–570.

32. Theodosis DT, Poulain DA. Contribution of astrocytes to activity-dependent structural plasticity in the adult brain. *Adv Exp Med Biol* 1999; 468:175–182.

33. Novikov LN, Novikova LN, Holmberg P, Kellerth J. Exogenous brain-derived factor regulates the synaptic composition of axonally lesioned and normal adult rat motoneurons. *Neuroscience* 2000; 100:171–181.

34. Hösli E, Hösli L, Schousboe A. Amino acid uptake. In: Federoff S, Vernadakis A,(eds.), *Astrocytes: Biochemistry, Physiology and Pharmacology of Astrocytes.* London: Academic Press, 1986; 133–153.

35. Kimelberg HK. Catecholamine and serotonin uptake in astrocytes. In Federoff S, Vernadakis A (eds.), *Astrocytes: Biochemistry, Physiology and Pharmacology of Astrocytes.* London: Academic Press, 1986; 107–131.

36. Williams KA, Hart DNJ, Fabre JW, Morris PJ. Distribution and quantitation of HLA-ABC and DR (Ia) antigens on human kidney and other tissues. *Transplantation* 1980; 29:274–279.

37. Wong GHW, Bartlett PF, Clark-Lewis I, Battye F, Schrader JW. Inducible expression of H-2 and Ia antigens on brain cells. *Nature (Lond)* 1984; 310:688–691.

38. Fierz W, Fontana A. The role of astrocytes in the interaction between the immune and nervous system. In: Federoff S, Vernadakis A (eds.), *Astrocytes: Cell Biology and Pathology of Astrocytes.* London: Academic Press, 1986; 203–229.

39. Panitch HS, Hirsch RL, Haley AS, Johnson KP. Treatment of multiple sclerosis with gamma interferon: Exacerbations associated with activtion of the immune system. *Neurology* 1987; 37:1097–1102.

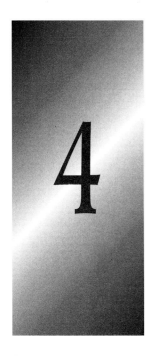

# 4 Molecular Structure of the Myelin Membrane

*Joyce A. Benjamins, Ph.D.*

Central nervous system (CNS) myelin is a specialized extension of the plasma membrane of the oligodendrocyte; it is characterized by a high ratio of lipids to proteins and enrichment in a relatively small number of proteins compared with plasma membranes and intracellular membranes. The prominence of myelin destruction in multiple sclerosis (MS) has catalyzed investigation over the past 50 years of the physical and molecular properties of the myelin membrane. The remarkable multilamellar structure, abundance of myelin in the CNS, and its ease of isolation have contributed to our ability to characterize its composition and to isolate genes coding for myelin proteins. This fundamental information is now being applied to the more complex issues of the functions of these lipids and proteins in myelin assembly and maintenance and in interactions of the various specialized myelin structures with the axons they ensheath.

Our base of knowledge about myelin has increased extensively since the first reports of isolation of the CNS myelin membrane in the 1960s, with 280 papers in 1970 and more than 1200 papers on myelin proteins and lipids published in 2000. A number of older books and reviews provide useful references for detailed background and information about the chemical composition, metabolic properties, and molecular structure of myelin (1–6). Several recent reviews provide excellent updates (7–9),

including the comprehensive review by Baumann and Pham Dinh (10). Space limitations prevent reference to all these original articles. This review focuses on summarizing the current knowledge about the molecular properties of the proteins and lipids of CNS myelin, the organization of these components in the various specialized domains of myelin, and the mechanisms regulating their synthesis and subsequent assembly into myelin. Comparisons with peripheral nervous system (PNS) myelin are included where relevant.

## CNS MYELIN PROTEINS: STRUCTURE AND FUNCTION

Early characterization of compact multilamellar myelin used X-ray diffraction and electron microscopy, followed by physical isolation of myelin on density gradients and identification of its biochemical composition. Subsequent analyses of regions of noncompacted myelin and associated paranodal and nodal specializations has relied on electron microscopy, freeze-fracture analysis, and immunocytochemistry. Our current knowledge of the localization of proteins within compact and noncompact myelin regions is summarized in Figure 4.1 (also see Figure 2.5C). More recently, analysis with magnetic resonance imaging (MRI) has added to our understanding of alterations in myelin during development and disease

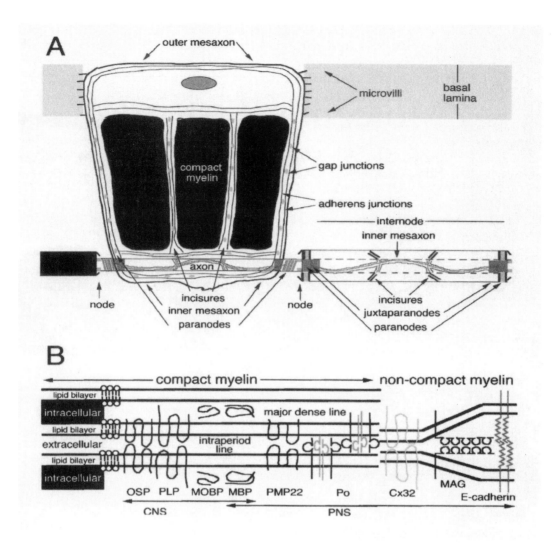

**FIGURE 4.1**

Schematic view of a myelinated axon in the PNS and proteins of CNS and PNS myelin. **A.** One myelin Schwann cell was unrolled to show the incisures and paranodes, regions of noncompact myelin. Adherens junctions are depicted as two continuous lines, with gap junctions depicted as ovals between the rows of adherens junctions. **B.** CNS and PNS contain overlapping and distinct sets of proteins. In the CNS, compact myelin contains PLP, OSP, MOBP, and MBP; in the PNS, compact myelin contains P0, PMP 22 and MBP. In the CNS, components of noncompact myelin are not yet defined; in PNS, noncompact myelin contains E-cadherin, MAG, and Cx32. Note that P0 and MAG have extracellular immunoglobulinlike domains (semicircles) and that PLP, PMP-22, OSP, and Cx32 have 4 transmembrane domains. CNS, central nervous system; Cx32, connexin 32; MAG, myelin-associated glycoprotein; MBP, myelin basic protein; MOBP, myelin-associated oligodendrocytic basic protein; OSP, oligodendrocyte-specific protein (claudin 11); PLP, proteolipid protein; PMP-22, peripheral myelin protein-22; PNS, peripheral nervous system; P0, P zero glyoprotein. (Reprinted with permission from Arroyo EJ, Scherer SS. On the molecular architecture of myelinated fibers. *Histochem Cell Biol* 2000; 113:1–18. ©2000 Springer-Verlag.)

(also see Chapter 15) (11). Structure–function relationships have received increasing focus with the characterization of the effects of mutations on these various myelin structures in human genetic diseases and transgenic mice.

Analysis of white versus gray matter showed that regions enriched with myelin and axons have lower water content and higher lipid content than other regions. In humans, approximately 35 percent of the dry weight of brain is composed of myelin, with about 40 percent of the brain lipid in myelin (12). Subsequent isolation of the lipid-rich compact myelin membrane on density gradients allowed extensive characterization of its composition (12,13). Thus, myelin contains 40 percent water compared with 80 percent in gray matter. The ratio of lipid to protein is 70:30 compared with 35:65 in most other membranes. The two major classes of CNS myelin proteins, myelin basic proteins (MBPs) and proteolipid proteins (PLPs), were first isolated by chemical extraction of brain or isolated myelin. With the development of sodium dodecyl sulfate (SDS) gel electrophoresis, and 2-dimensional polyacrylamide gel electrophoresis (PAGE) to separate membrane proteins, a more complex picture appeared. Typical SDS gel patterns of proteins in isolated CNS and PNS myelin from rat and human are shown in Figure 4.2 (8). Exact proportions of various proteins are difficult to estimate due to differences in binding of dyes used to stain the gels (14). However, based on extraction and gel staining, the MBPs and PLPs are clearly the most abundant families, together constituting 60 to 80 percent of the total myelin proteins. Patterns change during development, with higher molecular weight proteins more prominent in myelin isolated from developing brain as opposed to

mature brain (14). In mice, MBPs constitute about 30 percent of the myelin proteins at day 30, increasing to 35 percent in the adult. PLP increases from 21 to 28 percent, and DM-20 increases from 8 to 10 percent over that same period. Immunoreactivity to antibodies and application of gene cloning have identified a number of less abundant proteins in myelin that were not detected or identified by gel electrophoresis. Complete sequences of the messenger RNAs and proteins of numerous genes coding for myelin-enriched proteins are known. Models for 3-dimensional structures of several of the proteins have been proposed based on sequence data, homology searching (15), and X-ray crystallography in the case of P0 glycoprotein of PNS myelin (16). Properties of the more abundant myelin proteins and many of the less abundant ones identified to date are summarized in Table 4.1.

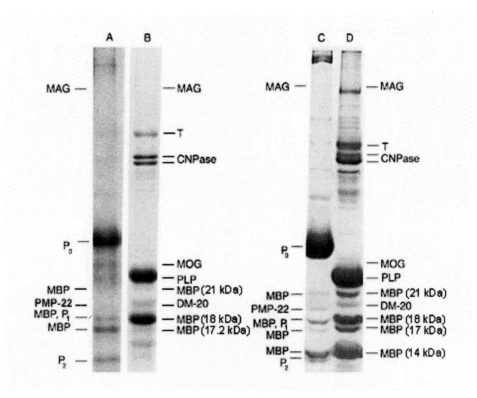

**FIGURE 4.2**

Profiles of human and rat myelin from PNS and CNS after separation by polyacrylamide gel electrophoresis in the presence of sodium dodecyl sulfate and stained with Coomassie blue. **A.** Human PNS. **B.** Human CNS. **C.** Rat PNS. **D.** Rat CNS. See Table 4.1 for the molecular weights of the proteins. The 25-kd MOG protein is probably the faint band just above PLP in CNS myelin, which is most apparent in D. CNPase is a tight doublet, with the lower and upper bands referred to as CNP1 and CNP2, respectively. MAG stains too faintly to be seen on the gel but is found just above the prominent band in D in CNS myelin, which is probably the 96-kd subunit of $Na^+,K^+$-ATPase. CNPase, cyclic nucleotide phosphohydrolase; CNS, central nervous system; DM-20, splice variation of PLP; MAG, myelin-associated glycoprotein; MBP, myelin basic protein; MOG, myelin oligodendrocytic glycoprotein; PLP, proteolipid protein; PMP-22, peripheral myelin protein-22; PNS, peripheral nervous system; P0, P zero glycoprotein; T, tubulin in CNS myelin. (Reprinted with permission from Morell P, Quarles RH. Gel electrophoresis of myelin proteins in the presence of sodium dodecyl sulfate (SDS). In: Siegel GJ, ed. *Basic Neurochemistry: Molecular, Cellular and Medical Aspects,* 6th ed. Philadelphia: Lippincott-Raven; 1999:80 ©1999 LIppincott-Raven.)

TABLE 4.1
### Major Proteins Of CNS and PNS Myelin

| Protein | Molecular Weight (kD) | Isoelectric Point | Description |
|---|---|---|---|
| MBP | H: 21.5, 20.2, 18.5, 17.2<br>M: 21.5, 18.5, 17, 14 | >10.6 | • Protein associated with the cytoplasmic surface of myelin membrane (major dense line); role in compaction of myelin layers and cytoskeletal organization<br>• Induces experimental allergic encephalomyelitis (autoimmune demyelination: model of MS). |
| PLP | 30 | 9.2 | • Very hydrophobic; soluble in organic solvents; transmembrane protein, spanning bilayer four times<br>• May be a proton channel<br>• Highly conserved among species, indicating functional importance<br>• Major CNS myelin protein compromising 30% of total protein<br>• Minor component < 1% in Schwann cells in PNS<br>• Mutations identified in PMD (CNS demyelination); deletions also show PNS phenotype |
| DM-20 | 25 | | • Splice variant of PLP |
| CNPase 1, 2 | 46, 48 | 9.7 | • Associated with cytoskeleton in oligodendroglia and other cells; in noncompact myelin; GTP-binding sites; possible role in targeting of MBP to compact myelin |
| MAG | 110 (apoproteins 67, 72) | Acidic (3–4) | • Minor component; related to cell adhesion molecules and immunoglobulin gene family; binds to integrins<br>• Localized to lamella nearest to axon and in cytoplasmic loops; important in myelin–axon interactions |
| P0 glycoprotein (PNS) | 30 (apoprotein 23) | | • Glycoprotein comprising 50–60 percent of total protein in PNS myelin<br>• Homology with immunoglobulin gene superfamily<br>• PNS myelin compaction |
| P2 protein (PNS) | 13.5 | | • Induces experimental allergic neuritis (PNS) (autoimmune demyelination of PNS; model of Guillain-Barre syndrome)<br>• Fatty acid binding protein |
| PMP-22 (PNS) | 22 | | • Transmembrane protein; spans bilayer four times; may be a pore or channel<br>• Mutations identified in Charcot-Marie-Tooth disease, an inherited peripheral neuropathy |
| MOG | 25 | | • Interacts with MBP in compact myelin |
| MOBP | 8.7, 9.7, 11.7 | | • In compact myelin at the cytoplasmic surface |
| MOSP | 48 | | • Associated with the cytoskeleton in noncompact regions of myelin |
| OSP | 22 | | • Tight junction protein in CNS radial component; 7 percent of CNS myelin protein; structure similar to PMP-22 |
| OMgP | 120 | | • GPI-anchored glycoprotein; HNK-1 epitope; paranodal location |
| MAL | 17 | | • Hydrophobic protein; may stabilize lipid protein domains |
| NI35/250 | 35, 220 | | • Nogo proteins rich in CNS myelin but poor in PNS myelin; inhibit axonal outgrowth |

GPI, glycosylphosphatidylinositol; H, human; M, mouse; MAG, myelin-associated glycoprotein; MOSP, myelin/oligodendrocyte-specific protein; MS, multiple sclerosis; OMgp, olidodendrocyte–myelin glycoprotein; PMD, Pelizaeus-Merzbacher disease; MAL, myelin and lymphocyte protein.

## Myelin Basic Proteins

MBPs constitute approximately 30 percent of the myelin proteins and were first identified by extraction of brain or myelin with dilute acidic or salt solutions (17,18). See Campagnoni and Skoff (9) for a comprehensive review of the structure, distribution, and possible functions of the products of the MBP gene.

The "classic" MBPs are characterized by a high content of basic amino acids and low molecular weights, from 14000 to 21000 kd. They are located as peripheral proteins on the cytoplasmic surface of the myelin membrane, at the major dense line (Figure 4.1). These proteins share many sequence similarities, and are encoded by a single messenger (mRNA) with seven exons that are alternatively spliced to produce several variants (9,19). All MBPs identified to date contain the first and last exons in their mRNAs and thus share the same amino acid sequences at their amino and carboxy ends. The most prominent MBP species in human myelin is the 18.5-kd isoform, corresponding to amino acids coded from classic exons 1 and 3–7 (corresponding to Golli-MBP exons 5 and 7–11; see below). MBPs can be modified post-translationally, giving rise to a large number of species differing in charge (20,21). These modifications include phosphorylation, deimidation, citrullination, and loss of the carboxy terminal (C-terminal) arginine.

At present, functional differences arising from the sequence variations and post-translational modifications are under investigation. Mutant mice deficient in MBP show loose packing of myelin lamellae at the major dense line, in keeping with its cytoplasmic location. However, increasing compaction of myelin with age does not appear to be related exclusively to a given MBP isoform because the 18.5-kd species is most abundant in adult human myelin, but the 14-kd species is most abundant in adult mice (3,6). Further, the 14-kd form of MBP is sufficient to restore myelin compaction when expressed in *shiverer* mice lacking MBP (22). Different MBP species have different distributions within the cell, with 14- and 18.5-kd isoforms localized primarily to the plasma membrane (23) and 17- and 21.5-kd isoforms (classic exon 2-containing isoforms) found diffusely in the cytoplasm and transported into the nucleus (24). The phosphate groups on MBP show a rapid turnover (25), postulated to occur in compact myelin and regions of myelin membrane exposed to cytoplasm in paranodal loops or incisures. Myelin isolated from the brains of some patients with MS show a less mature pattern of charge microheterogeneity compared with non-MS tissue, raising the possibility of an association with cause or effect in MS (20,26).

The presence of MBP or derived peptides in cerebrospinal fluid (CSF) serves as a marker for acute myelin damage in MS and other types of neural injury, such as stroke (27). The MBP peptide 80-89 is the predominant species in CSF. The levels of MBP peptides in CSF increase rapidly during acute relapse of MS, but not in chronic or progressive stages of disease or optic neuritis. Levels of MBP peptides in urine appear to correlate with progression of disease rather than with acute demyelination.

Injection of MBP or peptides containing portions of MBP sequence gives rise to the autoimmune disease experimental allergic encephalomyelitis (EAE), a model for MS (28) (see Chapter 6). The use of defined, overlapping peptides has allowed epitope mapping of this immune response, with variations in encephalitogenic potency of a given peptide between species and even between different strains of rats or mice. Many aspects of this disease mimic characteristics of MS, especially with regard to the immune-mediated demyelination that occurs. Induction of EAE is not exclusive to MBP. Injection of PLP, myelin oligodendrocytic glycoprotein (MOG), and several other myelin proteins also give rise to EAE, but MBP has been the most studied model. The use of MBP to induce EAE and the ability of some peptides to suppress disease provided the basis for exploring the use of a random sequence of basic amino acids to suppress disease, first in animal models and then, with some success, in MS (29) (see Chapter 9).

Murine mutants deficient in MBP have demonstrated several functions for these proteins. *Shiverer* mutant mice have a deletion of the last five exons of the MBP gene, resulting in lack of MBP, hypomyelination, and abnormally compacted CNS myelin (30–32). Introducing the normal MBP gene into *shiverer* mice to provide 25 to 50 percent of the normal MBP levels restores myelin compaction (33,34). *Shiverer* oligodendrocytes in vivo and in vitro showed altered cytoskeletal structures and microprocesses (35–37). Phosphorylation of axonal cytoskeleton and neuronal gene expression also were altered in *shiverer* CNS (38). PNS myelin shows normal compaction which is thought to be due to P0 glycoprotein rather than to MBP in PNS myelin. However, the PNS has a 2- to 3-fold increase in the numbers of Schmidt-Lantermann incisures (39), and expression of myelin-associated glycoprotein (MAG) and the incisure-associated connexin 32 are increased, apparently at the post-transcriptional level (40). Myelin-deficient mice (shi^mld) showed markedly reduced expression of MBP due to duplication and inversion of a large portion of the MBP gene (41). These mice showed a mosaic pattern of compact and noncompact myelin. Only those two spontaneous MBP mutations in mice and one in rat (42) have been identified, in contrast to the multiple mutations, duplications, and deletions found for PLP in humans and rodents (see below). Deletions of the entire MBP gene occur as part of a large chromosomal inversion in 18q syndrome in humans (43); symptoms include mental retardation and white matter changes, which may be due in part to the loss of MBP gene products.

The MBP gene contains four exons in addition to those coding for the classic forms of MBP (44). A transcription start site 70 kb upstream from the two start sites for the classic MBP isoforms gives rise to the Golli-MBP family of proteins, with two major proteins, J37 and BG21, and a minor isoform, TP8, identified to date.

The Golli-MBP transcripts and proteins have been detected in oligodendroglial and neuronal populations, specifically granule, hippocampal, and cortical neurons throughout development (45,46). In oligodendroglia, Golli-MBP proteins are targeted to the nucleus and cell body but not into the processes or compact myelin in vivo or in vitro (47). The Golli-MBP products are also expressed in thymus, primarily in T cells (44,48), prompting analysis of the role of these gene products in the development of tolerance and susceptibility of various strains of mice to EAE (49,50). The possible role of the Golli-MBP gene in susceptibility to MS has been examined in two different patient populations, with different results (51,52). Analysis of 151 MS families from Finland and Sweden suggested a role for the Golli-MBP locus in MS susceptibility. Another study from France examined a polymorphic (CA) repeat within the Golli-MBP locus but found no evidence for linkage of the gene to MS susceptibility in 191 families studied.

Because of the shared sequences between Golli-MBPs and the classic MBPs, some of the changes in mutant and transgenic mice attributed to classic MBPs will need to be re-examined to determine the specific contributions of the various products of this complex gene (9). For example, the *shiverer* mouse expresses no classic MBP proteins but does express one Golli isoform, BG21, which contains Golli sequences and classic MBP amino acids 1 to 57.

## Myelin Proteolipid Proteins

The two major integral membrane proteins of compact CNS myelin are myelin PLP and its splice isoform DM-20. These proteins are characterized by an abundance of hydrophobic amino acids and were first isolated from brain by extraction with chloroform-methanol, commonly used to extract lipids (53). The molecular weights of PLP and DM-20 are 30 kd and 25 kd, respectively, with slightly lower apparent molecular weights on SDS gels (25 kd and 20 kd, respectively). Like MBPs they are quite basic (Table 4.1). PLP and DM-20 in human and mouse are completely conserved in amino acid sequence and display 92 percent homology in the mRNA sequences in the upstream regulatory and 5'-noncoding regions (54). They form tetraspan structures in the membrane, with the carboxy and amino ends facing the cytoplasm.

PLP and DM-20 together comprise about 40 percent of CNS myelin proteins; both proteins are found at low levels in Schwann cells. They were not detected in PNS myelin (55); but a recent study has identified PLP in compact myelin with immunogold labeling and electron microscopy (56). Levels of DM-20 are high relative to PLP in the CNS in early development, but the ratio of PLP to DM-20 is about 5:1 in adult myelin. PLP and DM-20 are splice isoforms, with PLP mRNA containing 7 exons and DM-20 missing exon 3b, resulting in a 35 amino acid deletion in the cytoplasmic loop of PLP (57).

PLP and DM-20 are acylated at selected cysteine residues with thioester linkages to long-chain fatty acids (58–60). The fatty acids show a more rapid turnover than the protein moiety, with respective half-lives of 3 days versus 1 month (59). Deacylation of PLP in situ has demonstrated that the fatty acids on PLP play a role in stabilizing compaction of the myelin lamellae (61). PLP is also glycated nonenzymatically, with the majority of sites on extracytoplasmic domains. In hyperglycemic conditions, i.e., in diabetic mice, nonenzymatic glycosylation on extracytoplasmic domains of PLP was increased, suggesting a relation to CNS complications in diabetes (62).

As found for MBP, PLP is encephalitogenic, and injection of the protein gives rise to autoimmune demyelination in rodents (63–65). Epitope clusters within residues 40–70, 100–119, and 178–209 have been identified as encephalitogenic in mice (66). Increased immune responses to several PLP peptides have been identified in some MS patients (67–69). In mice, thioacylation of selected PLP peptides increases their immunogenicity and encephalitogenicity, suggesting that acylation contributes to the immunopathogenesis in mice and in MS (70).

Many mutations in the PLP gene have been identified in Pelizaeus-Merzbacher disease (PMD) and spastic paraplegia in humans, and in numerous mouse mutants; for recent comprehensive reviews, see (9,71,72). The mutations include deletions, frameshifts, point mutations, and duplications at a variety of sites throughout the gene. The human mutations are cataloged at http://www.med.wayne/edu/neurology.plp.html. Duplications of the PLP gene account for approximately 75 percent of the PMD mutations, with point mutations and deletions accounting for the remainder. These mutations and the studies in PLP overexpressing and knockout mice suggest multiple functions for PLP and DM-20 (9). These functions include subtle effects on myelin compaction (73), and major effects on oligodendrocyte proliferation, differentiation and survival (74–76), metabolism, and regulation of vesicle transport (77). Axon–glia communication, axonal integrity, and in some cases CNS axonal conductance velocities also are affected (78,79). Null mutants display a mild phenotype; in one family with PMD, a null mutation was associated with peripheral neuropathy, indicating for the first time a critical function for PLP in peripheral nerves (56). Overexpression of PLP, including duplications, leads to marked effects on myelination and oligodendrocyte survival, demonstrating a toxic role for the protein if not tightly regulated (75). Various mutations give rise to mild or severe phenotypes, with the jimpy and TJ6 mutations, both frameshifts, giving rise to the most severe phenotype in mice and humans. Transfection of nonglial cells with various PLP and DM-20 mutations has shown some correlations between phenotypic severity of PLP mutants in vivo and alterations in transport of PLP and DM-20 in nonglial cells in vitro. Those studies demonstrated a regulatory role for DM-20 in the transport of PLP and provided tools for dissecting the effects of expression of altered PLP proteins (76,77,80,81).

Novel isoforms of the PLP gene containing an additional exon were characterized recently (82). The exon is located between exons 1 and 2; referred to as *exon 1.1*, the exon codes for an additional 12 amino acid leader sequence. The proteins, termed *srPLP* and *srDM-20*, are found in the cell bodies but not in the processes of neurons and oligodendroglia and are seen in presumed precursors of these cells in the subventricular zone in newborn and adult mice. Other members of the gene family include M6A and M6B, with about 50 percent sequence identity to DM-20 (83); both are expressed in neurons, with M6B also found in oligodendroglia and myelin.

## Cyclic Nucleotide Phosphohydrolase

These proteins were originally identified as part of the "Wolfgram" fraction, myelin components remaining after the extraction of PLP and basic protein from myelin (84). They comprise a small portion, approximately 5 percent, of myelin proteins. The two most common isoforms are 46 and 48 kd, which arise due to two different translational start sites (85). They are also enriched in photoreceptor cells, another cell type that produces large amounts of highly organized plasma membrane (86), and are found ubiquitously in a number of cell types. The proteins are associated with cytoskeletal elements in oligodendroglial cytoplasm and membrane sheets (87,88), and are especially prominent at the growing edges of these membrane sheets in culture. In vivo, cyclic nucleotide phosphohydrolase (CNP) proteins are associated primarily with cytoplasmic loops rather than with compact myelin.

The proteins can hydrolyze 2'3'-cyclic nucleotides, but whether this enzymatic activity plays a role in the function of CNP is not known. CNP, primarily CNP1, associates with membranes via isoprenylation (89). CNP has binding sites for guanosine triphosphate (GTP) and has sequences similar to those of the GTP-binding domains of the Ras family (90); how this relates to its function in myelination is not known.

Transgenic mice expressing six times the normal levels of CNP support evidence from in vitro studies that CNP functions in the expansion of membranes during myelination (91). Aberrant membrane expansions and myelin without major dense lines suggest that CNP functions in the regulation of myelin membrane assembly and targeting of MBP to compact myelin.

## Myelin-Associated Glycoprotein

First identified by their lectin-binding properties, MAG proteins are the most prominent glycoproteins in CNS myelin but constitute only about 1 percent of the total myelin protein (92). In the PNS, P0 glycoprotein is the predominant glycoprotein, with MAG comprising only 0.1 percent of total myelin protein. Much interest has focused on MAG due to its localization in the CNS on the abaxonal surface, i.e., on the innermost myelin wrap adjacent to the axon (93) (see Figure 2.5C). The two MAG proteins are members of the super immunoglobulin family and are highly glycosylated, bearing the HNK-1 epitope. The proteins run as a diffuse band with an apparent molecular weight of 100 kd on SDS-PAGE but as two species of 72 and 67 kd after deglycosylation. Small MAG arises by alternate splicing of exon 12, leading to a shorter cytoplasmic domain at the carboxy terminus, but with the extracellular domain and transmembrane domain identical to that of large MAG (94,95). A variety of functions have been proposed for MAG (96,97). Its localization, homology to neural cell adhesion molecule (N-CAM), and presence of the LN/HNK1 epitope (98,99) indicate a role in axonal and myelin recognition and signaling. L-MAG has been implicated in the regulation of fyn tyrosine kinase, which plays a role in the differentiation of oligodendrocytes and subsequent myelination. Further, myelin itself and specifically MAG inhibit axonal regeneration from adult neurons but promote axonal outgrowth from younger neurons of the same type (100). The switch from promotion to inhibition is mediated by decreases in levels of cyclic adenosine monophosphate and activity of protein kinase A (101).

Proteolytic cleavage of MAG near the transmembrane domain produces a soluble peptide termed *dMAG* (102). This soluble peptide is found in CSF and occurs in increased amounts in myelin from MS patients, suggesting an association with demyelination (103).

MAG-deficient and L-MAG mutant mice (104,105) show periaxonal alterations, decreased axonal diameter, axonal degeneration, and a variety of effects on myelination and myelin maintenance in the CNS and PNS. L-MAG appears to be the critical isoform for normal CNS myelination, whereas S-MAG is more critical for PNS.

## Myelin-Oligodendrocytic Glycoprotein

Like MAG, myelin oligodendrocytic glycoprotein (MOG) is a minor myelin protein that belongs to the superimmunglobulin gene family and bears the HNK1 epitope. However, in the CNS, MOG is found on the surface of oligodendrocytes and outer myelin wraps (106) rather than in the periaxonal spaces in the innermost wrap of myelin. MOG was first identified as a target antigen in the induction of EAE (107); thus far, it is a unique antigen for induction of autoimmune demyelination in that it causes both T-cell–mediated inflammation and antibody-mediated demyelination. Several studies in animal models pointed to a possible role for MOG in antibody-mediated demyelination in MS (108,109). Interestingly, the cow milk protein butyrophilin can augment induction or suppress disease in EAE initiated by MOG, apparently by molecular mimicry (110).

## Other Myelin Proteins

A number of other proteins enriched in myelin have been characterized, and in some cases the genes have been cloned. Many other proteins seen on PAGE remain to be characterized, especially several with high molecular weights. Baumann and Pham-Dinh (10) classified some of the identified proteins into the categories of (a) small basic proteins, including myelin-associated oligodendrocytic basic protein (MOBP) and P2 protein, a fatty acid–binding protein; (b) tetraspan proteins, including rat myelin and lymphocyte protein (rMAL or MVP17), plasmolipin, oligodendrocyte-specific protein (OSP or claudin 11), connexin 32 (Cx32), and tetraspan 2; and (c) other proteins, including oligodendrocyte-myelin glycoprotein (OMgp), myelin/oligodendrocyte-specific protein (MOSP), RIP antigen, neurofascin (NF155), and the NI-35/250, or Nogo, proteins. In addition, numerous receptors and enzymes have been identified in low but significant levels in highly purified myelin membrane fractions (see next section).

Two of these proteins are in compact myelin. MOBP is relatively abundant and has three low-molecular-weight isoforms generated by alternate splicing (111). Like MBP, MOBP is localized in compact myelin at the cytoplasmic surface (major dense line). This protein may play a role in regulating the diameter of myelinated axons since mice deficient in MOBP have myelinated axons of increased diameter. The hydrophobic myelin and lymphocyte protein (MAL), is also found in compact myelin; the protein associates with glycosphingolipids and may help stabilize protein lipid microdomains in myelin and apical epithelial membranes (112).

MOSP is a membrane protein on the surface of oligodendrocytes and myelin; it redistributes over cytoskeletal structures in myelin membrane sheets in the presence of MOSP antibody, indicating a role in membrane–cytoskeletal interactions (113). These cytoskeletal veins also contain CNPase and presumably represent the cytoplasmic loop regions in myelin. In contrast, MOG appears to interact with MBP in compact myelin regions because MOG redistributes over MBP domains in cultured oligodendroglial membrane sheets after interaction with MOG antibody.

Nogo proteins (NI-35/250) are transmembrane proteins, highly enriched in CNS but not in PNS myelin (114). The Nogo proteins actively inhibit and repulse axonal outgrowth in neuronal cultures, whereas antibodies to the proteins promote axonal regeneration after injury in vivo. The higher-molecular-weight protein, Nogo-A, has been cloned recently (115).

RIP antigen identifies two proteins of 23 and 160 kd; the epitope is found in oligodendroglia and myelin. The antibody identifying RIP antigen was raised to oligodendroglia from olfactory bulb. In at least one brain region, oligodendroglia that are positive for RIP and carbonic anhydrase II myelinate smaller-diameter axons, whereas oligodendroglia that are positive for RIP but negative for carbonic anhydrase II myelinate larger-diameter axons (116).

With regard to cytoskeletal components, isolated myelin contains actin and both subunits of tubulin (117). Three isoforms of $\alpha$ subunits and nine isoforms of $\beta$ subunits were identified by PAGE. The microtubule-associated protein 1B colocalizes with tubulin staining in cultured oligodendrocytes, and major and fine processes extend into membrane sheets (118). Based on disruption of actin filaments and microtubules in oligodendroglial membrane sheets, MBP is associated with microtubules and CNPase with actin filaments and microtubules (87,88,119). Further, isolated S-MAG binds to tubulin and slows the polymerization of tubulin to microtubules (120), whereas MBP binds to G and F actins and induces polymerization of G actin (121). These interactions may have relevance for myelin formation in vivo: microtubule alterations in the taiep rat led to accumulation of microtubules in oligodendrocyte cell bodies, hypomyelination, and progressive demyelination (122).

## Localization of Proteins in Incisures, Radial Components, and Paranodal and Nodal Regions of Myelin

As described for individual proteins in the previous section, MBP, PLP, and MOBP are localized to the compact regions of the myelin membrane, whereas CNPase and MAG are associated primarily with noncompact regions (Figure 4.1). In addition to this compartmentalization, other proteins are enriched in the several specialized structures within myelin.

Myelin specializations at the nodal and paranodal regions (7) (Figure 4.1; see also Figure 2.5C) are complex structures important for saltatory conduction and axon–glial interactions. On the axonal membrane, several proteins have been localized to the highly specialized nodal, paranodal, and juxtaparanodal regions of the axon. However, the proteins on the apposing paranodal and adaxonal myelin membranes are less well defined. At the node, the axolemma contains Na$^+$ channels, ankyrin G, neuronal cell adhesion molecule (Nr-CAM), the neurofascin NF186 and tensacins; Caspr (paranodin) and contactin are found in the adjacent paranodal axolemma, with OMgp; NF155 and the gap junction protein Cx32 are found in the apposing paranodal loops of CNS myelin. Caspr2, the K$^+$ channels Kv1.1 and 1.2, and an interacting B2 subunit are concentrated in the axonal juxtaparanodal region, whereas K$^+$ channels of unidentified subtype have been found on the apposing myelin membrane.

Both PNS and CNS myelin have incisures, thought to form a spiral pathway for diffusion of ions and small molecules directly across the wrapped myelin lamellae (7). PNS incisures have the structural components of "reflexive" adherens junctions and gap junctions, whereas CNS incisures do not (7). However, oligodendrocyte cell bodies and processes express the gap junction protein Cx32 (123). This protein is also found in paranodal loops of myelin ensheathing some subpopulations of axons (124). Cx32 null mice exhibit hypomyelination and marked decreases in γ-aminobutyric acidergic inhibitory synaptic transmission (125).

In addition to incisures, CNS myelin has a radial component that contains the tight junction protein OSP (126). It constitutes about 7 percent of the myelin protein and has 48 percent amino acid similarity to PMP-22 in the PNS (127). Earlier isolation from myelin of CNS radial component structures in a Triton-insoluble fraction showed enrichment in the 21.5- and 17-kd isoforms of MBP, CNPase, tubulin, and actin (128).

## Enzymes and Receptors in Myelin

Numerous enzymes and receptors are associated with or intrinsic to the myelin membrane. Early studies found little enzymatic activity, with the exception of the major myelin protein 2'3'-CNPase. However, more recent studies have identified a wide range of enzymatic activities in highly purified myelin fractions (129), in keeping with the origin of myelin as a specialized extension of the plasma membrane of the oligodendrocyte. The criteria for designating a given molecule as an intrinsic part of myelin were discussed in detail by Ledeen (129). Many enzymes involved in lipid synthesis or degradation have low but significant activity in myelin fractions, including enzymes that metabolize steroids, glycolipids, and phospholipids. Cholesterol ester synthetase and two cholesterol ester hydrolases are associated with myelin, in keeping with the appearance of cholesterol esters during active myelination and demyelination. Protein kinases and phosphatases, Na$^+$/K$^+$ ATPase, proteases including calpains, guanyl cyclase, G proteins, and enzymes involved in protein acylation and deacylation, transport processes, and second messenger signaling have been reported as myelin components. Of special interest, a fatty acyltransferase that catalyzes the removal of fatty acid from PLP is present in isolated myelin, suggesting local control of PLP acylation within myelin itself (130).

The enzyme N-acetyl aspartic acylase and its substrate N-acetyl aspartic acid (NAA) have been identified in oligodendrocytes and their precursors (131–133). Astrocytes are also highly enriched with this enzyme (134). The enzyme was recently identified in highly purified myelin itself (135). Mutations in the gene for aspartoacylase cause Canavan disease, an autosomal recessive disorder characterized by myelin loss without axonal loss and spongiform degeneration (137). NAA itself was proposed as a marker for neuronal loss and mitochondrial function (136) and is used widely as a marker for axonal integrity in myelinated and nonmyelinated axons, especially in MRI studies (138,139), although its function and sites of synthesis are still under investigation. NAA was identified in neurons and axons by immunocytochemical, high-performance liquid chromatographic, and nuclear magnetic resonance (NMR) methods (131,140,141). One current model suggests that NAA is synthesized primarily in neurons and transported extracellularly from neuronal cell bodies or axons to glia, where it serves in cell-specific signaling and is subsequently degraded (142). Until the gene for the synthetic enzyme is cloned and the enzyme localized, our picture of NAA metabolism remains incomplete.

With regard to receptors, high-affinity muscarinic cholinergic receptors and β-adrenergic receptors were found in myelin fractions, whereas α-adrenergic, serotoninergic, and dopaminergic receptors were not (143). However, a recent report has identified D3 dopaminergic receptors on oligodendrocyte precursors (144).

Several metabolic enzymes enriched in oligodendroglia are found in compact myelin. The enzyme carbonic anhydrase II is highly enriched in oligodendroglia at all stages of development (145) and also is found in myelin fractions (146). Both protein and message for glycerol phosphate dehydrogenase are greatly enriched in oligodendroglia (147), which is consistent with the demand for lipid synthesis for myelin formation and maintenance; one study reported significant levels of the enzyme in myelin itself (148). Glutamine synthetase is also enriched in oligodendroglia, as are glutamate transporters of the GLAST subtype (149). These findings suggest that oligodendroglia play a role in the glutamate/glutamine cycle, but the presence of these transporters in myelin has not been reported.

Most oligodendrocytes in white matter contain ferritin, transferrin, and transferrin receptors, in keeping with their high content of iron and the need for oxidative metabolism for lipid synthesis (150). In MS lesions, ferritin binding is lost in plaque and periplaque regions, whereas transferrin binding and transferrin receptors are retained in the periplaque region (151).

An increasing number of growth factors and cytokines are known to be synthesized and secreted by oligodendroglia. For example, oligodendroglia synthesize nerve growth factor (152). Because oligodendrocytes and possibly myelin have receptors for a number of these proteins, these agents might act in an autocrine manner as well as a paracrine manner with neurons, axons, and other glia. Oligodendroglia synthesize receptors for a number of growth factors and cytokines. Thus, nerve growth factor, PDGF, basic FGF, IGF-1, neurotrophin 3, glial growth factor, ciliary neurotrophic factor, GDNF, tumor necrosis factor α (TNF-α), transforming growth factor β, interleukins 2 and 6, and other factors interact with their corresponding receptors on oligodendrocytes or their precursors, as demonstrated functionally and in some cases by direct identification of the receptor (10). However, the presence of these receptors in myelin, either in compact myelin or specialized nodal or paranodal regions, has not been investigated in detail. The presence of neutral sphingomyelinase in myelin has led to the hypothesis that elevated levels of TNF-α in MS lesions interact directly with myelin, presumably with TNF receptors, activate sphingomyelinase, and thus disrupt myelin locally by destabilization of its structure (153).

## CNS Myelin Lipids

Myelin accounts for approximately 50 percent of the lipid in white matter and 30 percent of total brain lipid. Myelin is characterized by a high ratio of lipid to protein, with 70 to 75 percent lipid compared with 35 to 40 percent in other membranes and a higher proportion of glycolipids (Figure 4.3). The ratio of phospholipids to cholesterol to galactolipid is about 2:1:1 versus 3:1:0.3 in other membranes.

Myelin lipids are rich in ethanolamine plasmalogens and galactolipids, the latter containing very long chain hydroxy fatty acids (>22–26 C). Lipids producing the most dramatic increases during myelination include galactolipids, sphingomyelin, and triphosphoinositides (154). Interestingly, cholesterol esters and gangliosides show maximal rates of increase before myelination, suggesting an association with axon outgrowth and synaptogenesis.

There are no lipids localized exclusively to myelin, but galactocerebroside and its sulfated form, galactocerebroside sulfate (sulfatide), are greatly enriched with myelin compared to other membranes. These two lipids appear in oligodendrocytes at the stage of transition from proliferating progenitor cells to immature oligodendrocytes, marking a key step in differentiation of oligodendrocytes. The content of galactocerebroside and sulfatide in brain is proportional to the amount of myelin, and their rates of synthesis are proportional to the rate of myelination (155–157) and remyelination (158). Although the rate of galactocerebroside synthesis correlates well with the rates of accumulation of myelin, galactocerebroside, and MBP, there is less correspondence between the rate of myelination and the levels of the enzyme synthesizing galactocerebroside, the rate of MBP synthesis, or the rate of cholesterol synthesis.

Antibodies to galactolipids disrupt the normal differentiation program of oligodendrocytes (OLs) in culture, indicating that the galactolipids interact with endogenous ligands to regulate OL differentiation in vivo (159–162). Antibodies to galactocerebroside also inhibit myelination and cause demyelination in myelinating organotypic CNS cultures (163). In the PNS, monoclonal antibodies to galactocerebroside also inhibit myelin formation. Axons and Schwann cells associate in their normal 1:1 relationship and the mesaxon is formed, but elongation is prevented, apparently due to removal of surface galactocerebroside by internalization of antigen–antibody complexes (164). Whether a similar mechanism can block CNS myelination is not known.

Galactocerebroside sulfotransferase catalyzes the formation of sulfatide from its precursor sulfatide. Studies with antibodies specific for each of the two lipids found that galactocerebroside is expressed before sulfatide on the surface of oligodendroglia and Schwann cells in vivo and in vitro (165). Another sulfated molecule, a sulfated proteoglycan, termed pro-oligodendrocyte antigen (POA), is reactive with some monoclonal antibodies to sulfatide (159). POA appears on proliferating oligodendroglial precursors (166) and appears to play a role in regulating subsequent differentiation (159). Inhibition of protein and lipid sulfation with sodium chlorate does not inhibit maturation of oligodendrocytes in culture but does retard formation of processes and membrane sheets, suggesting a role for sulfatide in myelination (167).

The gene has been cloned for UDP-galactose ceramide galactosyl transferase, the enzyme that synthesizes galactocerebroside (168–170). Knockout mice deficient in this enzyme and thus in galactocerebroside and sulfatide (galactocerebroside sulfate) show multiple abnormalities and decreased life spans (171,172). Decreased myelination and structural alterations at the nodes and paranodes occur in the CNS (173). The ultrastructure of compact myelin is initially normal except for somewhat thinner sheaths, but the nodal regions have altered lengths, a number of heminodes, no transverse bands, and reversed lateral loops. A detailed study in PNS showed abnormal paranodes lacking the putative adhesion proteins Caspr2, contactin, and NF-155 (174). As the animals mature, tremor, ataxia, and spinal cord vacuolization occur, along with a block in saltatory conduction in the CNS. These changes point to essential roles for galactolipids in oligodendrocytes and Schwann cells in the formation and maintenance of correct nodal regions and axon–glial interactions (see section on Myelin Assembly). Glucosyl ceramide

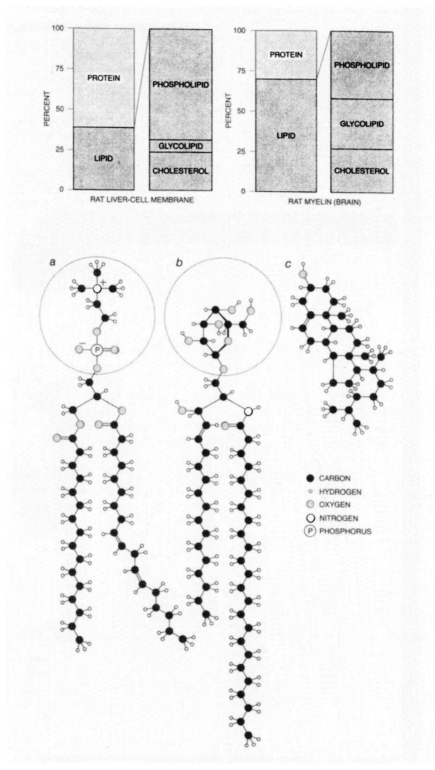

**FIGURE 4.3**

Distribution and structures of the major lipid classes in myelin. Molecular content of myelin and that of a more typical cell-surface membrane are compared by weight. In myelin the lipids are dominant over protein. Three lipids in myelin are diagrammed, representing the 3 classes of lipids shown in the bar graphs. **a.** Phosphatidyl choline is a phospholipid. **b.** Galactocerebroside is the most prominent glycolipid in myelin. A double bond between carbon atoms bends a tail of phosphatidyl choline; double bonds are not common in glycolipids, but hydroxy fatty acids are prominent in myelin galactolipids. **c.** The third molecule is cholesterol. (Reprinted with permission from Morell P, Norton WT. Myelin. *Sci Am* 1980: 242:106.)

and its sulfated product are synthesized in increased amounts in the mutant animals and appear to be able to substitute for the galactolipids in the initiation and wrapping of CNS myelin but not in the formation of the specialized nodal regions interacting with axons.

Cholesterol is a major lipid component of myelin and rich in myelin compared with other membranes (Figure 4.3) (12,175). This sterol decreases fluidity in compact myelin regions, serves as precursor to neurosteroids, and is postulated to regulate ion permeability and the function of myelin proteins in adhesion or channel formation (175). Almost all of the cholesterol in brain is synthesized locally, with only a small contribution from circulating cholesterol (176,177). Inhibition of cholesterol synthesis retards myelination in spinal cord cultures (178) and in vivo (175). Impairment of cholesterol synthesis may be a factor in the forebrain demyelination seen in a genetic mouse model of phenylketonuria (PKU) (179). Further, elevated levels of phenylalanine decreased cholesterol synthesis in a glioma cell line, supporting the possibility that selected populations of oligodendroglia respond to elevated phenylalanine levels by decreased cholesterol synthesis and subsequent demyelination. A portion of cholesterol in the oligodendroglial plasma membrane associates with cytoskeletal structures in the myelin-like membranes elaborated by cultured oligodendroglia (180), and this association is altered by activating signaling pathways in response to binding of filipin or antibodies to galactocerebroside or MOSP. Cholesterol has recently been identified as covalently bound to the transcription factor sonic hedgehog, a critical factor for differentiation of oligodendroglial progenitors (181). The addition of cholesterol to Hedgehog transcription factors increases anchoring to cells, and the removal of cholesterol regulates the release and long-range signaling of these factors (182).

Notably, cholesterol esters are a hallmark of early myelination, demyelination, and remyelination, as initially identified in histologic specimens by the Marchi stain (183) and subsequently confirmed by biochemical analysis (184). The cholesterol esters may function to sequester cholesterol for subsequent reuse in myelin assembly, although one recent study on the PNS indicated that it is required for axonal regeneration but not for remyelination (185). Under conditions of decreased exogenous cholesterol, Schwann cells upregulated de novo cholesterol deposition, whereas axons were more dependent on cholesterol reuse. Cholesterol released by astrocytes and bound to apolipoprotein E stimulated synapse formation in cultured neurons (186,187). Whether oligodendrocytes or myelin release cholesterol that functions in this way in normal or pathologic situations, is not known.

Gangliosides are less rich in myelin than in synapses, constituting 0.7 to 2.5 μg sialic acid/mg protein in rat myelin (12), compared with 0.8 μg sialic acid/mg protein in neuronal cell bodies and 9.0 μg sialic acid/mg protein in synaptic endings, calculated assuming 70 percent lipid in myelin and 40 percent water (188). Among the gangliosides in myelin, GM1 ganglioside is more prominent than the polysialyl gangliosides. GM1 ganglioside has a high affinity for MBP, and binding of GM1 to MBP–calmodulin complexes releases calmodulin (189); whether this interaction occurs in myelin is not known. GM4 ganglioside (sialylated galactocerebroside) is enriched in human and rodent myelin but not in bovine myelin (190). GD3 ganglioside, cross-reactive with the A2B5 antibody, is found in oligodendrocyte precursors. Interestingly, exogenous GM3 gangliosides enhanced differentiation of cultured oligodendrocytes (191).

Lipids in the myelin bilayer show an asymmetric distribution, in keeping with lipids in most cell membranes (192,193). The glycolipids, including galactolipids and gangliosides, are thought to be in the external bilayer in addition to most of the phosphatidyl choline and sphingomyelin. Phospholipids in the internal bilayer, or cytoplasmic surface, include phospatidyl ethanolamine, both diacyl and plasmalogen forms, phosphatidyl serine, and probably phosphatidyl inositol and the related phosphoinositides. In some cell types, an adenosine triphosphate–dependent translocase can transport phosphatidyl serine and phosphatidyl ethanolamine, but not phosphatidyl choline, from the outer to inner lipid layer of the membrane (194); whether this occurs in myelin is not known. The active site of the enzyme synthesizing sulfatide, galactocerebroside sulfotransferase, is thought to face the lumenal surface of the endoplasmic reticulum and Golgi apparatus and thus the extracellular surface of the plasma membrane and myelin. However, the active site of the enzyme synthesizing its precursor, galactocerebroside, may face the cytoplasmic surface of the endoplasmic reticulum, and thus the intracellular surface of the plasma membrane and myelin, by analogy with the UDP-glucuronyl transferases, members of the same gene family (195). How galactocerebroside is subsequently enriched on the lumenal surface of the endoplasmic reticulum or on the extracellular surface of the plasma membrane, and how this asymmetry is regulated during myelination and remyelination is not known.

## STRUCTURAL–MOLECULAR RELATIONSHIPS

### Interactions among Lipids and Proteins in the Myelin Membrane

Several studies have addressed the issue of micro-organization and interaction of lipids with proteins in the myelin membrane (192,196). Lactoperoxidase iodination of proteins in the intact dorsal column of the spinal cord provided the first evidence that MBP is at the cytoplasmic surface of the myelin membrane (corresponding to the major dense line), with at least a portion of PLP at the external surface (197). This was confirmed by immunocytochemistry and analysis of the structure, synthesis and transport of these proteins (see section on Myelin Assembly). Even though a number of studies reported an association of the ganglioside GM1 with MBP in artificial mixtures, this association was not demonstrated directly in the myelin membrane or oligodendroglia. Photoactivated cross-linking of cholesterol or a phosphatidyl choline analog in cultured oligodendroglia associated PLP with cholesterol but not with the phospholipids (198).

Recent interest has focused on glycosphingolipid/ cholesterol-enriched microdomains, or "rafts," in organizing membrane structure. Insolubility in cold Triton X-100 is frequently used as a criterion of the association of lipids and proteins in rafts. Several investigators showed that a large fraction of the proteins in isolated myelin is soluble in Triton X-100, including PLP/DM-20, MBP, MAG, and MOG (199–202). Only CNPase and a portion of MOG were associated with the glycolipids-enriched Triton-insoluble fraction, suggesting that PLP was not associated with lipid rafts. A recent study extracted myelin with the milder detergent CHAPS and found a CHAPS-insoluble fraction containing PLP/DM-20, MAG, and MOG (203). This fraction was isolated from cultured oligodendroglia and myelin. The investigators proposed that this is a specialized raft in myelinating glia, a model supported by examining intracellular transport of PLP (see next section).

Immunocytochemical studies reported the colocalization of several components in myelin or the extensive membrane sheets elaborated by rodent oligodendroglia in culture (87,88,119). Dynamic interactions among myelin lipids and proteins were demonstrated in a series of studies with the use of an antibody to galactocerebroside (204). Whereas this glycolipid was evenly distributed on the membrane surface as identified in lightly fixed cells, the antibody redistributed the glycolipid into large "islands," or domains, on the surface. This surface reorganization of the lipid was accompanied by redistribution of MBP and CNPase and depolymerization of tubulin, demonstrating associations among these components within the membrane. These events were accompanied by an influx of calcium, indicating that the interaction of the antibody with galactocerebroside initiated signaling across the membrane (205). A recent study showed that liposomes containing galactocerebroside and sulfatide also altered distribution of galactocerebroside and MBP and induced depolymerization of microtubules and actin in oligodendroglial sheets (206). The investigators suggested that the effects were due to interactions between galactocerebroside and sulfatide in opposing plasma membranes.

## Assembly of CNS Myelin

Two recent reviews integrated the extensive literature on myelin assembly in the context of current concepts of membrane trafficking (207,208). Metabolic studies, summarized below, reported several different mechanisms for transporting and targeting myelin proteins and lipids from their sites of synthesis to compact myelin or to the specialized regions of noncompact myelin. Kramer et al. (208) summarized evidence for transport of various myelin proteins via directed transport, transcytosis, regulated exocytosis, or lipid rafts. In directed transport, as characterized in polarized endothelial cells, myelin components would be presorted in the trans-Golgi network and then targeted to various myelin domains in vesicles, with specificity and fusion mediated by rab GTPases and SNARES. In transcytosis, vesicles move between distinct membrane domains, with a single secretory path to the plasma membrane, followed by endocytosis, resorting via endosomal rab GTPases, and recycling to the growing myelin membrane. Regulated exocytosis, as defined in detail for synaptic vesicle release, involves fusion of preformed vesicles with the plasma membrane via specific SNAPs and SNARES, in response to a specific signal, perhaps axonal contact or ionic signaling in the case of myelin assembly. In the lipid raft model, regions of membrane greatly enriched with phospholipids, galactolipids, and specific proteins are preassembled in the Golgi and then directed in vesicles via the cytoskeleton toward the axon, where the rafts coalesce into large myelin domains. These mechanisms are interrelated and not necessarily exclusive; a given protein may use one or more of these pathways depending on the cell type, state of differentiation, or presence of axons or growth factors. Thus, specific myelin proteins may exhibit basolateral sorting in one situation but apical sorting in another (208).

In addition to sorting of integral membrane proteins, cytoplasmic- or membrane-associated proteins are targeted by other mechanisms yet to be identified. For example, mRNA for MBP and ribosomal machinery are transported into oligodendroglial processes, thereby providing a mechanism for synthesizing this protein as needed "on demand" for myelin compaction at a site of assembly (209). Enzymes for synthesizing and modifying lipids are found also within purified compact myelin fractions, thereby providing a mechanism for adding or remodeling lipids locally within assembling myelin. Post-translational modification of myelin proteins in situ also may play a role in targeting proteins to build or remodel specialized regions of myelin.

MBPs are synthesized on free ribosomes (210), and appear within minutes after synthesis in the myelin membrane (211). Subsequent studies reported transport of mRNA for MBP from the oligodendroglial cell bodies and into the processes (209), mediated at least in vitro by astroglial contact (6,212). The transport of the mRNA requires microtubules and kinesin (213).

PLP is synthesized on membrane-bound ribosomes (210), acylated in a pre-Golgi compartment (214), and transported through the Golgi to myelin by a vesicular, microtubule-dependent process (214,215). PLP and DM-20 show a delay of about 45 min between synthesis and appearance in myelin (211,216). Examination of the association of PLP with CHAPS-insoluble rafts during intracellular transport in oligodendroglia associated PLP with rafts after leaving the endoplasmic reticulum but before leaving the Golgi (203). Further, cholesterol and galactocerebroside were required for PLP to associate with these lipid-rich complexes.

A series of studies has characterized the transport of PLP and DM-20 in nonoligodendroglial cell lines transfected with normal and mutant forms of the two proteins (77). Normal DM-20 can restore normal transport of some mutant PLPs to the plasma membrane, indicating interactions between these two proteins in trafficking from the endoplasmic reticulum to the plasma membrane (and presumably myelin). Several studies suggested that PLP and sulfatide are cotransported in vesicles based on similar kinetics (211), inhibition by colchicine (215) and monensin (217), and association in complexes. Hypomyelination and decreased myelin stability in the CGT knockout mouse was attributed in part to an interference with transport of PLP into myelin due to the absence of galactocerebroside and sulfatide (200,218). However, other observations suggested that PLP transport does not depend entirely on sulfatide. First, a considerable amount of myelin of normal periodicity formed in the CGT knockout mouse. Second, PLP was transported to the plasma membrane in cultured oligodendroglia in normal amounts, even though sulfatide synthesis was inhibited by 85 percent with sodium chlorate (201).

Several previous studies addressed the synthesis and transport of lipids into myelin, but the underlying mechanisms are less well understood than those for proteins. Analysis of the kinetics of lipid entry into compact myelin fractions found two classes, those lipids appearing in myelin immediately upon synthesis and those showing a delay of 30 to 45 min, similar to that seen for PLP (219,220). Galactocerebroside and most phospholipids showed no delay between synthesis and appearance in myelin, consistent with synthesis by enzymes within myelin itself or very rapid membrane flow or transport from nonmyelin sites of synthesis. However, sulfatide and ethanolamine plasmalogen showed a delay in entry, indicative of independent mechanisms regulating the assembly of these two lipids into myelin compared with the other lipids. Subsequent studies confirmed previous findings that galactocerebroside is synthesized in myelin and in endoplasmic reticulum and Golgi-enriched fractions, whereas sulfatide is synthesized primarily in Golgi-enriched fractions (221). Further, its transport was

blocked by monensin (214) and colchicine (215), whereas that of galactocerebroside was not, supporting a pathway through Golgi and dependence on microtubules for sulfatide transport. Studies on ganglioside transport were more difficult to interpret because disruption of Golgi with monensin inhibited ganglioside synthesis per se but also blocked transport into myelin of the major complex gangliosides, with the exception of GM2 and GM3 gangliosides (222).

## Regulation of Myelination

The stages in differentiation of oligodendroglia and the resulting myelination were identified through a combination of morphologic, immunocytochemical, and molecular studies in vivo and in vitro (223). Transcriptional regulation of this differentiation is not understood in detail, but an increasing number of transcription factors has been identified as critical at various stages of the myelination program (224). Oligodendroglial-specific transcription factors of the bHLH family, Olig1 and Olig2 were identified recently (225,226). These transcription factors are thought to be involved in very early lineage decisions, appear in oligodendroglial progenitors, and continue to be expressed in mature oligodendrocytes. Another transcription factor, Sox10, had the same developmental profile; in the CNS it was expressed predominantly in cells of the oligodendroglia lineage but in contrast to Olig1 and Olig2, Sox10 is expressed in a variety of cells outside the CNS (227). The cyclic adenosine monophosphate–inducible POU protein SCIP (228,229) is expressed early in proliferating cells in the OL lineage, then downregulated as differentiation to a myelinating phenotype begins (230). Sox4 and Sox11 show a similar developmental profile (231). The zinc-finger protein MyT-1 was expressed transiently as SCIP went down and expression of myelin proteins began (232). The transcription factor peroxisome proliferator-activator receptor was found in immature OLs and showed a pattern of expression similar to that of MyT-1 during OL maturation (233). GtX, a homeodomain transcription factor, was upregulated as terminal differentiation occurred and continued to be expressed in the mature OL phenotype (234). Binding sites for SCIP, MyT-1, and GtX were found in the promoter regions of the MBP and PLP genes (234), but the functional relevance of these binding sites in the OL is not known. Oligodendroglia upregulated expression of myelin gene expression in vitro in the absence of axons, but axonal contact was required for the high levels of gene expression accompanying initiation and maintenance of the extensive multilamellar wraps of myelin (235).

The key area of focus for future investigations is the role of axon–oligodendroglia interactions in the initiation of myelination and maintenance of axonal and myelin integrity (236,237). Molecular dissection of the structure and function of nodal specializations and of the process of myelin formation, coupled with advances in brain imaging, will provide new strategies for treating white matter diseases during development and adulthood.

## Acknowledgments

Research from our laboratory presented in this chapter was supported by funding from the NIH and NMSS. I thank Dr. Robert Skoff for insightful discussion and Diane Studzinski for expert preparation of the manuscript, reference list, and figures.

# References

1. Morell P, (ed.), *Myelin*. New York: Plenum Press; 1984.
2. Martenson RE. *Myelin: Biology and Chemistry*. Boca Raton: CRC Press; 1992.
3. Benjamins JA, Morell P, Hartman BK, Agrawal HC. Central nervous system myelin. In: Lajtha A (ed.), *Handbook of Neurochemistry*, 2nd ed. New York: Plenum Press; 1984, 361–415.
4. Benjamins JA, Smith MA. Metabolism of myelin. In: Morell P (ed.), *Myelin*, 2nd ed. New York: Plenum Press; 1984; 225–258.
5. Benjamins JA Protein metabolism of oligodendroglial cells in vivo. In: Norton WT (ed.), *Oligodendroglia*. New York: Plenum Press; 1984; 87–124.
6. Campagnoni AT, Macklin WB. Cellular and molecular aspects of myelin protein gene expression. *Mol Neurobiol* 1988; 2:41–89.
7. Arroyo EJ, Scherer SS. On the molecular architecture of myelinated fibers. *Histochem Cell Biol* 2000; 113:1–18.
8. Morell P, Quarles RH. Myelin formation, structure and biochemistry. In: Siegel GJ (ed.), *Basic Neurochemistry: Molecular, Cellular and Medical Aspects*, 6th ed. Philadelphia: Lippincott-Raven; 1999; 69–93.
9. Campagnoni AT, Skoff RP. The pathobiology of myelin mutants reveal novel biological functions of the MBP and PLP genes. *Brain Pathol* 2001; 11:74–91.
10. Baumann N, Pham-Dinh D. Biology of oligodendrocyte and myelin in the mammalian central nervous system. *Physiol Rev* 2001; 81:871–927.
11. Barkovich AJ. Concepts of myelin and myelination in neuroradiology. *Am J Neuroradiol* 2000; 21:1099–1109.
12. Norton WT, Cammer W. Isolation and characterization of myelin. In: Morell P (ed.), *Myelin*, 2nd ed. New York: Plenum Press; 1984; 147–195.
13. Norton WT. Isolation of myelin from nerve tissue. In: Fleischer L (ed.), *Methods in Enzymology*. New York: Academic Press; 1974; 435–444.
14. Morell P, Greenfield, S, Constanino-Ceccarini E, Wisniewski H. Changes in the protein composition of mouse brain myelin during development. *J Neurochem* 1972; 19:3.
15. Inouye H, Kirschner DA. Folding and function of the myelin proteins from primary sequence data. *J Neurosci Res* 1991; 28:1–17.
16. Shapiro L, Doyle JP, Hensley P, Colman DR, Hendrickson WA. Crystal structure of the extracellular domain from P0, the major structural protein of peripheral nerve myelin. *Neuron* 1996; 17:435–449.
17. Einstein ER, Dalal KB, Csejtey J. Increased protease activity and changes in basic proteins and lipids in multiple sclerosis plaques. *J Neurol Sci* 1970; 11:109–121.
18. Martenson RE, Deibler GE, Kies MW, Levine S, Alvord EC Jr. Myelin basic proteins of mammalian and submammalian vertebrates: Encephalitogenic activities in guinea pigs and rats. *J Immunol* 1972; 109:262–270.
19. Kamholz J, de Ferra F, Puckett C, Lazzarini R. Identification of three forms of human myelin basic protein by cDNA cloning. *Proc Natl Acad Sci USA*. 1986; 83:4962–4966.
20. Moscarello MA, Brady GW, Fein DB, Wood DD, Cruz TF. The role of charge microheterogeneity of basic protein in the formation and maintenance of the multilayered structure of myelin: A possible role in multiple sclerosis. *J Neurosci Res* 1986; 15:87–99.
21. Wood DD, Moscarello MA. The isolation, characterization, and lipid-aggregating properties of a citrulline containing myelin basic protein. *J Biol Chem* 1989; 264:5121–5127.
22. Kimura M, Sato M, Akatsuka A, Nozawa-Kimura S, Takahashi R, Yokoyama M, et al. Restoration of myelin formation by a single type of myelin basic protein in transgenic *shiverer* mice. *Proc Natl Acad Sci USA* 1989; 86:5661–5665.
23. Allinquant B, Staugaitis SM, D'Urso D, Colman DR. The ectopic expression of myelin basic protein isoforms in *Shiverer* oligodendrocytes: Implications for myelinogenesis. *J Cell Biol* 1991; 113:393–403.
24. Pedraza L, Fidler L, Staugaitis SM, Colman DR. The active transport of myelin basic protein into the nucleus suggests a regulatory role in myelination. *Neuron* 1997; 18:579–589.
25. DesJardins KC, Morell P. Phosphate groups modifying myelin basic proteins are metabolically labile; methyl groups are stable. *J Cell Biol* 1983; 97:438–446.
26. Moscarello MA, Wood DD, Ackerley C, Boulias C. Myelin in multiple sclerosis is developmentally immature. *J Clin Invest* 1994; 94:146–154.
27. Whitaker JN. Myelin basic protein in cerebrospinal fluid and other body fluids. *Mult Scler* 1998; 4:16–21.
28. Swanborg RH. Experimental autoimmune encephalomyelitis in rodents as a model for human demyelinating disease. *Clin Immunol Immunopathol* 1995; 77:4–13.
29. Bornstein MB, Miller AI, Teitelbaum D, Arnon R, Sela M. Multiple sclerosis: Trial of a synthetic polypeptide. *Ann Neurol* 1982; 11:317–319.
30. Dupouey P, Jacque C, Bourre JM, Cesselin F, Privat A, Baumann N. Immunochemical studies of myelin basic protein in *shiverer* mouse devoid of major dense line of myelin. *Neurosci Lett* 1979; 12:113–118.
31. Mikoshiba K, Aoki E, Tsukada Y. 2'-3'-cyclic nucleotide 3'-phosphohydrolase activity in the central nervous system of a myelin deficient mutant. *Shiverer. Brain Res* 1980; 192:195–204.
32. Doolittle DP, Baumann N, Chernoff G. Allelism of two myelin deficiency mutations in the mouse. *J Hered* 1981; 72:285.
33. Readhead C, Popko B, Takahashi N, Shine HD, Saavedra RA, Sidman RL, et al. Expression of a myelin basic protein gene in transgenic *shiverer* mice: Correction of the dysmyelinating phenotype. *Cell* 1987; 48:703–712.
34. Shine HD, Readhead C, Popko B, Hood L, Sidman RL. Morphometric analysis of normal, mutant, and transgenic CNS: Correlation of myelin basic protein expression to myelinogenesis. *J Neurochem* 1992; 58:342–349.
35. Wolf MK, Billings-Gagliardi S. Quaking *shiverer* double mutant mice: Morphological phenotypes support possible dual actions of the *shiverer* locus. *Brain Res* 1988; 461:257–273.
36. Dyer CA, Philibotte TM, Billings-Gagliardi S, Wolf MK. Cytoskeleton in myelin-basic-protein-deficient *shiverer* oligodendrocytes. *Dev Neurosci* 1995; 17:53–62.
37. Dyer CA, Phillbotte T, Wolf MK, Billings-Gagliardi S. Regulation of cytoskeleton by myelin components: Studies on *shiverer* oligodendrocytes carrying an Mbp transgene. *Dev Neurosci* 1997; 19:395–409.
38. Brady ST, Witt AS, Kirkpatrick LL, de Waegh SM, Readhead C, Tu PH, et al. Formation of compact myelin is required for maturation of the axonal cytoskeleton. *J Neurosci* 1999; 19:7278–7288.
39. Gould RM, Byrd AL, Barbarese E. The number of Schmidt-Lanterman incisures is more than doubled in *shiverer* PNS myelin sheaths. *J Neurocytol* 1995; 24:85–98.
40. Smith-Slatas C, Barbarese E. Myelin basic protein gene dosage effects in the PNS. *Mol Cell Neurosci* 2000; 15:343–354.
41. Popko B, Puckett C, Hood L. A novel mutation in myelin-deficient mice results in unstable myelin basic protein gene transcripts. *Neuron* 1988; 1:221–225.
42. O'Connor LT, Goetz BD, Kwiecien JM, Delaney KH, Fletch AL, Duncan ID. Insertion of a retrotransposon in Mbp disrupts mRNA splicing and myelination in a new mutant rat. *J Neurosci* 1999; 19:3404–3413.

43. Loevner LA, Shapiro RM, Grossman RI, Overhauser J, Kamholz J. White matter changes associated with deletions of the long arm of chromosome 18 (18q- syndrome): A dysmyelinating disorder? *AJNR Am J Neuroradiol* 1996; 17:1843–1848.

44. Campagnoni AT, Pribyl TM, Campagnoni CW, et al. Structure and developmental regulation of Golli-mbp, a 105-kilobase gene that encompasses the myelin basic protein gene and is expressed in cells in the oligodendrocyte lineage in the brain. *J Biol Chem* 1993; 268:4930–4938.

45. Landry CF, Ellison JA, Pribyl TM, Campagnoni C, Kampf K, Campagnoni AT. Myelin basic protein gene expression in neurons: Developmental and regional changes in protein targeting within neuronal nuclei, cell bodies, and processes. *J Neurosci* 1996; 16:2452–2462.

46. Landry CF, Pribyl TM, Ellison JA, Givogri MI, Kampf K, Campagnoni CW, et al. Embryonic expression of the myelin basic protein gene: Identification of a promoter region that targets transgene expression to pioneer neurons. *J Neurosci* 1998; 18:7315–7327.

47. Givogri MI, Bongarzone ER, Schonmann V, Campagnoni AT. Expression and regulation of Golli products of MBP gene during in vitro development of oligodendrocytes. *J Neurosci Res*. In 2001; 66: 679–690.

48. Feng JM, Givogri IM, Bongarzone ER, Campagnoni C, Jacobs E, Handley VW, et al. Thymocytes express the golli products of the myelin basic protein gene and levels of expression are stage dependent. *J Immunol* 2000; 165:5443–5450.

49. Huseby ES, Goverman J. Tolerating the nervous system: A delicate balance. *J Exp Med* 2000; 191:757–760.

50. Givogri MI, Bongarzone ER, Campagnoni AT. New insights on the biology of myelin basic protein gene: The neural–immune connection. *J Neurosci Res* 2000; 59:153–159.

51. Tienari PJ, Kuokkanen S, Pastinen T, et al. Golli-MBP gene in multiple sclerosis susceptibility. *J Neuroimmunol* 1998; 81:158–167.

52. Coppin H, Ribouchon MT, Bausero P, et al. No evidence for transmission disequilibrium between a new marker at the myelin basic protein locus and multiple sclerosis in French patients. *Genes Immunol*. 2000; 1:478–482.

53. Folch J, Lees MB. Proteolipids, a new type of tissue lipoproteins, their isolation from brain. *JBiol Chem* 1951; 191:807–817.

54. Macklin WB, Campagnoni CW, Deininger PL, Gardinier MV. Structure and expression of the mouse myelin proteolipid protein gene. *J Neurosci Res* 1987; 18:383–394.

55. Puckett C, Hudson L, Ono K, et al. Myelin-specific proteolipid protein is expressed in myelinating Schwann cells but is not incorporated into myelin sheaths. *J Neurosci Res* 1987; 18:511–518.

56. Garbern JY, Cambi F, Tang XM, et al. Proteolipid protein is necessary in peripheral as well as central myelin. *Neuron* 1997; 19:205–218.

57. Nave KA, Lai C, Bloom FE, Milner RJ. Splice site selection in the proteolipid protein (PLP) gene transcript and primary structure of the DM-20 protein of central nervous system myelin. *Proc Natl Acad Sci USA* 1987; 84:5665–5669.

58. Bizzozero OA, Good LK. Myelin proteolipid protein contains thioester-linked fatty acids. *J Neurochem* 1990; 55:1986–1992.

59. Bizzozero OA, Good LK. Rapid metabolisim of fatty acids covalently bound to myelin proteolipid protein. *J Biol Chem* 1991; 266:17092–17098.

60. Weimbs T, Stoffel W. Proteolipid protein (PLP) of CNS myelin: Positions of free, disulfide-bonded, and fatty acid thioester-linked cysteine residues and implications for the membrane topology of PLP. *Biochemistry* 1992; 31:12289–12296.

61. Bizzozero OA, Bixler HA, Davis JD, Espinosa A, Messier AM. Chemical deacylation reduces the adhesive properties of proteolipid protein and leads to decompaction of the myelin sheath. *J Neurochem* 2001; 76:1129–1141.

62. Weimbs T, Stoffel W. Topology of CNS myelin proteolipid protein: Evidence for the nonenzymatic glycosylation of extracytoplasmic domains in normal and diabetic animals. *Biochemistry* 1994; 33:10408–10415.

63. Hashim GA, Wood DD, Moscarello MA. Myelin lipophilin-induced demyelinating disease of the central nervous system. *Neurochem Res* 1980; 5:1137–1145.

64. Cambi F, Lees MB. Chronic experimental allergic encephalomyelitis in guinea pigs: Immunologic studies on the two major myelin proteins. *Cell Immunol* 1984; 86:567–574.

65. Yoshimura T, Kunishita T, Sakai K, Endoh M, Namikawa T, Tabira T. Chronic experimental allergic encephalomyelitis in guinea pigs induced by proteolipid protein. *J Neurol Sci* 1985; 69:47–58.

66. Greer JM, Sobel RA, Sette A, Southwood S, Lees MB, Kuchroo VK. Immunogenic and encephalitogenic epitope clusters of myelin proteolipid protein. *J Immunol* 1996; 156:371–379.

67. Johnson D, Hafler DA, Fallis RJ, et al. Cell-mediated immunity to myelin-associated glycoprotein, proteolipid protein, and myelin basic protein in multiple sclerosis. *J Neuroimmunol* 1986; 13:99–108.

68. Sobel RA, Greer JM, Kuchroo VK. Minireview: Autoimmune responses to myelin proteolipid protein. *Neurochem Res* 1994; 19:915–921.

69. Tuohy VK. Peptide determinants of myelin proteolipid protein (PLP) in autoimmune demyelinating disease: a review. *Neurochem Res* 1994; 19:935–944.

70. Greer JM, Denis B, Sobel RA, Trifilieff E. Thiopalmitoylation of myelin proteolipid protein epitopes enhances immunogenicity and encephalitogenicity. *J Immunol* 2001; 166:6907–6913.

71. Dimou L, Klugmann M, Werner H, Jung M, Griffiths IR, Nave KA. Dysmyelination in mice and the proteolipid protein gene family. *Adv Exp Med Biol* 1999; 468:261–271.

72. Garbern J, Cambi F, Shy M, Kamholz J. The molecular pathogenesis of Pelizaeus-Merzbacher disease. *Arch Neurol* 1999; 56:1210–1214.

73. Klugmann M, Schwab MH, Puhlhofer A, Schneider A, et al. Assembly of CNS myelin in the absence of proteolipid protein. *Neuron* 1997; 18:59–70.

74. Knapp PE, Skoff RP. A defect in the cell cycle of neuroglia in the myelin deficient jimpy mouse. *Brain Res* 1987; 432:301–306.

75. Yang X, Skoff RP. Proteolipid protein regulates the survival and differentiation of oligodendrocytes. *J Neurosci* 1997; 17:2056–2070.

76. Southwood C, Gow A. Molecular pathways of oligodendrocyte apoptosis revealed by mutations in the proteolipid protein gene. *Microsc Res Tech* 2001; 52:700–708.

77. Gow A, Friedrich VL Jr, Lazzarini RA. Many naturally occurring mutations of myelin proteolipid protein impair its intracellular transport. *J Neurosci Res* 1994; 37:574–583.

78. Boison D, Stoffel W. Disruption of the compacted myelin sheath of axons of the central nervous system in proteolipid protein-deficient mice. *Proc Natl Acad Sci USA* 1994; 91:11709–11713.

79. Griffiths I, Klugmann M, Anderson T, et al. Axonal swellings and degeneration in mice lacking the major proteolipid of myelin. *Science* 1998; 280:1610–1613.

80. Thomson CE, Montague P, Jung M, Nave KA, Griffiths IR. Phenotypic severity of murine Plp mutants reflects in vivo and in vitro variations in transport of PLP isoproteins. *Glia* 1997; 20:322–332.

81. Gow A, Southwood CM, Lazzarini RA. Disrupted proteolipid protein trafficking results in oligodendrocyte apoptosis in an animal model of Pelizaeus-Merzbacher disease. *J Cell Biol* 1998; 140:925–934.

82. Bongarzone ER, Campagnoni CW, Kampf K, et al. Identification of a new exon in the myelin proteolipid protein gene encoding novel protein isoforms that are restricted to the somata of oligodendrocytes and neurons. *J Neurosci* 1999; 19:8349–8357.

83. Yan Y, Lagenaur C, Narayanan V. Molecular cloning of M6: Identification of a PLP/DM20 gene family. *Neuron* 1993; 11:423–431.

84. Wolfgram F. A new proteolipid fraction of the nervous system. I. Isolation and amino acid analyses. *J Neurochem* 1966; 13:461–470.

85. O'Neill RC, Minuk J, Cox ME, Braun PE, Gravel M. CNP2 mRNA directs synthesis of both CNP1 and CNP2 polypeptides. *J Neurosci Res* 1997;50:248-257.

86. Kohsaka S, Nishimura Y, Takamatsu K, Shimai K, Tsukada Y. Immunohistochemical localization of 2',3'-cyclic nucleotide 3'-phosphodiesterase and myelin basic protein in the chick retina. *J Neurochem* 1983; 41:434–439.

87. Wilson R, Brophy PJ. Role for the oligodendrocyte cytoskeleton in myelination. *J Neurosci Res* 1989; 22:439–448.
88. Dyer CA, Benjamins JA. Organization of oligodendroglial membrane sheets: II. Galactocerebroside:antibody interactions signal changes in cytoskeleton and myelin basic protein. *J Neurosci Res* 1989; 24:212–221.
89. Braun PE, De Angelis D, Shtybel WW, Bernier L. Isoprenoid modification permits 2',3'-cyclic nucleotide 3'- phosphodiesterase to bind to membranes. *J Neurosci Res* 1991; 30:540–544.
90. Braun PE, Horvath E, Yong VW, Bernier L. Identification of GTP-binding proteins in myelin and oligodendrocyte membranes. *J Neurosci Res* 1990; 26:16–23.
91. Yin X, Peterson J, Gravel M, Braun PE, Trapp BD. CNP overexpression induces aberrant oligodendrocyte membranes and inhibits MBP accumulation and myelin compaction. *J Neurosci Res* 1997; 50:238–247.
92. Quarles RH, McIntyre LJ, Pasnak CF. Lectin-binding proteins in central-nervous-system myelin. Binding of glycoproteins in purified myelin to immobilized lectins. *Biochem J* 1979; 183:213–221.
93. Trapp BD, Andrews SB, Cootauco C, Quarles R. The myelin-associated glycoprotein is enriched in multivesicular bodies and periaxonal membranes of actively myelinating oligodendrocytes. *J Cell Biol* 1989; 109:2417–2426.
94. Lai C, Brow MA, Nave KA, et al. Two forms of 1B236/myelin-associated glycoprotein, a cell adhesion molecule for postnatal neural development, are produced by alternative splicing. *Proc Natl Acad Sci USA* 1987; 84:4337–4341.
95. Salzer JL, Holmes WP, Colman DR. The amino acid sequences of the myelin-associated glycoproteins: Homology to the immunoglobulin gene superfamily. *J Cell Biol* 1987; 104:957–965.
96. Meyer-Franke A, Barres B. Axon myelination. Myelination without myelin-associated glycoprotein. *Curr Biol* 1994; 4:847–850.
97. Filbin MT. The muddle with MAG. *Mol Cell Neurosci* 1996; 8:84–92.
98. McGarry RC, Helfand SL, Quarles RH, Roder JC. Recognition of myelin-associated glycoprotein by the monoclonal antibody HNK-1. *Nature* 1983; 306:376–378.
99. Poltorak M, Sadoul R, Keilhauer G, Landa C, Fahrig T, Schachner M. Myelin-associated glycoprotein, a member of the L2/HNK-1 family of neural cell adhesion molecules, is involved in neuron-oligodendrocyte and oligodendrocyte-oligodendrocyte interaction. *J Cell Biol* 1987; 105:1893–1899.
100. Qiu J, Cai D, Filbin MT. Glial inhibition of nerve regeneration in the mature mammalian CNS. *Glia* 2000; 29:166–174.
101. Cai D, Qiu J, Cao Z, McAtee M, Bregman BS, Filbin MT. Neuronal cyclic AMP controls the developmental loss in ability of axons to regenerate. *J Neurosci* 2001; 21:4731–4739.
102. Stebbins JW, Jaffe H, Moller JR. Characterization of myelin-associated glycoprotein (MAG) proteolysis in the human central nervous system. *Neurochem Res* 1998; 23:1005–1010.
103. Moller JR, Yanagisawa K, Brady RO, Tourtellotte WW, Quarles RH. Myelin-associated glycoprotein in multiple sclerosis lesions: A quantitative and qualitative analysis. *Ann Neurol* 1987; 22:469–474.
104. Li C, Tropak MB, Gerlai R, et al. Myelination in the absence of myelin-associated glycoprotein. *Nature* 1994; 369:747–750.
105. Fujita N, Kemper A, Dupree J, et al. The cytoplasmic domain of the large myelin-associated glycoprotein isoform is needed for proper CNS but not peripheral nervous system myelination. *J Neurosci* 1998; 18:1970–1978.
106. Brunner C, Lassmann H, Waehneldt TV, Matthieu JM, Linington C. Differential ultrastructural localization of myelin basic protein, myelin/oligodendroglial glycoprotein, and 2',3'-cyclic nucleotide 3'- phosphodiesterase in the CNS of adult rats. *J Neurochem* 1989; 52:296–304.
107. Lebar R, Lubetzki C, Vincent C, Lombrail P, Boutry JM. The M2 autoantigen of central nervous system myelin, a glycoprotein present in oligodendrocyte membrane. *Clin Exp Immunol* 1986; 66:423–434.

108. Stefferl A, Brehm U, Linington C. The myelin oligodendrocyte glycoprotein (MOG): A model for antibody- mediated demyelination in experimental autoimmune encephalomyelitis and multiple sclerosis. *J Neural Transm* 2000; 58(Suppl):123–133.
109. Berger T, Reindl M. Immunopathogenic and clinical relevance of antibodies against myelin oligodendrocyte glycoprotein (MOG) in Multiple Sclerosis. *J Neural Transm* 2000; 60(Suppl):351–360.
110. Stefferl A, Schubart A, Storch M, et al. Butyrophilin, a milk protein, modulates the encephalitogenic T cell response to myelin oligodendrocyte glycoprotein in experimental autoimmune encephalomyelitis. *J Immunol* 2000; 165:2859–2865.
111. Yamamoto Y, Mizuno R, Nishimura T, et al. Cloning and expression of myelin-associated oligodendrocytic basic protein. A novel basic protein constituting the central nervous system myelin. *J Biol Chem* 1994; 269:31725–31730.
112. Frank M, van der Haar ME, Schaeren-Wiemers N, Schwab ME. rMAL is a glycosphingolipid-associated protein of myelin and apical membranes of epithelial cells in kidney and stomach. *J Neurosci* 1998; 18:4901–4913.
113. Dyer CA, Matthieu JM. Antibodies to myelin/oligodendrocyte-specific protein and myelin/oligodendrocyte glycoprotein signal distinct changes in the organization of cultured oligodendroglial membrane sheets. *J Neurochem* 1994; 62:777–787.
114. Huber AB, Schwab ME. Nogo-A, a potent inhibitor of neurite outgrowth and regeneration. *Biol Chem* 2000; 381:407–419.
115. Chen MS, Huber AB, van der Haar ME, et al. Nogo-A is a myelin-associated neurite outgrowth inhibitor and an antigen for monoclonal antibody IN-1. *Nature* 2000; 403:434–439.
116. Butt AM, Ibrahim M, Ruge FM, Berry M. Biochemical subtypes of oligodendrocyte in the anterior medullary velum of the rat as revealed by the monoclonal antibody Rip. *Glia* 1995; 14:185–197.
117. de Nechaud B, Wolff A, Jeantet C, Bourre JM. Characterization of tubulin in mouse brain myelin. *J Neurochem* 1983; 41:1538–1544.
118. Fischer I, Konola J, Cochary E. Microtubule associated protein (MAP1B) is present in cultured oligodendrocytes and co-localizes with tubulin. *J Neurosci Res* 1990; 27:112–124.
119. Dyer CA, Benjamins JA. Organization of oligodendroglial membrane sheets. I: Association of myelin basic protein and 2',3'-cyclic nucleotide 3'-phosphohydrolase with cytoskeleton. *J Neurosci Res* 1989; 24:201–211.
120. Kursula P, Lehto VP, Heape AM. The small myelin-associated glycoprotein binds to tubulin and microtubules. *Brain Res Mol Brain Res* 2001; 87:22–30.
121. Boggs JM, Rangaraj G. Interaction of lipid-bound myelin basic protein with actin filaments and calmodulin. *Biochemistry* 2000; 39:7799–7806.
122. Song J, O'Connor LT, Yu W, Baas PW, Duncan ID. Microtubule alterations in cultured taiep rat oligodendrocytes lead to deficits in myelin membrane formation. *J Neurocytol* 1999; 28:671–683.
123. Nagy JI, Rash JE. Connexins and gap junctions of astrocytes and oligodendrocytes in the CNS. *Brain Res Brain Res Rev* 2000; 32:29–44.
124. Li J, Hertzberg EL, Nagy JI. Connexin32 in oligodendrocytes and association with myelinated fibers in mouse and rat brain. *J Comp Neurol* 1997; 379:571–591.
125. Sutor B, Schmolke C, Teubner B, Schirmer C, Willecke K. Myelination defects and neuronal hyperexcitability in the neocortex of connexin 32-deficient mice. *Cereb Cortex* 2000; 10:684–697.
126. Gow A, Southwood CM, Li JS, et al. CNS myelin and sertoli cell tight junction strands are absent in Osp/claudin-11 null mice. *Cell* 1999; 99:649–659.
127. Bronstein JM, Popper P, Micevych PE, Farber DB. Isolation and characterization of a novel oligodendrocyte-specific protein. *Neurology* 1996; 47:772–778.
128. Karthigasan J, Kosaras B, Nguyen J, Kirschner DA. Protein and lipid composition of radial component-enriched CNS myelin. *J Neurochem* 1994; 62:1203–1213.
129. Ledeen R. Enzymes and receptors of myelin. In: Martenson RE (ed.), *Myelin: Biology and Chemistry*. Boca Raton: CRC Press, 1992; 531–570.

130. Bizzozero OA, Leyba J, Nunez DJ. Characterization of prote-olipid protein fatty acylesterase from rat brain myelin. *J Biol Chem* 1992; 267:7886–7894.

131. Urenjak J, Williams SR, Gadian DG, Noble M. Proton nuclear magnetic resonance spectroscopy unambiguously identifies different neural cell types. *J Neurosci* 1993; 13:981–989.

132. Baslow MH, Suckow RF, Sapirstein V, Hungund BL. Expression of aspartoacylase activity in cultured rat macroglial cells is limited to oligodendrocytes. *J Mol Neurosci* 1999; 13:47–53.

133. Bhakoo KK, Pearce D. In vitro expression of N-acetyl aspartate by oligodendrocytes: Implications for proton magnetic resonance spectroscopy signal in vivo. *J Neurochem* 2000; 74:254–262.

134. Bhakoo KK, Craig TJ, Styles P. Developmental and regional distribution of aspartoacylase in rat brain tissue. *J Neurochem* 2001; 79:211–220.

135. Chakraborty G, Mekala P, Yahya D, Wu G, Ledeen RW. Intraneuronal N-acetylaspartate supplies acetyl groups for myelin lipid synthesis: Evidence for myelin-associated aspartoacylase. *J Neurochem* 2001; 78:736–745.

136. Baslow MH. Canavan's spongiform leukodystrophy: A clinical anatomy of a genetic metabolic CNS disease. *J Mol Neurosci* 2000; 15:61–69.

137. Clark JB. N-acetyl aspartate: A marker for neuronal loss or mitochondrial dysfunction. *Dev Neurosci* 1998; 20:271–276.

138. Bjartmar C, Kidd G, Mork S, Rudick R, Trapp BD. Neurological disability correlates with spinal cord axonal loss and reduced N-acetyl aspartate in chronic multiple sclerosis patients. *Ann Neurol* 2000; 48:893–901.

139. Pendlebury ST, Lee MA, Blamire AM, Styles P, Matthews PM. Correlating magnetic resonance imaging markers of axonal injury and demyelination in motor impairment secondary to stroke and multiple sclerosis. *Magn Reson Imaging* 2000; 18:369–378.

140. Anderson KJ, Borja MA, Cotman CW, Moffett JR, Namboodiri MA, Neale JH. N-acetylaspartylglutamate identified in the rat retinal ganglion cells and their projections in the brain. *Brain Res* 1987; 411:172–177.

141. Simmons ML, Frondoza CG, Coyle JT. Immunocytochemical localization of N-acetyl-aspartate with monoclonal antibodies. *Neuroscience* 1991; 45:37–45.

142. Baslow MH. Functions of N-acetyl-L-aspartate and N-acetyl-L-aspartylglutamate in the vertebrate brain: role in glial cell-specific signaling. *J Neurochem* 2000; 75:453–459.

143. Larocca JN, Cervone A, Ledeen RW. Stimulation of phosphoinositide hydrolysis in myelin by muscarinic agonist and potassium. *Brain Res* 1987; 436:357–362.

144. Bongarzone ER, Howard SG, Schonmann V, Campagnoni AT. Identification of the dopamine D3 receptor in oligodendrocyte precursors: Potential role in regulating differentiation and myelin formation. *J Neurosci* 1998; 18:5344–5353.

145. Ghandour MS, Vincendon G, Gombos G, et al. Carbonic anhydrase and oligodendroglia in developing rat cerebellum: A biochemical and imunohistological study. *Dev Biol* 1980; 77:73–83.

146. Cammer W, Fredman T, Rose AL, Norton WT. Brain carbonic anhydrase: Activity in isolated myelin and the effect of hexachlorophene. *J Neurochem* 1976; 27:165–171.

147. Cheng JD, Espinosa de los Monteros A, de Vellis J. Glial- and fat-specific expression of the rat glycerol phosphate dehydrogenase-luciferase fusion gene in transgenic mice. *J Neurosci Res* 1997; 50:300–311.

148. Cammer W, Snyder DS, Zimmerman TR Jr, Farooq M, Norton WT. Glycerol phosphate dehydrogenase, glucose-6-phosphate dehydrogenase, and lactate dehydrogenase: Activities in oligodendrocytes, neurons, astrocytes, and myelin isolated from developing rat brains. *J Neurochem* 1982; 38:360–367.

149. Domercq M, Sanchez-Gomez MV, Areso P, Matute C. Expression of glutamate transporters in rat optic nerve oligodendrocytes. *Eur J Neurosci* 1999; 11:2226–2236.

150. Connor JR, Menzies SL. Relationship of iron to oligodendrocytes and myelination. *Glia* 1996; 17:83–93.

151. Hulet SW, Powers S, Connor JR. Distribution of transferrin and ferritin binding in normal and multiple sclerotic human brains. *J Neurol Sci* 1999; 165:48–55.

152. Byravan S, Foster LM, Phan T, Verity AN, Campagnoni AT. Murine oligodendroglial cells express nerve growth factor. *Proc Natl Acad Sci USA* 1994; 91:8812–8816.

153. Ledeen RW, Chakraborty G. Cytokines, signal transduction, and inflammatory demyelination: Review and hypothesis. *Neurochem Res* 1998; 23:277–289.

154. Wells MA, Dittmer JC. A comprehensive study of the postnatal changes in the concentration of the lipids of developing rat brain. *Biochemistry* 1967; 6:3169.

155. Costantino-Ceccarini E, Morell P. Quaking mouse: In vitro studies of brain sphingolipid biosynthesis. *Brain Res* 1971; 29:75–84.

156. McKhann GM, Ho W. The in vivo and in vitro synthesis of sulphatides during development. *J Neurochem* 1967; 14:717–724.

157. Muse ED, Jurevics H, Toews AD, Matsushima GK, Morell P. Parameters related to lipid metabolism as markers of myelination in mouse brain. *J Neurochem* 2001; 76:77–86.

158. Jurevics H, Hostettler J, Muse ED, et al. Cerebroside synthesis as a measure of the rate of remyelination following cuprizone-induced demyelination in brain. *J Neurochem* 2001; 77:1067–1076.

159. Bansal R, Gard AL, Pfeiffer SE. Stimulation of oligodendrocyte differentiation in culture by growth in the presence of a monoclonal antibody to sulfated glycolipid. *J Neurosci Res* 1988; 21:260–267.

160. Bansal R, Pfeiffer SE. Reversible inhibition of oligodendrocyte progenitor differentiation by a monoclonal antibody against surface galactolipids. *Proc Natl Acad Sci USA* 1989; 86:6181–6185.

161. Bansal R, Pfeiffer SE. Regulation of gene expression in mature oligodendrocytes by the specialized myelin-like membrane environment: Antibody perturbation in culture with the monoclonal antibody R-mAb. *Glia* 1994; 12:173–179.

162. Bansal R, Winkler S, Bheddah S. Negative regulation of oligodendrocyte differentiation by galactosphingolipids. *J Neurosci* 1999; 19:7913–7924.

163. Raine CS, Johnson AB, Marcus DM, Suzuki A, Bornstein MB. Demyelination in vitro. Absorption studies demonstrate that galactocerebroside is a major target. *J Neurol Sci* 1981; 52:117–131.

164. Ranscht B, Wood PM, Bunge RP. Inhibition of in vitro peripheral myelin formation by monoclonal anti-galactocerebroside. *J Neurosci* 1987; 7:2936–2947.

165. Ranscht B, Clapshaw PA, Price J, Noble M, Seifert W. Development of oligodendrocytes and Schwann cells studied with a monoclonal antibody against galactocerebroside. *Proc Natl Acad Sci USA* 1982; 79:2709–2713.

166. Bansal R, Stefansson K, Pfeiffer SE. Proligodendroblast antigen (POA), a developmental antigen expressed by A007/O4-positive oligodendrocyte progenitors prior to the appearance of sulfatide and galactocerebroside. *J Neurochem* 1992; 58:2221–2229.

167. Bansal R, Pfeiffer SE. Inhibition of protein and lipid sulfation in oligodendrocytes blocks biological responses to FGF-2 and retards cytoarchitectural maturation, but not developmental lineage progression. *Dev Biol* 1994; 162:511–524.

168. Bosio A, Binczek E, Stoffel W. Functional breakdown of the lipid bilayer of the myelin membrane in central and peripheral nervous system by disrupted galactocerebroside synthesis. *Proc Natl Acad Sci USA* 1996; 93:13280–13285.

169. Coetzee T, Li X, Fujita N, Marcus J, Suzuki K, Francke U, et al. Molecular cloning, chromosomal mapping, and characterization of the mouse UDP-galactose: ceramide galactosyltransferase gene. *Genomics* 1996; 35:215–222.

170. Schulte S, Stoffel W. UDP galactose: ceramide galactosyltransferase and glutamate/aspartate transporter. Copurification, separation and characterization of the two glycoproteins. *Eur J Biochem* 1995; 233:947–953.

171. Marcus J, Dupree JL, Popko B. Effects of galactolipid elimination on oligodendrocyte development and myelination. *Glia* 2000; 30:319–328.

172. Popko B, Dupree JL, Coetzee T, Suzuki K. Genetic analysis of myelin galactolipid function. *Adv Exp Med Biol* 1999; 468:237–244.

173. Dupree JL, Coetzee T, Suzuki K, Popko B. Myelin abnormalities in mice deficient in galactocerebroside and sulfatide. *J Neurocytol* 1998; 27:649–659.

174. Poliak S, Gollan L, Salomon D, et al. Localization of Caspr2 in myelinated nerves depends on axon-glia interactions and the generation of barriers along the axon. *J Neurosci* 2001; 21:7568–7575.

175. Snipes GJ, Suter U. Cholesterol and myelin. *Subcell Biochem* 1997; 28:173–204.

176. Edmond J, Korsak RA, Morrow JW, Torok-Both G, Catlin DH. Dietary cholesterol and the origin of cholesterol in the brain of developing rats. *J Nutr* 1991; 121:1323–1330.

177. Jurevics H, Morell P. Cholesterol for synthesis of myelin is made locally, not imported into brain. *J Neurochem* 1995; 64:895–901.

178. Kim SU. Effects of the cholesterol biosynthesis inhibitor ay9944 on organotypic cultures of mouse spinal cord. Retarded myelinogenesis and induction of cytoplasmic inclusions. *Lab Invest* 1975; 32:720–728.

179. Shefer S, Tint GS, Jean-Guillaume D, et al. Is there a relationship between 3-hydroxy-3-methylglutaryl coenzyme a reductase activity and forebrain pathology in the PKU mouse? *J Neurosci Res* 2000; 61:549–563.

180. Lintner RN, Dyer CA. Redistribution of cholesterol in oligodendrocyte membrane sheets after activation of distinct signal transduction pathways. *J Neurosci Res* 2000; 60:437–449.

181. Pringle NP, Yu WP, Guthrie S, et al. Determination of neuroepithelial cell fate: Induction of the oligodendrocyte lineage by ventral midline cells and sonic hedgehog. *Dev Biol* 1996; 177:30–42.

182. Ingham PW. How cholesterol modulates the signal. *Curr Biol* 2000; 10:R180–183.

183. Adams CWM. Histochemistry of lipids. In: Adams CWM (ed.), *Neurohistochemistry*. New York: Elsevier Publishing Company, 1965, 6–66.

184. Kinney HC, Karthigasan J, Borenshteyn NI, Flax JD, Kirschner DA. Myelination in the developing human brain: Biochemical correlates. *Neurochem Res* 1994; 19:983–996.

185. Goodrum JF, Brown JC, Fowler KA, Bouldin TW. Axonal regeneration, but not myelination, is partially dependent on local cholesterol reutilization in regenerating nerve. *J Neuropathol Exp Neurol* 2000; 59:1002–1010.

186. Barres BA, Smith SJ. Neurobiology. Cholesterol—making or breaking the synapse. *Science* 2001; 294:1296–1297.

187. Mauch DH, Nagler K, Schumacher S, et al. CNS synaptogenesis promoted by glia-derived cholesterol. *Science* 2001; 294:1354–1357.

188. Ledeen RW. Ganglioside structures and distribution: Are they localized at the nerve ending? *J Supramol Struct* 1978; 8:1–17.

189. Chan KF, Robb ND, Chen WH. Myelin basic protein: Interaction with calmodulin and gangliosides. *J Neurosci Res* 1990; 25:535–544.

190. Cochran FB Jr, Yu RK, Ledeen RW. Myelin gangliosides in vertebrates. *J Neurochem* 1982; 39:773–779.

191. Yim SH, Farrer RG, Hammer JA, Yavin E, Quarles RH. Differentiation of oligodendrocytes cultured from developing rat brain is enhanced by exogenous GM3 ganglioside. *J Neurosci Res* 1994; 38:268–281.

192. Braun PE. Molecular organization of myelin. In: Morell P (ed.), *Myelin*. New York: Plenum Press, 1984; 97–116.

193. Agranoff BW, Benjamins JA, Hajra AK. Lipids. In: Siegel GJ (ed.), *Basic Neurochemistry*. Philadelphia: Lippincott-Raven, 1999; 47–68.

194. Devaux PF. Protein involvement in transmembrane lipid asymmetry. *Annu Rev Biophys Biomol Struct* 1992; 21:417–439.

195. Radominska-Pandya A, Czernik PJ, Little JM, Battaglia E, Mackenzie PI. Structural and functional studies of UDP-glucuronosyltransferases. *Drug Metab Rev* 1999; 31:817–899.

196. Boggs JM, Moscarello MA. Structural organization of the human myelin membrane. *Biochim Biophys Acta* 1978; 515:1–21.

197. Poduslo JF, Braun PE. Topographical arrangement of membrane proteins in the intact myelin sheath. Lactoperoxidase incorproation of iodine into myelin surface proteins. *J Biol Chem* 1975; 250:1099–1105.

198. Simons K, Toomre D. Lipid rafts and signal transduction. *Nat Rev Mol Cell Biol* 2000; 1:31–39.

199. Pereyra PM, Horvath E, Braun PE. Triton X-100 extractions of central nervous system myelin indicate a possible role for the minor myelin proteins in the stability in lamellae. *Neurochem Res* 1988; 13:583–595.

200. Kramer EM, Koch T, Niehaus A, Trotter J. Oligodendrocytes direct glycosyl phosphatidylinositol-anchored proteins to the myelin sheath in glycosphingolipid-rich complexes. *J Biol Chem* 1997; 272:8937–8945.

201. van der Haar ME, Visser HW, de Vries H, Hoekstra D. Transport of proteolipid protein to the plasma membrane does not depend on glycosphingolipid cotransport in oligodendrocyte cultures. *J Neurosci Res* 1998; 51:371–381.

202. Kim T, Pfeiffer SE. Myelin glycosphingolipid/cholesterol-enriched microdomains selectively sequester the non-compact myelin proteins CNP and MOG. *J Neurocytol* 1999; 28:281–293.

203. Simons M, Kramer EM, Thiele C, Stoffel W, Trotter J. Assembly of myelin by association of proteolipid protein with cholesterol- and galactosylceramide-rich membrane domains. *J Cell Biol* 2000; 151:143–154.

204. Dyer CA, Benjamins JA. Antibody to galactocerebroside alters organization of oligodendroglial membrane sheets in culture. *J Neurosci* 1988; 8:4307–4318.

205. Dyer CA, Benjamins JA. Glycolipids and transmembrane signaling: Antibodies to galactocerebroside cause an influx of calcium in oligodendrocytes. *J Cell Biol* 1990; 111:625–633.

206. Boggs JM, Wang H. Effect of liposomes containing cerebroside and cerebroside sulfate on cytoskeleton of cultured oligodendrocytes. *J Neurosci Res* 2001; 66:242–253.

207. de Vries H, Hoekstra D. On the biogenesis of the myelin sheath: Cognate polarized trafficking pathways in oligodendrocytes. *Glycoconj J* 2000; 17:181–190.

208. Kramer EM, Schardt A, Nave KA. Membrane traffic in myelinating oligodendrocytes. *Microsc Res Tech* 2001; 52:656–671.

209. Ainger K, Avossa D, Diana AS, Barry C, Barbarese E, Carson JH. Transport and localization elements in myelin basic protein mRNA. *J Cell Biol* 1997; 138:1077–1087.

210. Colman DR, Kreibich G, Frey AB, Sabatini DD. Synthesis and incorporation of myelin polypeptides into CNS myelin. *J Cell Biol* 1982; 95:598–608.

211. Benjamins JA, Iwata R, Hazlett J. Kinetics of entry of proteins into the myelin membrane. *J Neurochem* 1978; 31:1077–1085.

212. Colombatti A, Bonaldo P, Ainger K, Bressan GM, Volpin D. Biosynthesis of chick type VI collagen. I. Intracellular assembly and molecular structure. *J Biol Chem* 1987; 262:14454–14460.

213. Carson JH, Worboys K, Ainger K, Barbarese E. Translocation of myelin basic protein mRNA in oligodendrocytes requires microtubules and kinesin. *Cell Motil Cytoskeleton* 1997; 38:318–328.

214. Townsend LE, Benjamins JA. Effects of monensin on post-translational processing of myelin proteins. *J Neurochem* 1983; 40:1333–1339.

215. Bizzozero OA, Pasquini JM, Soto EF. Differential effect of colchicine upon the entry of proteins into myelin and myelin related membranes. *Neurochem Res* 1982; 7(11):1415–1425.

216. Benjamins JA, Jones M, Morell P. Appearance of newly synthesized protein in myelin of young rats. *J Neurochem* 1975; 24:1117–1122.

217. Townsend LE, Benjamins JA, Skoff RP. Effects of monensin and colchicine on myelin galactolipids. *J Neurochem* 1984; 43:139–145.

218. Coetzee T, Suzuki K, Popko B. New perspectives on the function of myelin galactolipids. *Trends Neurosci* 1998; 21:126–130.

219. Benjamins JA, Fitch J, Radin NS. Effects of ceramide analogs on myelinating organ cultures. *Brain Res* 1976; 102:267–281.

220. Benjamins JA, Iwata R. Kinetics of entry of galactolipids and phospholipids into myelin. *J Neurochem* 1979; 32:921–926.

221. Benjamins JA, Hadden T, Skoff RP. Cerebroside sulfotransferase in Golgi-enriched fractions from rat brain. *J Neurochem* 1982; 38:233–241.

222. Farrer RG, Benjamins JA. Entry of newly synthesized gangliosides into myelin. *J Neurochem* 1992; 58:1477–1484.

223. de Vellis J, Carpenter E. Developments. In: *Basic Neurochemistry: Molecular, Cellular and Medical Aspects*, 6th ed. Philadelphia: Lippincott-Raven; 1999: 537–563.

224. Wegner M. Expression of transcription factors during oligodendroglial development. *Microsc Res Tech* 2001; 52:746–752.

225. Lu QR, Yuk D, Alberta JA, et al. Sonic hedgehog–regulated oligodendrocyte lineage genes encoding bHLH proteins in the mammalian central nervous system. *Neuron* 2000; 25:317–329.

226. Zhou Q, Wang S, Anderson DJ. Identification of a novel family of oligodendrocyte lineage-specific basic helix-loop-helix transcription factors. *Neuron* 2000; 25:331–343.

227. Kuhlbrodt K, Herbarth B, Sock E, Hermans-Borgmeyer I, Wegner M. Sox10, a novel transcriptional modulator in glial cells. J *Neurosci* 1998; 18:237–250.

228. Monuki ES, Kuhn R, Weinmaster G, Trapp BD, Lemke G. Expression and activity of the POU transcription factor SCIP. *Science* 1990; 249:1300–1303.

229. Monuki ES, Weinmaster G, Kuhn R, Lemke G. SCIP: A glial POU domain gene regulated by cyclic AMP. *Neuron* 1989; 3:783–793.

230. Collarini EJ, Kuhn R, Marshall CJ, Monuki ES, Lemke G, Richardson WD. Down-regulation of the POU transcription factor SCIP is an early event in oligodendrocyte differentiation in vitro. *Development* 1992; 116:193–200.

231. Kuhlbrodt K, Herbarth B, Sock E, Enderich J, Hermans-Borgmeyer I, Wegner M. Cooperative function of POU proteins and SOX proteins in glial cells. *J Biol Chem* 1998; 273:16050–16057.

232. Armstrong RC, Kim JG, Hudson LD. Expression of myelin transcription factor I (MyTI), a "zinc-finger" DNA- binding protein, in developing oligodendrocytes. *Glia* 1995; 14:303–321.

233. Granneman J, Skoff R, Yang X. Member of the peroxisome proliferator-activated receptor family of transcription factors is differentially expressed by oligodendrocytes. *J Neurosci Res* 1998; 51:563–573.

234. Awatramani R, Scherer S, Grinspan J, et al. Evidence that the homeodomain protein Gtx is involved in the regulation of oligodendrocyte myelination. *J Neurosci* 1997; 17:6657–6668.

235. Macklin WB, Weill CL, Deininger PL. Expression of myelin proteolipid and basic protein mRNAs in cultured cells. *J Neurosci Res* 1986; 16:203–217.

236. Bjartmar C, Yin X, Trapp BD. Axonal pathology in myelin disorders. *J Neurocytol* 1999; 28:383–395.

237. Morell P, Norton WT. Myelin. *Sci Am* 1980; 242:88–90, 92, 96 passim.

# II

# EXPERIMENTAL ASPECTS
# OF DEMYELINATION

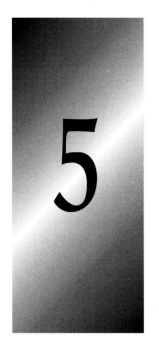

# 5

# The Nature of Immunologic Privilege in the Central Nervous System

*Zsuzsa Fabry, Ph.D.*
*Matyas Sandor, Ph.D.*
*Diane Sewell, Ph.D.*
*Emily Reinke*

The central nervous system (CNS) has been regarded as an immunologically privileged site because of the existence of several anatomic and physiologic protective mechanisms. This view was formulated based on the relative hospitality of the brain toward transplanted allografts that survive for longer periods than transplants in other tissues (1). However, the concept of immunologic privilege has evolved. Our view has become more complex as new information with regard to communication between the immune and the nervous systems has become available; it has become evident that these bidirectional interactions are augmented further under pathologic conditions (2). Nevertheless, it is well appreciated that there is a unique microenvironment in the CNS involving factors that have a profound influence on resident cell populations and their ability to modulate an immune response in the nervous tissue. Some of these factors have a suppressive effect that can prevent or limit the initiation of inflammatory responses in the CNS (2). However, activated lymphocytes invading the CNS can release proinflammatory mediators altering the balance in the negative modulation of immunity in the CNS. Thus, the balance between pro- and anti-inflammatory factors in the CNS determining the localization, intensity, and course of immune responses in the brain differs from that in the peripheral nervous system. As a result, an overwhelming invasion of activated lympho-cytes can create a predominantly proinflammatory local environment in the CNS leading to immune-mediated diseases of the nervous tissue.

Analysis of local CNS factors showed that multiple mechanisms are responsible for maintaining immunologic privilege in the CNS (Table 5.I). These include an immunologic barrier manifested by the absence of draining lymph nodes and lack of immune surveillance; the limited expression of major histocompatibility (MHC) class I and class II molecules in the brain parenchyma, the lack of resident professional antigen-presenting cells, and limited expression of costimulatory molecules; and an active suppression of immune responses in the CNS. This immunologic barrier is localized behind the most prominent element involved in keeping the immune-privileged status of the CNS, i.e., the blood–brain barrier (BBB), which provides anatomic and physiologic blockades.

The consensus is that these multiple mechanisms together shape the anti-inflammatory environment in the CNS and strongly inhibit immune responses in the nervous tissues. However, over the past few decades the issue of immune privilege has been complicated by many experiments indicating that the CNS itself may have an innate immune system capable of regulating adaptive immune responses. Moreover, it has been demonstrated, in a properly functioning BBB, that lymphocytes can readily enter the brain at sites of inflammatory reactions. Further, it was demonstrated that activated T-cells (3,4) and even

**TABLE 5.1**

*Local Multiple Factors in the CNS Responsible for Maintaining Immunologic Privilege in the Nervous Tissue*

**Anatomic barrier:**
- Isolation of CNS behind the BBB

**Immunologic barrier:**
- Absence of draining lymph nodes and lymphoid circulation in the CNS
- Lack of immune surveillance in the brain
- Limited expression of MHC class I and class II molecules in the brain parenchyma
- Lack of professional, fully competent APCs
- Limited expression of costimulatory molecules in the CNS
- Active suppression of immune responses in the CNS

APC, antigen-presenting cell; BBB, blood–brain barrier; CNS, central nervous system; MHC, major histocompatibility complex.

naive T-lymphocytes (5) can migrate across the healthy BBB; thus the normal, noninflamed CNS is accessible to immune cells. More recently, it was shown that there are pathways for the lymphatic drainage of interstitial fluid and proteins from the brain (6–8) and that this drainage results in antibody production in cervical lymph nodes (9–12). In addition, protein antigens can be collected in the cervical lymph nodes after intracerebral administration of antigens and induce T-cell activation in the periphery (13).

In this chapter we discuss the current view of immunologic privilege in the CNS, and we promote an active regulatory role of the BBB in immune responses. Undoubtedly, the immune system has to protect and defend the CNS from pathogens and insults and, hence, have access to the CNS; however, immune system functions must be highly regulated in this unique tissue to avoid destruction of sensitive and irreplaceable neurons. We take a careful look at this fine regulation by focusing on the 1) BBB and the nature of immunologic privilege in the CNS, 2) normal immune surveillance and pathologic traffic of lymphocytes into the CNS tissue, and 3) role of antigen-presenting cells in the brain tissue, with special interest in macrophages and microglia.

## BBB AND THE NATURE OF IMMUNOLOGIC PRIVILEGE IN THE CNS

### Traditional View of the BBB

The concept of the BBB was born more than a century ago, when Paul Ehrlich (14,15) and Edwin Goldman (16) intravenously injected water-soluble dyes and observed that the dyes were selectively excluded from the brain tis-

sue. This was the first demonstration of a highly regulated and restrictive structure between the peripheral system and the CNS, with a mission to separate the brain from the rest of the body. Since those early studies our knowledge about the BBB has significantly deepened. Using horseradish peroxidase as a tracer, Reese and Karnovsky (17) demonstrated the fine structure of the BBB and indicated that it is located at the level of the vascular endothelial cells. They suggested that the presence of the BBB correlated well with the existence of tight interendothelial junctions and the lack of micropinocytosis in the brain endothelial cells. The presence of tight junctions severely restricts the paracellular flux and the lack of any significant number of endocytotic vesicles limits the transcellular flux across the BBB (18). A very selective intracellular transport system permits the passage of a limited number of specifically transported nutrients such as glucose and amino acids and some transcytosed larger molecules, such as transferrin, across the BBB (19–21).

The currently accepted theory is that cerebral microvessels possess different morphologic and enzymatic properties compared with the microvessels of other organs (22,23). For example, cerebral endothelial cells synthesize multidrug-resistance protein P-glycoprotein, or mdr 1a (also called mdr3), that actively transports a variety of low-molecular-weight toxic molecules out of the brain to the circulation (24). Cerebral endothelium also has specific transport systems for delivering nutrients from the circulation into the nervous tissue, including the glucose transporter Glut-1 and a set of amino acid transporters (19,25,26). The unique properties of brain endothelial cells are also reflected by the expression of specific cell surface molecules on the BBB. One of these molecules, the HT7 antigen, which is a highly glycosylated 45- to 52-kDa protein, was reported to be localized to brain endothelial cells, kidney epithelial cells, and erythroblasts. Based on the nucleotide sequence, it was demonstrated that HT7 is a novel glycoprotein with two C2-like immunoglobulin-related domains, one transmembrane, domain and a cytoplasmic tail (27). Recent results demonstrated that HT7, neurothelin, gp42, basigin, and OX-47 are probably different names for the same glycoprotein in different species; therefore, in this text we designate these molecules "neurothelin" (28,29). Besides these BBB markers, other molecules have been suggested to be expressed highly, although not selectively, at the BBB. These markers include CD71/transferrin receptor (30) and platelet-derived growth factor receptor (19). During their differentiation, cerebral endothelial cells not only acquire specific markers but also lose molecules that are otherwise present on noncerebral endothelial cells such as MECA 32 and VE-cadherin (31,32).

Undoubtedly, the most prominent characteristic of cerebral endothelial cells is their capability to form tight junctions leading to the formation of a metabolic and

## APICAL JUNCTIONAL COMPLEX

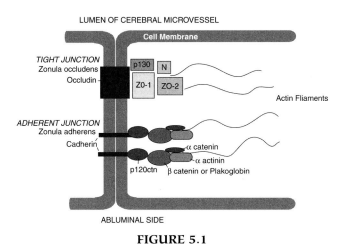

**FIGURE 5.1**

The crucial structural aspects of the molecular basis of apical junctional complex assembly. Tight junctions and adherent junctions form between endothelial cells in the central nervous system.

physical barrier that under normal conditions is a stringent gatekeeper for hematopoietic cells (Figure 5.1).

This is in contrast to endothelial cells in non-neural tissues, where activated blood cells can easily cross the vessel wall. In lymphoid organs, naive lymphocytes continually recirculate from blood to lymph nodes and back to blood through specialized endothelia composed of large, cuboidal cells known as high endothelial venules (HEV). Interestingly, such HEV-like vessels can develop in the CNS during inflammatory processes (33).

Over the years, several laboratories have developed long-term cultures of brain microvessel endothelial cells (34–41). In vitro BBB migration assays also characterized the mechanisms of leukocyte migration across the BBB (42,43). Several adhesion molecules and immune mediators were found to be produced by brain endothelial cells (43–49). Based on our studies and research from other laboratories, we must consider the vascular wall endothelial cells in the brain as "gatekeepers" for T-cell traffic into the CNS.

Tight junctions represent the major component of the "gatekeeper" function of the BBB. Morphologically, BBB tight junctions are similar to epithelial tight junctions, but there are essential differences between these structures. For example, in contrast to tight junctions in epithelial systems, structural and functional characteristics of tight junctions in endothelial cells are highly sensitive to several mediators. Many molecular components of tight junctions have been identified and characterized including claudins, occludin, zonula occludens molecules, such as ZO-1, ZO-2, ZO-3, cingulin, and 7H6 (Figure 5.1) (50). Some signaling pathways involved in tight junction regulation have

also been identified, and the involvement of G-proteins, serine, threonine, and tyrosine kinases, extra- and intracellular calcium levels, and cyclic adenosine monophosphate levels have been demonstrated. Common to most of these pathways is the modulation of cytoskeletal elements. In addition, cross-talk between components of the tight junction and the adherent junctions (cadherin-catenin system) has been demonstrated. It is generally accepted that tight junctions are particularly developed in cerebral endothelial cells in strong association with cytoskeletal elements (51). Through this cytoskeletal association, the tight junction and the adherent junction form a functional unit termed the *apical junctional complex*. The crucial aspects of the molecular basis of tight junction regulation and assembly are shown in Figure 5.1.

Developmentally, cerebral microvessels derive from the meningeal vessels and invade the brain by angiogenesis. Traditionally, astrocytes were thought to contribute to the important microenvironmental factors in inducing the development of the BBB and tight junction formation (52). The role of astrocytes in the induction of endothelial cells to adopt a brain phenotype has become more controversial recently. Structurally, the cell types that are closest to endothelial cells are astrocytes and glia limitans, a network of astrocyte foot processes that form a tight sheath surrounding brain and spinal cord microvessels (Figure 5.2). However, this glia limitans sheath is absent in the meningeal vessels and choroid plexus; despite the absence of this sheath, there are tight junctions between the choroid plexus endotrelial cells.

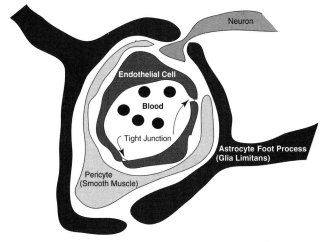

**FIGURE 5.2**

A network of astrocyte foot processes (glia limitans) form a tight sheath surrounding the endothelial cells in brain and spinal cord microvessels. Tight junctions form between brain microvessel endothelial cells leading to the formation of a metabolic and physical barrier. Perivascular cells and occasional neural endings surround the cerebral microvessels.

The importance of astrocytes in inducing the endothelial barrier characteristics was first demonstrated by Stewart and Wiley (53). Soluble factors of astrocyte origin also were proposed to upregulate neurothelin expression in endothelial cells of chorioallantoic vessels (54). However, pial vessels, which have high electrical resistance, are not connected with astrocytic endfeet in the same uniform manner (55). Based on this observation, the full brain endothelial cell phenotype is probably induced by several factors and possibly by cells other than astrocytes. One of these cell types might be the neuron, because different nerve endings are found in the vicinity of brain capillaries (Figure 5.2) (56). Recently, glial cell line–derived neutrophic factor was demonstrated to induce barrier function of endothelial cells of brain origin (57) with the use of a cAMP-dependent pathway (58). However, despite this extensive effort, the detailed mechanism of tight junction assembly and its regulation is not fully understood.

There are variations in the level of BBB restriction in different areas of the CNS. This indicates a microenvironmental regulation of brain microvessel permeability in areas of the CNS involved in neuroendocrine feedback. One of the most important of these areas is the capillaries of the hypothalamus tuber cinereum, where rich and close connections between the endothelial cells and neurons result in the formation of a fenestrated endothelial cell wall, allowing the free diffusion of releasing and inhibitory hormones into the circulation. The absence of BBB at the area postrema has an opposite result, allowing the diffusion of materials from the blood to the brain tissue, thereby providing an important area of the brain for neuroendocrine feedback mechanisms. These areas, also termed *circumventricular organs*, not only lacked a BBB but also are deficient in the expression of the neurothelin BBB marker (59).

The expression of neurothelin protein and glucose transporter correlates with BBB function (59). In the brain parenchyma, where a characteristic BBB exists, ZO-1 was localized in discrete, continuous lines along blood vessels. However, the ependymal cells in the ventricular walls displayed a more punctate pattern of ZO-1 distribution, indicative of discontinuous tight junctions (60). In two of the circumventricular organs, the median eminence and the subfornical organ, many capillaries lack detectable ZO-1 immunoreactivity. These data demonstrate a distribution of ZO-1 in CNS parenchyma outside the circumventricular organs that is consistent with an organization of tight junctions preventing free paracellular exchange of substances between blood and brain parenchyma but allowing continuity between cerebrospinal fluid (CSF) and the neuronal environment (60). The localization and distribution of ZO-1 are good indicators of disrupted BBB. We demonstrated that ZO-1 is localized in discrete, continuous lines along blood ves-

sels in the intact, healthy brain parenchyma, but a more punctate pattern of ZO-1 distribution indicates more discontinuous tight junctions in areas of traumatic injuries (Figure 5.3). Further, redistribution of ZO-1 molecule indicates leakiness in the BBB, as illustrated by extravasation of serum proteins such as fibrinogen (Figure 5.3). The "leakiness" or disruption of the BBB is presumed to be associated with the cellular infiltration into the brain or at least with the facilitated migration of blood-borne cells across the BBB.

## The Importance of the BBB in Maintaining Immune Privilege in the CNS

In general, we associate an intact BBB with healthy, normal brain tissue. It is widely assumed that the BBB in an intact stage is impermeable to large compounds such as antibodies and cells. However, antibodies against amyloid-β peptide crossed the BBB to act directly in the CNS (61). Further, the immune surveillance of CNS by activated T-cells has been suggested. Despite these observa-

ZO-1 Distribution and Fibrinogen Extravasation

ZO-1 Stain
Intact Vascular Endothelium

ZO-1 Stain
Disrupted Vascular Endothelium

Localized Fibrinogen Stain
Intact Vascular Endothelium

Diffuse Fibrinogen Stain
Disrupted Vascular Endothelium

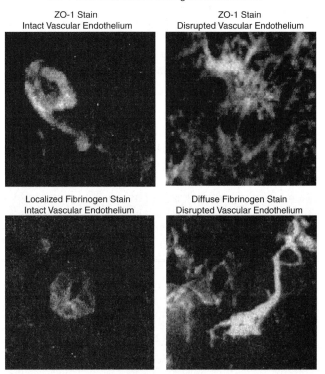

**FIGURE 5.3**

ZO-1 is localized in discrete, continuous lines along blood vessels in the intact, healthy brain parenchyma; however, a more punctate pattern of ZO-1 distribution indicates more discontinuous tight junctions at areas of traumatic injury. Extravasation of serum proteins such as fibrinogen indicates "leakiness" or disruption of the blood–brain barrier.

tions, the disruption of the BBB is associated with pathologic conditions. Any mechanism that physically destroys the BBB will open the barrier. This could occur in traumatic or surgical injury, infarction, or hemorrhage. In such circumstances, inflammatory agents are delivered to the site of the injury in a prompt, nonspecific way.

### BBB Opening in Infectious Diseases

Several infectious diseases may influence the permeability of BBB, leading to the disruption of this barrier. In bacterial or fungal meningitis, the infectious agent itself might produce agents that open or destroy the BBB (62,63). Viral infection may affect the BBB via its effects on the cells it infects. It was recently proposed that monocytes can gain access to the CNS through disruptions in BBB tight junctions, which occur in human immunodeficiency virus (HIV) encephalitis (HIVE) in association with an accumulation of activated, HIV-1–infected, perivascular macrophages and serum protein extravasation (64). It was also demonstrated that the expression of tight junction-associated proteins (occludin and ZO-1) is significantly altered in basal ganglia tissue from macaques infected with simian immunodeficiency virus (SIV) that have developed encephalitis (SIVE) (65). When compared with noninfected macaques and SIV-infected macaques without encephalitis, cerebral vessels from macaques with SIVE showed fragmentation and decreased immunoreactivity for both tight junction proteins. These alterations were associated spatially with the accumulation of perivascular macrophages. In addition, perivascular extravasation of fibrinogen, a plasma protein, and a change from a strong linear staining pattern to a more irregular pattern of the glucose transporter GLUT-1, a metabolic BBB marker, were observed in regions with vascular tight junction protein alterations. These findings demonstrate that tight junction disruption occurs in SIVE in association with perivascular macrophage accumulation. Although the exact mechanism of this disruption in BBB integrity is not fully understood, it is obvious that these disruptions could serve as portals for additional accumulation of perivascular macrophages in SIVE.

### BBB Opening in Autoimmune Diseases

In different autoimmune CNS diseases the disruption of the BBB involves inflammatory mediators, which result in activation of the cells of the BBB. This activation eventually leads to the cellular infiltration of leukocytes. The most direct evidence for increased BBB permeability by immune mediators is demonstrated using *in vitro* models of BBB. These immune mediators include chemotactic agents, cytokines, prostaglandins, reactive oxygen species, proteolytic enzymes released by leukocytes, and nitric oxide (66) (Table 5.2). In multiple sclerosis (MS),

visible disruptions of the BBB leading to MS lesions can be demonstrated by gadolinium-enhanced magnetic resonance imaging (MRI). These lesions are associated with the progression of disease. The most important inflammatory mediators inducing disruption in the BBB are listed in Table 5.2.

Some growth or angiogenic factors, although they are not inflammatory, may also modulate immune responses in the CNS by opening the BBB. One of these mediators, vascular endothelial growth factor (VEGF), has been shown to open the BBB and play a role in tumor vascularization in the CNS (67).

In summary, alterations in the BBB integrity are the results of a complex interplay involving several mediators and cellular components. The BBB is crucial in CNS homeostasis and is an important factor in maintaining immune privilege in the CNS.

## T LYMPHOCYTES IN THE CNS

In the previous section we outlined the importance of the BBB and its importance for maintaining the immunologic privilege in the CNS. In this section we discuss the nature of immune surveillance in the CNS under normal and pathologic conditions and the mechanisms of lymphocyte migration and survival in the brain parenchyma.

It is well appreciated that normal traffic and inflammatory recruitment of leukocytes to sites of inflammation in many tissues comprise a highly controlled process involving specificity to the endothelial cell wall and a series of orchestrated regulatory steps (68,69). It is also well established that nonactivated T-cells continuously recirculate through the blood and secondary lymphoid organs. This basal state of lymphocyte recirculation is changed after the introduction of antigen into the host

**TABLE 5.2**
*Inflammatory Mediators That Can Affect the BBB*

| INFLAMMATORY MEDIATOR | ALTERATIONS IN THE BBB | REFERENCE |
|---|---|---|
| TNF-α | Increased BBB permeability | 240 |
| | Adhesion molecule upregulation | 239 |
| IL-1β | Decreased TEER | 237 |
| IL-6 | Decreased TEER | 237 |
| | Downregulated plasma membrane–associated tyrosine phosphatase activity in brain endothelial cells | 238 |

BBB, blood—brain barrier; IFN-γ, interferon-γ; IL, interleukin; TEER, transendothelial electrical resistance; TNF-α, tumor necrosis factor-α.

(Figure 5.4). Blood-borne antigens will direct recirculating lymphocytes into the spleen and result in the transient trapping of these cells in that organ (70,71). Peripherally located antigens, such as subcutaneous pathogens or mucosal antigens, which drain into regional lymph nodes, induce migration of circulating lymphocytes to those lymph nodes and peripheral inflammatory sites (72,73). The seminal work of Cserr and Knopf demonstrated that antigens from the CNS can be delivered from the brain to regional lymph nodes through cerebrospinal and brain interstitial fluids (9–12,74–77). Several routes, including through the arachnoid villi into blood of the dural sinus and along routes adjacent to cranial and spinal nerves, accomplish this efflux of lymphatic drainage from the brain. After injection of radiolabeled protein into the CNS, a significant fraction of this tracer can be detected in the cervical lymph nodes in a short time (9) (summarized in Figure 5.4). Our laboratory has demonstrated that, after pigeon cytochrome C (PCC) Alexa 568® injection into the CNS, most of the labeled antigen is localized around the injection site in the first 2 hours after injection. However, starting at 4 hours after injection, MAC-1–positive cells (e.g., macrophage or microglia) that ingested some of the PCC antigen can be detected in the brain parenchyma. In addition, 8 hours after injection, PCC antigen can be detected in the cervical lymph nodes (13), indicating peripheral presentation of CNS antigens.

A change in T-cell trafficking is due to the fact that activated effector cells arising from interaction with antigen have localization properties different from naive T-cells do (78). Activated T-cells migrate poorly to lymph nodes or to mucosal lymphoid tissues, but accumulate effectively at sites of inflammation (72,79,80). This is due to the enhanced ability of activated T-cells to adhere to locally activated endothelium (81–83). The approximately 1 percent of surviving memory T-cell pool generated from the effector T-cell population after encounters with antigen disseminate widely late in a primary immune response in different tissues, enabling the host to respond rapidly to a secondary challenge with antigen regardless of its site of entry (84,85). Altogether, this differential migrating pattern is due mostly to the fact that naive, activated/effector and memory cells express different sets of adhesion molecules (86–89). To understand the migration requirement for T-cells in the CNS, it is important to consider the factors governing this process. In Table 5.3, we summarize those adhesion molecules, activation markers, and chemokine receptors that are expressed on resting (naive) or activated (effector) and memory T-cells and regulate their migration into tissues.

The process of leukocyte emigration into inflammatory sites is generally called *recruitment*. The basic mechanisms of leukocyte recirculation, homing, and recruitment, are very similar and focused on the interac-

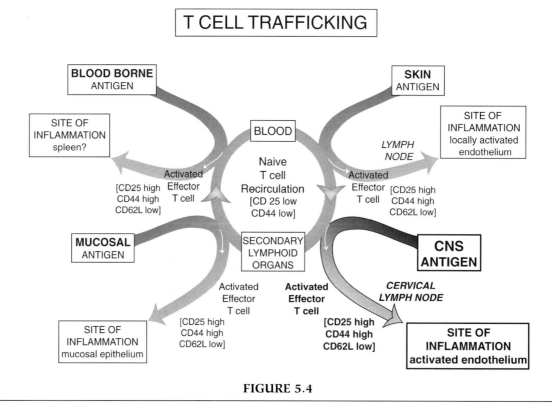

**FIGURE 5.4**

T-cell recirculation during naive and activated stages. CNS, central nervous system; IL-2R, interleukin-2 receptor.

**TABLE 5.3**
*Surface Molecules on Naive, Activated/Eeffector, and Memory T-cell Subsets*

| SURFACE MOLECULES | NAIVE CD4+ T-CELLS | ACTIVATED/EFFECTOR CD4+ T-CELLS | MEMORY CD4+ T-CELLS |
|---|---|---|---|
| CD3 | + | + | + |
| CD4 | + | + | + |
| TCR | + | + | + |
| CD45RA | + | − | − |
| CD45RO | − | + | + |
| CD69 | − | + | − |
| CD25 (IL–2Rα P55) | − | + | ++ |
| CD11a (LFA–1) | + | ++ | ++ |
| CD11b (MAC–1) | − | − | ± |
| CD18 (β2 integrin) | + | + | ++ |
| CD44 | + | ++ | ++ |
| CD62L (L-selectin) | ++ | − | + |
| CD29/CD49d (VLA–4) | + | ++ | + |
| CXCR4 | +++ | ++ | + |
| CCR4 | ± | ++ | ± |
| CCR6 | ± | + | + |
| CXCR3 | − | + | ++ |
| CCR1 | − | ± | + |
| CCR3 | − | − | + |
| CCR5 | − | ± | ++ |
| CXCR7 | + | − | ++ |

tion between leukocytes and endothelial cells. Leukocyte extravasation is highly regulated and viewed as an active process requiring several sequential events:

1. Tethering by selectin–carbohydrate adhesion mocules
2. Activation by chemokines and their G-protein–linked receptors
3. Arrest and transmigration mediated by integrin–immunoglobulin adhesion molecule interactions
4. Activation–dependent arrest

These sequential steps mediating leukocyte adhesion to the endothelial wall in extracerebral and cerebral tissues are illustrated in Figure 5.5.

Several mechanisms might also contribute to regulation of leukocyte recruitment in different tissues. They include the expression and regulation of adhesion molecules, the local availability of chemokines, and the activation stage of the leukocytes. This general mechanism of leukocyte recruitment into tissues has been reviewed in great detail in (69,90).

The currently accepted theory is that activated T-cells of any specificity can cross the BBB, but only those with specificity for CNS antigens are retained in the brain parenchyma (3,4,91,92). One proposed hypothesis for T-cell entry into the CNS in experimental autoimmune encephalomyelitis (EAE; an experimental animal model of MS) is as follows. Once the activated CNS antigen-specific T-cell binds to the endothelium, whether by leukocyte functional antigen-1/intercellular adhesion molecule-1 (LFA-l/ICAM-l) interaction or selectin binding, the T-cells induce upregulation of VCAM-I on the endothelium by producing interferon-γ (IFN-γ) and tumor necrosis factor-α (TNF-α), and then the VLA-4–expressing T-cells bind to the newly induced VCAM-I and enter the CNS (93,94). As the cells migrate deeper and deeper into the extracellular matrix and then into the tissue, they gradually downregulate the expression of VLA-4 and LFA-1 adhesion molecules (93–95). The migration of myelin basic protein (MBP)–specific T-cells seems to involve the entire effector population, resulting in a practically complete depletion of the effector cells from the periphery (96). Chemokines produced by neural cells can be responsible for the induction of T-cell migration into the CNS (97).

It is very interesting that paracellular permeability is altered during the migration of leukocytes across the apical junction complex and that the apical junction complex plays an important role in the regulation of leukocyte transmigration (or extravasation) through the endothelium and epithelium. Evidence suggests that important cell–cell adhesive events between transmigrat-

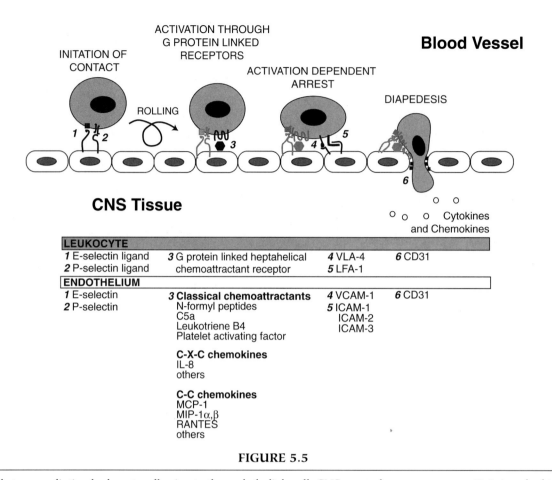

**FIGURE 5.5**

Sequential steps mediating leukocyte adhesion to the endothelial wall. CNS, central nervous system; IL-8, interleukin-8.

ing leukocytes and the apical junction complex and subsequent signaling events result in the facilitation of the passage of cells through the paracellular space (98).

### Adhesion Molecule Expression on Nonactivated and Inflamed Brain Endothelium

Different adhesion molecules are involved in lymphocyte migration into the CNS. The expression of these molecules is tightly regulated on resting and activated BBB (42,43,99,100) (Figure 5.6).

In vivo immunocytochemical studies have demonstrated upregulated expression of ICAM-1 (CD54) and MECA-325 (a marker of lymph node high endothelial venules) on inflamed CNS endothelial cells, (33,101–103) indicating highly facilitated trafficking of T lymphocytes into the CNS. From EAE experiments it is clear that the VLA-4/VCAM-1 adhesion molecule pair is important in brain inflammatory reactions. Monoclonal antibody to the $\alpha4\beta1$ integrin (VLA-4, CD49d-CD29) was used successfully to prevent experimentally induced inflammation of CNS in rats. Some lines of evidence point to the possibility that loss of the encephalitogenic potential of MBP-

specific CD4$^+$ T-cell clones corresponds to the reduced capacity of these T-cell clones to migrate into the brain (93). VLA-4 expression is also required for proteolipid protein (PLP)-specific T-cells to be encephalitogenic, although this requirement can be bypassed by pretreating the recipient animal with pertussis toxin or irradiation, both of which probably act by increasing vascular permeability and facilitating entry into the CNS (104). Others have also demonstrated little or no effect of anti–VLA-4 treatment on passively transferred EAE, but have found inhibition of this treatment in an actively induced EAE model (101,105).

ICAM-1/LFA-1 also may play an important role in activated leukocyte migration across the BBB. ICAM-1 is expressed on CNS vessels in EAE, and its expression coincides with inflammatory cell infiltration. Our laboratory also demonstrated that ICAM-1 expression is upregulated on murine and human brain microvessel cells following inflammatory cytokine treatment (42,47).

Selective recruitment of proinflammatory autoimmune T-helper (Th1) cells, as opposed to anti-inflammatory Th2 cells, might offer an additional level of immune regulation at the BBB. It has been demonstrated

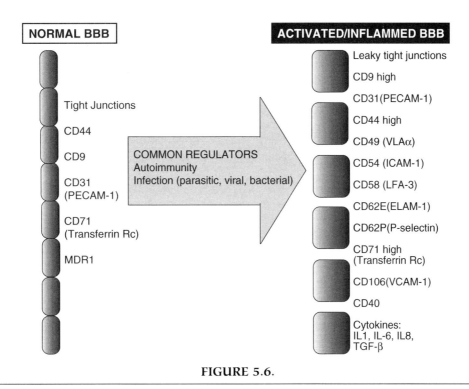

**FIGURE 5.6.**

Different adhesion molecules are involved in lymphocyte migration into the central nervous system. The expression of these molecules is tightly regulated on resting and activated BBB. BBB, blood–brain barrier; IL, interleukin; TGF-β, transforming growth factor β.

that only Th1 cells can efficiently enter inflamed sites in the CNS in Th1-dominated disease models such as EAE (106). It has been further demonstrated that Th1 cells but not Th2 cells are able to bind to P-selectin and E-selectin (106). Engelhart et al. presented dissenting evidence to this model by showing that E-selectin and P-selectin are not involved in recruitment of inflammatory cells across the BBB (107).

In addition, data suggest a role for PECAM-1/CD31 in T-cell accumulation in the brain. PECAM-1/CD31 is a 130-kd molecule that is expressed on the surface of circulating platelets, monocytes, neutrophils, and different T-cell subsets. It is also a major constituent of endothelial cell intercellular junctions. Platelet endothelial cell adhesion molecule-1 (PECAM-1/CD31) was originally assigned to the immunoglobulin Ig–like adhesion molecule family. Recently it has been suggested that PECAM-1/CD31 functions as an inhibitory receptor, serving to attenuate tyrosine kinase–mediated signaling pathways (108,109). PECAM-1/CD31 inhibits the T-cell receptor (TCR)–mediated release of calcium from intracellular stores and may also function to shut down the mitogen-activated protein kinase pathway in cells after serum stimulation (108,109). The role of PECAM-1/CD31 in Lewis rats in EAE induction was also studied by Williams et al. (110). They concluded that the administration of anti–PECAM-1/CD31 antibody does not result in a delay

in the onset of clinical signs or of weight loss, nor does it decrease the incidence and severity of disease. In vitro, migration across activated monolayers of brain microvessel endothelial cells, but not across untreated endothelium, is significantly blocked by antibodies to PECAM-1/CD31 and E-selectin (111). Thus, the role of PECAM-1/CD31 in T-cell accumulation in the brain remains controversial.

Our laboratory has focused on the role of PECAM-1/CD31 molecule in the accumulation of antigen-specific T-cells in the CNS. Trafficking of antigen-specific T-cells into the CNS is an important initiating step in inflammation in the brain. Despite extensive knowledge about the role of adhesion molecules in T-cell migration across peripheral vessels, the mechanism of the entry of antigen-specific T-cells into the CNS is not known. To study this, antigen specific T-cells were tracked in an in vivo migration assay using TCR transgenic mice having 95 percent of T-cells specific for a defined antigen, PCC (13). TCR transgenic mice were cannulated intraventricularly and PCC antigen was infused into the ventricles of the brain. Upon PCC infusion into the CNS, CSF was sampled through the cannulas and the number of transgenic $\alpha/\beta$ TCR$^+$ V$\beta$3$^+$ MAC1$^-$ cells in the CSF was characterized in the presence or absence of anti-adhesion molecule reagents. We found that antibodies against VCAM-1 (CD106), VLA-4 (CD49d/CD29), ICAM-1 (CD54), and LFA-1 (CD11a/CD18) did not influence the increased number of antigen-specific T-cells in the CSF. However, anti–PECAM-1 (CD31) antibody or PECAM-Ig chimeric protein inhibited the trafficking of α/β TCR$^+$ Vβ3$^+$ MAC1$^-$ cells into the CNS when injected intravenously. The expression of PECAM-1/CD31 was also upregulated on antigen-specific T-cells in a time-dependent manner with antigenic stimulation in vitro. Hence, PECAM-1/CD31 may play an important role in regulating antigen-specific T-cells trafficking in CNS inflammatory diseases (112).

In summary, the BBB plays a very important role in maintaining the immune privileged status of the CNS. In pathologic conditions, the integrity of the BBB can be breached and the inflamed brain endothelial cells can play an important role in regulating the migration of leukocytes via adhesion molecules into the CNS parenchyma.

## Normal Immune Surveillance and Pathologic Traffic of Immune Cells into the CNS

It is generally accepted that nonactivated T-cells are excluded from the CNS and, upon their activation, they gain access to the brain tissue (3,4). However, recent experiments in sheep demonstrated that naive lymphocytes infused directly into the blood could circulate through the CSF (113). Further, it was demonstrated that naive T-cells can traffic to the CNS without prior activation in MBP TCR transgenic animals. Interestingly, it was also suggested that naive MBP-specific T-cells do not trigger autoimmunity when they traffic to the CNS because they undergo tolerance induction within the brain (5). Therefore, we also have to consider that, even if nonactivated autoimmune T-cells could gain access to the brain parenchyma, they would be eliminated or functionally inhibited very rapidly in the CNS due to the absence of costimulatory molecules and major histocompatibility antigens in the CNS (Figure 5.7).

The circulation of naive, autoreactive T-cells through the CNS represents a potential hazard for autoimmunity; therefore, it must be tightly controlled. However, the circulation of non–CNS specific naive T-cells through the CNS could be an important part of the normal surveillance of CNS. Nevertheless, activated T-cells probably have a competitive advantage over naive T-cells crossing the BBB. Under certain conditions, the number of activated T-cells in the periphery could decrease, allowing more naive T-cells into the CNS (5).

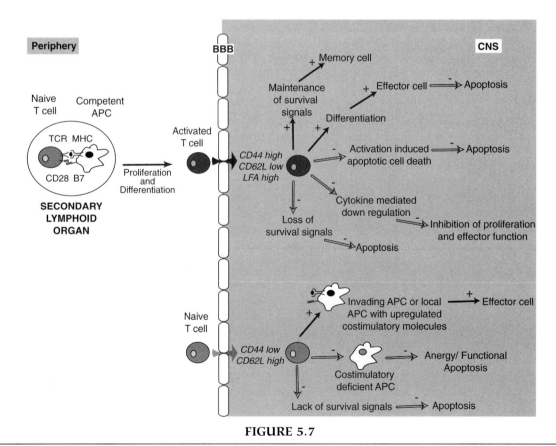

**FIGURE 5.7**

The entry and fate of T-cells in the CNS. APC, antigen-presenting cell; BBB, blood–brain barrier; CNS, central nervous system; MHC, major histocompatibioity complex; TCR, T-cell receptor.

The idea that only activated T-cells gain access to the CNS is supported by several studies. Mobley et al. demonstrated that T-cells with CD44high L-selectin–low phenotype (activated effector cells) can accumulate in the CNS of mice with viral encephalitis (114,115). A distinctive lymphocyte phenotype in chronically inflamed brain was also suggested by Engelhardt et al. (116). In their experiments, a model of chronic inflammation induced by injection of heat-killed *Corynebacterium parvum* into mouse brain cortex was used. Inflammatory T-cells isolated from injection sites express much higher levels of CD44, and LFA-1, and lower levels of CD45RB (features commonly associated with activated cells). Further, these cells are L-selectin or α6-integrin negative and bind to VCAM-1 but not to MAdCAM-1. Altogether, these data suggest the existence of a distinct activated phenotype of CNS-infiltrating T-cells.

In summary, it is more generally accepted that, unlike naive T (L-selectin$^{high}$, CD44$^{low}$) and resting memory (CD44$^{intermediate}$, L-selectin$^{intermediate}$) cells, activated T-cell blasts (CD44$^{high}$, L-selectin$^{low}$) readily penetrate the BBB and enter the noninflamed CNS. The activation of these CNS infiltration T-cells is initiated in the peripheral secondary lymphoid organs (summarized in Figure 5.7). Subsequently, as a consequence of a subsequent antigen recognition, the neuroantigen specific T-cells are retained and the nonspecific cells exit the CNS (4,117) or are eliminated by apoptosis inducing mechanisms. Driven by antigen recognition, the antigen-specific T-cells secrete cytokines and induce a delayed-type hypersensitivity–like reaction, inducing the migration of monocytes/macrophages to the inflammatory site. Once chronic inflammatory lesions have developed, endothelial cells of the BBB form HEV-like structures. The noninflamed CNS, the acutely inflamed CNS, and the chronically inflamed CNS might require different mechanisms of T-cell entry and survival. T-cells entering the parenchyma and the perivascular compartment might survive differentially in the CNS (117).

## Th1 and Th2 Subsets of CD4$^+$ Helper T-cells in the Brain

Different migration patterns for Th1 and Th2 cells have also been suggested. Two distinct subsets of T-cells have been identified among long-term, cloned T-cell lines (118). Th1 clones secrete IFN-γ, interleukin-2 (IL-2), TNF-α, and TNF-β and promote cytotoxicity and delayed type hypersensitivity reactions. In contrast, Th2 clones produce IL-4, IL-5, IL-10, IL-13, and TGF-β and promote B-cell activation, antibody production, immune suppressor functions, and immediate hypersensitivity reactions (Figure 5.8). Th1 and Th2 clones also differ in their requirements for antigen presentation, because B cells preferentially stimulate Th2 clones, whereas adher-

ent T-cell-cells (macrophages/dendritic cells) preferentially stimulate Th1 clones (119).

Multiple lines of evidence indicate that Th1 cells cause EAE. Merrill and colleagues (120–122) characterized the lymphocytes infiltrating into the brain and spinal cord in synthetic myelin peptide-induced EAE and found that these cells were predominantly CD4$^+$ Th cells secreting IL-2 and IFN-γ. This suggests Th1-type cell activation in this in vivo model.

Khoury et al. associated oral tolerance to MBP and natural recovery from EAE with upregulation of IL-4 and TGF-β cytokines; infusion of anti-TNF or anti-IL-12 antibodies prevented EAE (123). Khoruts et al. also showed that adoptive transfer of neuroantigen-specific Th2 cell lines never resulted in EAE (124,125). These studies show the potential importance of activation of different T-cell subsets in CNS inflammatory diseases.

## Antigen-Specific T-Cell Migration and Accumulation in the CNS

It is widely accepted that antigen-specific T-cells play a crucial role in autoimmune attacks in the CNS such as those seen in EAE. Understanding the mechanism of entry of these cells into the CNS could lead us to selectively target and inactivate them for therapeutic purposes. Antigen specificity also plays a crucial role in the retention phase of T-cells in the CNS. In this phase, antigen-specific T-cells are selectively retained and probably further activated and induced to proliferate in the CNS parenchyma. This phase is highly regulated by the presence of antigen. It is followed by the recruitment of leukocytes from the circulation to the site of the initial inflammation. Although there is copious information on the importance of adhesion molecules and chemokines in the recruitment phase of CNS inflammation, the adhesion molecules and chemokines governing the initial T-cell entry into the CNS have not been defined. A major obstacle in studying the T-cell–mediated autoimmune process is the technical difficulty of studying these T-cells in vivo. The frequency of antigen-specific T-cells is below the detection limits of standard T-cell assays. Novel technical advances, such as transgenic technology and enzyme linked immunospot (ELISPOT) assay, allow us to study antigen-specific T-cells in the CNS.

Two groups have created MBP TCR transgenic mice to study the development of CNS autoimmune reactions. In one model, Vα2.3 transgenic mice were crossed with transgenic animals that contain the functionally rearranged Vβ8.2 containing the TCR gene to generate mice expressing completely transgenic TCRs (H-2u αβ) (126). Spontaneous EAE can develop in these mice if they are housed in nonsterile facilities. The second model was generated by crossing MBP-specific TCR transgenic mice and RAG-1–deficient mice to

## CD4+ T CELL DIFFERENTIATION

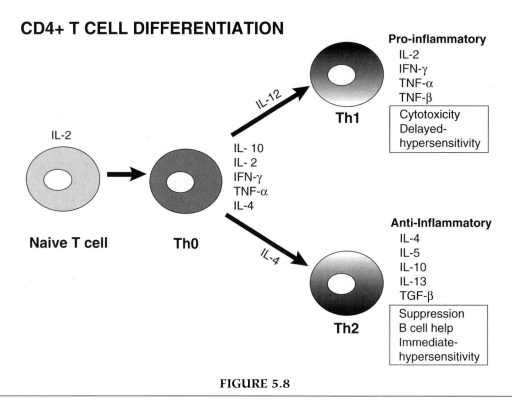

**FIGURE 5.8**

Two distinct subsets of T-cells have been identified among long-term, cloned T cell lines. Th1 clones secrete IFN-γ, IL-2, TNF-α, and TNF-β and promote cytotoxicity and delayed-type hypersensitivity reactions. In contrast, Th2 clones produce interleukins IL-4, IL-5, IL-10, IL-13, and TGF-β and promote B-cell activation, antibody production, immune suppressor functions, and immediate hypersensitivity reactions. IL, interleukin; IFN-γ, interferon-γ; TGF-β, transforming growth factor β; TNF, tumor necrosis factor; Th, T helper cell.

obtain lines that have only T-cells expressing the MBP-specific transgenic TCR (127). All of these mice developed spontaneous EAE within 12 months. This study shows that neither a diverse set of CD4$^+$ T-cell diversity, CD8$^+$ T-cell diversity nor B cells or γδ T-cells are required for the generation of EAE lesions and clinical symptoms.

To study this problem, we used AND TCR transgenic mice as a source of monoclonal T-cells with known antigen specificity to PCC residues 88 to 104 (128,129). We can readily monitor the accumulation of a small number of antigen-specific T-cells in the CSF by using monoclonal antibodies to their specific TCRs (Vα11 or Vβ3)and flow cytometry. Using this model, intraventricular delivery of PCC antigen resulted in the strongest antigen-specific T-cell accumulation in the CSF. Intraventricular delivery of PCC antigen could also activate antigen-specific T-cells in the peripheral blood, which is consistent with the current hypothesis that activated T-cells migrate in and out of the CNS. However, although injection of PCC antigen into the peripheral sites strongly activated the peripheral antigen-specific T-cells, the antigen-specific T-cell accumulation in the CSF was only modestly increased. This latter observation points to the

importance of antigen localization in the initiation phase of CNS inflammation (13).

In summary, several mediators regulate normal surveillance and pathologic T-cell migration into the CNS. These factors include adhesion molecules, chemokines, inflammatory mediators, and the localization of antigen.

In this section we discussed the importance of adhesion molecules, some inflammatory mediators, and the localization of antigen in this process. The role of chemokines in T-cell recruitment into the CNS is discussed elsewhere in this book. In the next section we focus on the importance of antigen-presenting cells in the CNS in maintaining T-cell survival in the nervous tissue.

### ANTIGEN PRESENTATION IN THE CNS BY CNS-RESIDENT-CELLS

We previously discussed the mechanism for T-cell trafficking across the BBB into the brain parenchyma. In this section we consider the immune regulatory functions of CNS-resident T-cells in regulating T-cell activation and survival in the CNS compartment. We focus on the antigen presentation properties of resident T-cells within the

CNS parenchyma (glial cells: microglia, astroglia) and resident cells at the vascular interface (endothelium, pericytes, and perivascular macrophages). Although dendritic cells (DCs) have been demonstrated to orchestrate the decision-making process in the induction of adaptive immune responses and T-cell activation in the periphery, their role in the CNS has been rather controversial. On the one hand, it was clearly demonstrated in mice that DCs can efficiently present MBP[Ac1-11] to antigen-specific T-cells in the periphery, resulting in the induction of EAE (130). On the other hand, although the presence of DCs in the CNS had been suggested (131,132), the issue is still being debated in the current literature. For the sake of simplicity, the presence or absence of DCs in the CNS will not be discussed further in this chapter.

### Antigen-specific Activation of T-cells

To understand the properties of antigen-presenting cells (APCs) in the CNS, first we discuss what is known about T-cell interactions with APCs in general. The $\alpha/\beta$ T-cells very rarely recognize free antigen, and their antigen recognition involves an interaction of the T-cell receptor (TCR) with fragments of antigen bound to class I or class II MHC molecules on the surface of an APC. MHC class I–restricted T-cells are almost exclusively CD8[+] (cytotoxic/suppressor) phenotypes, whereas class II–restricted T-cells are CD4[+] T phenotypes (133–136). The TCR is a disulfide-linked heterodimer made up of two chains, either $\alpha$ and $\beta$ chains on $\alpha/\beta$ T-cells or $\gamma$ and

$\delta$ chains on $\gamma/\delta$ T cells (137–140). The TCR repertoire is formed during thymic development with the use of different gene segments: the variable (V), diversity (D), joining (J), and constant (C) regions (141). These gene segments are randomly rearranged; after positive and negative selection, each individual mature T-cell has a single specificity when it leaves the thymus. The variable regions of the $\alpha/\beta$ TCR determine this specificity, and MHC-bound peptides are successfully generated by the very efficient APCs, such as dentritic cells and macrophages, as a result of their ability to phagocytose and endocytose and process pathogens and cellular debris (142). In addition to antigen presentation in the context of MHC molecules, secondary signals are required for the successful activation of peripheral T-cells. These secondary signals are provided by costimulatory molecules (Figure 5.9).

Several costimulatory molecules play an important role in T-cell activation. The presence or absence of costimulatory molecules on APCs strongly influences the outcome of T-cell antigen recognition (143,144). If costimulators are present, antigen presentation results in cytokine gene expression and T-cell proliferation. These activated T-cells are then capable of responding to subsequent antigen exposure. In contrast, in the absence of costimulatory molecules, suboptimal or no IL-2 gene expression occurs and the Th1 cells do not proliferate (143,144). The subsequent attempts at activation of these T-cells might show that these cells are in a long-lived anergic stage. Once anergized, helper T lymphocytes produce

## T CELL- APC INTERACTIONS

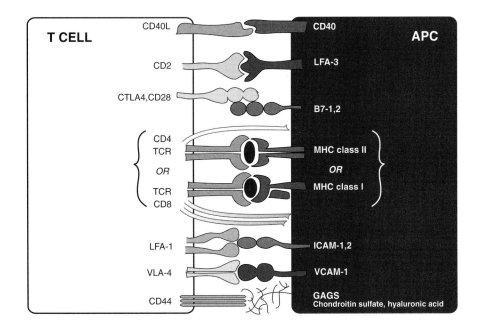

**FIGURE 5.9**

Antigen presentation in the context of MHC molecules. Secondary signals also are required for the successful activation of naive T-cells. Costimulatory molecules provide these secondary signals. APC, antigen-presenting cell; MHC, major histocompatibility complex; TCR, T-cell receptor.

no detectable IL-2 and reduced levels of IL-3 and IFN-γ in response to stimulation via the TCR complex and yet continue to proliferate in response to exogenous IL-2.

At least five distinct adhesion molecules present on APCs: B7-1 (CD80), B7-2 (CD86), ICAM-1 (CD54), LFA-3 (CD58), and VCAM-1 (CD106) have been individually shown to costimulate T-cell activation (145–150). These molecules interact with their counter-receptors on T-cells (Figure 5.9). The most well studied costimulatory receptor–ligand pair involves the B7-CD28/CTLA-4 system (151–153). Interruption of this signaling pathway with CD28 antagonists not only suppresses the immune response but in some cases also induces antigen-specific tolerance. However, the CD28/B7 system is increasingly complex due to the identification of multiple receptors and ligands with positive and negative signaling activities (154).

B7-1 was found to be the ligand for CD28 costimulatory molecule by Gimmi et al. (155). Constitutive expression of murine B7-1 mRNA was detected in hematopoietic cells of B-cell but not of T-cell origin. A second counterreceptor of CD28, termed B7-2, has been discovered and cloned (156). Although only 26 percent homologous to B7-1, B7-2 also costimulates IL-2 production and T-cell proliferation. Unlike B7-1, B7-2 messenger RNA is not constitutively expressed in unstimulated B-cells. It is likely that B7-2 provides a critical early costimulatory signal in determining whether the T-cell will contribute to an immune response or become anergic. A third counterreceptor, called CTLA-4, has been demonstrated for B7-1 and B7-2 (156). CTLA-4 is an adhesion receptor expressed on activated T-cells. Surface expression of CTLA-4 seems to be a tightly regulated event, with transient expression on activated T-cells peaking 48 to 72 hours after activation (157). The amino acid sequence of CTLA-4 is related to CD28, and it shares several features with CD28. A recent study found that CD28 and CTLA-4 are coexpressed at the mRNA level on activated T-cells but only CD28 is expressed on resting T-cells. Several studies have indicated that CTLA-4 serves as a negative regulator of T-cell activation (157–160). Interference with the B7 costimulatory signal, using CTLA-4Ig, resulted in a profound decrease in IL-2 production and significantly decreased lymphoproliferative and antibody responses by primed lymph node cells from rats with experimental autoimmune myasthenia gravis when stimulated with AChR in vitro (161). Systemic administration of CTLA-4Ig in EAE suppressed clinical disease and was effective even when CTLA-4Ig was delayed until day 10 postimmunization, a time when pathology is evident (162). Immunohistologic studies showed that CTLA-4Ig therapy suppresses the inflammatory response with inhibition of Th1 (IL-2 and IFN-γ) and sparing of Th2 (IL-4, IL-10, and IL-13) cytokines in the CNS (162). Together these studies support an essential role for B7-CD28/CTLA-4 costimulatory molecules in CNS autoimmunity.

It is generally accepted that autoimmune T-cells are stimulated in the periphery, enter the CNS, and likely need to encounter APCs at the target site for a secondary restimulation. Their fate in the CNS depends on this interaction (Figure 5.10). Absence of antigen or APCs could lead to the elimination of these T-cells from the brain parenchyma and, hence, termination of the immune response. However, their secondary restimulation could result in further activation and survival of these cells. Activated autoimmune T-cells in the CNS could induce the recruitment of mononuclear cells into the brain parenchyma, thereby inducing a broad inflammatory reaction and destruction of the myelin sheath (Figure 5.10). Throughout this process, autoimmune T-cells encounter residential cells of the BBB and then interact with resident APCs in the brain parenchyma. In the following paragraphs we outline the role of APCs in these interactions in more detail.

### Antigen Presentation at the BBB

Endothelial cells are potentially very important APCs in vivo because of their cumulative large surface area and anatomic location. The antigen-presenting capacity of brain capillary endothelial cells has been the subject of several investigations leading to quite divergent conclusions. It has been demonstrated by several laboratories that vascular cerebral endothelial cells can be induced to express class II molecules and acquire the capacity to activate CD4+ T-cells in vitro (163,164). Further, murine brain endothelial cells have been reported to process and present MBP antigen to T-cells (165). Pryce et al. (166) demonstrated that brain endothelial cells are poor stimulators of T-cell proliferation despite antigen-specific interactions between Th cells and endothelial cells. Others have shown that brain capillary endothelial cells from mouse and guinea pig act as APCs for the presentation of MBP to CD4+ T-cells but not for purified digested or whole ovalbumin (167,168). Bourdoulous et al. (169) found that IFN-γ–activated rat brain microvessel endothelial cells expressing MHC class II molecules in the presence of MBP, stimulate proliferation of a syngeneic CD4+ T-cell line.

Our laboratory found that murine brain microvessel endothelial cells and smooth muscle/pericytes (SM/P) express class II I-A molecules (170,171) and selectively induce the antigen-specific activation of different Th1 and Th2 CD4+ T-cell clones (172). Th1 and Th2 cell clones that were specific for the same peptide antigen in the context of the same class II allotype were used. SM/P preferentially activated Th1 cell clones, whereas endothelial cells activated Th2 cell clones better, as reflected by cell proliferation and production of IL-2 by SM/P-activated

# CNS AUTOIMMUNITY

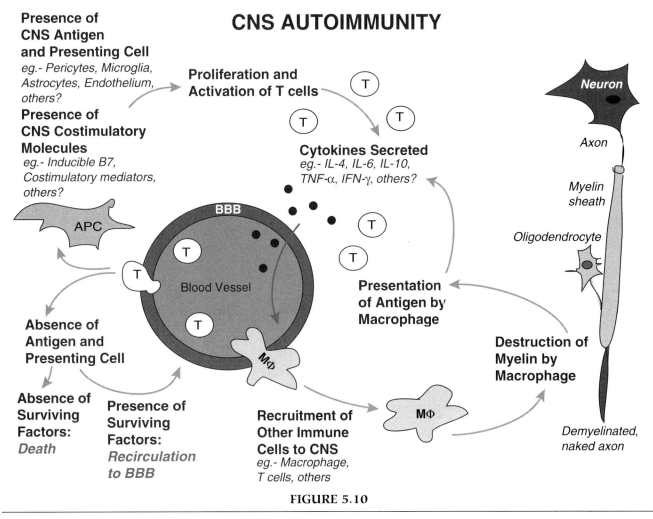

**FIGURE 5.10**

The mechanism of CNS autoimmunity. BBB, blood–brain barrier; CNS, central nervous system; IFN-γ, interferon-γ; IL, interleukin; TNF-α, tumor necrosis factor-α, Mφ, macrophage.

Th1 clones and IL-4 by endothelial cell activated Th2 clones. Because Th1 cells are the harmful effector cells in CNS autoimmunity, we proposed an active role for BBB endothelial cells in maintaining the BBB integrity by downregulating Th1 activity. Interestingly, we also demonstrated that there is no expression of CD80 (B7-1) on the surface of brain microvessel endothelial cells; however, with LPS stimulation, CD86 (B7-2) proteins can be detected on the surface of these cells (Figure 5.11 A and B). B7-2, but not B7-1, expression was also detected in vivo on brain microvessel endothelial cells at aseptic cerebral injury sites in mouse brain (Figure 5.11C).

To study further whether Th1 cells can be partly stimulated or anergized by brain microvessel endothelial cells, D1.1/Th1 cells were cocultured with IFN-γ–activated brain microvessel endothelial cells in the presence of their respective antigen (rabbit immunoglobulin) for 48 hours and then restimulated with splenic APCs and antigen. After 48 hours of restimulation with splenic APCs and antigen,

proliferation and production of IL-2 and IFN-γ by the Th1 cells was measured. Figure 5.12 shows that Th1 clones did not proliferate and produced very little IL-2 or IFN-γ when brain microvessel endothelial cells were used as primary stimulators. However, despite the observed lack of proliferation and cytokine production of Th1 cell in coculture with brain microvessel endothelial cells and antigen, endothelial cells induced functional changes in D1.1 Th1 clones. This was demonstrated by the expression of the p55 subunit of the IL-2R (CD25) subunit in Th1 cells (Figure 5.13). These results indicated that the costimulatory pathways activated by endothelial cells of the BBB can selectively inhibit Th1-type cell activation at the entry site of the brain parenchyma.

In summary, BBB cells clearly can contribute to brain inflammation by actively participating in immune responses via production of cytokines, expression of adhesion molecules, and inhibition of antigen-specific immune responses in the nervous tissue.

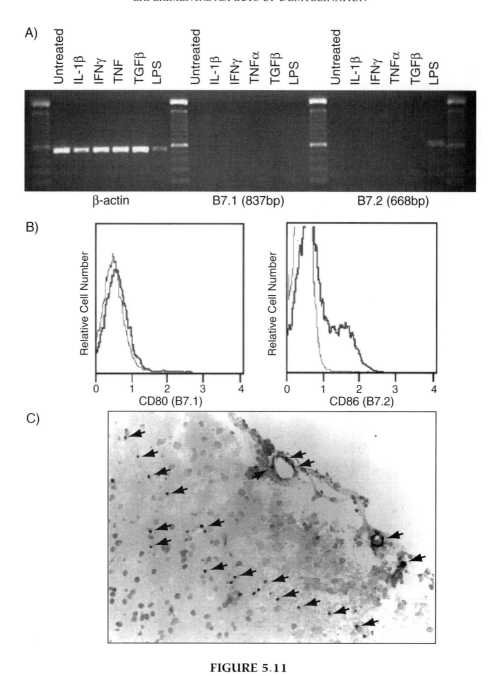

**FIGURE 5.11**

**A.** B7-1 and B7-2 gene expression in brain microvessel cells. B7-1 and B7-2 gene expressions were determined by reverse transcription–polymerase chain reaction analysis of mRNA isolated from brain microvessel cells. Each increment in the control ladder is 100 bp. **B.** CD80 (B7-1) and CD86 (B7-2) costimulatory molecule expression on a brain microvessel endothelial cell. Brain microvessel endothelial cells, $1 \times 10^6$, were stimulated with LPS for 24 hours. After this treatment, direct flow cytofluorimetry analysis was carried out using 4 μg, R-PE conjugated anti-mouse B7/BB1 (1G10) or B7-2 (GL1) monoclonal antibody/million cells. As a control, isotype matched rat immunoglobulin G 2a was used (thin line). **C.** Immunohistochemical localization of a B7-2 (CD86) costimulatory molecule at the site of freeze injury in murine brain. IFN-γ, interferon-γ; IL, interleukin; LPS, lipopolysaccharide; TGF-β, transforming growth factor-β; TNF, tumor necrosis factor.

Much less controversy arises about the important role of perivascular microglia/macrophages in shaping CNS autoimmunity. In general, perivascular microglia/macrophages are difficult to differentiate from resident microglia; however, this was elegantly achieved in bone marrow chimeric animals by Hickey and Kimura (173). These cells were capable of phagocytosis and constitutively expressed high levels of class II antigen (174,175).

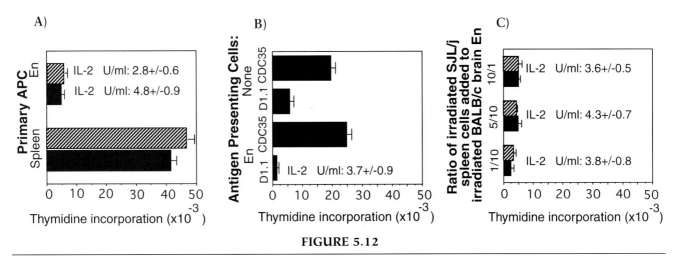

**FIGURE 5.12**

**A.** Subsequent antigen stimuli of D1.1 Th1 CD4(+) cell clone using syngeneic splenocytes as APCs. Applying anti-CD3 simulation (**B**) or allogeneic splenocytes (**C**) did not result in proliferation or lymphokine production by the D1.1 cells. D1.1 cells were cocultured with interferon–activated brain En cells plus antigen (rabbit immunoglobulin) for 48 hours (solid bars ) and then reactivated with secondary stimulus ( hatched bars). After 48 hours of proliferation, IL-2 lymphokine production by the T-cell clone was measured. APC, antigen-presenting cell; En, endothelial cell; IL, interleukin.

Further, using irradiated bone marrow chimeras in CD45-congenic rats, highly purified populations of microglia and nonmicroglial but not CNS-associated macrophages (CD45$^{high}$ CD11b/c$^+$) were isolated from the adult CNS. The minority CD45$^{high}$ CD11b/c$^+$ transitional macrophage population, and not the resident microglia, constituted the effective APCs for EAE by activating CD4$^+$ MBP-reactive T-cells (176). The depletion of systemic macrophage results in the depletion of the perivascular microglia/macrophage population and leads to the inhi-bition of the onset of EAE (177). Due to the important location of these cells and their ability to induce immune response, we must consider these cells to be the most important APCs at the BBB.

## Antigen Presentation in the Brain Parenchyma by Residential APCs

Undoubtedly, the local regulatory mechanism that defines the outcome of immune responses in the brain

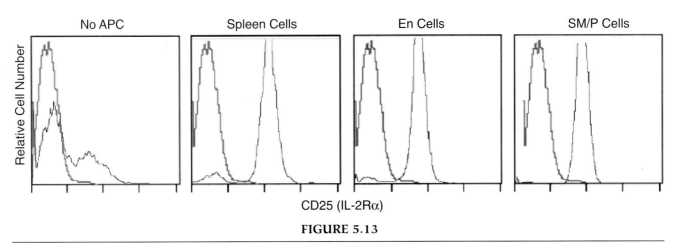

**FIGURE 5.13**

Splenocytes, brain microvessel En, and SM/P antigen presentation to D1.1 cells upregulate expression of the IL-2Ra chain on the T-cells. D1.1 cells were cocultured with APC in the presence of antigen for 48 hours. Viable T-cells were harvested, stained for expression of the p55 subunit of IL-2R using the 7D4 monoclonal antibody, and analyzed by flow cytometry. Fluoresence histogram of cells incubated with a primary rat anti-CD8 antibody was used as a control (thick line). APC, antigen-presenting cell; En, endothelial cell; IL-2Rα, interleukin-2 receptor-α; SM/P, smooth muscle/pericytes.

parenchyma must be closely studied to influence these reactions. Remarkably, this area of research has been the subject of great interest in the past few years, but also an area of great controversy. This controversy has been driven by several conflicting results demonstrating the antigen-presenting properties of two different types of CNS-resident glial cells, microglia and astrocytes.

Much of the available information suggests that microglia cells are of mesodermal origin and that they represent the resident macrophages, the most efficient APC in the CNS. The mesodermal origin of microglia has been a rather controversial issue. Some investigators claim that microglia originate from neuroectodermal matrix cells together with the macroglia, although most believe that microglial cells are of mesodermal origin and probably belong to the monocyte/macrophage cell line. It has been also suggested that these cells are derived from pericytes or from invasion of monocytes in early development into the CNS (178). The current view is that microglia cells are of mesodermal origin and probably belong to the monocyte cell lineage. Developing microglial cells probably enter the CNS from the blood, through the ventricular space or the meninges (179). After their migration into the developing CNS, microglial cells are distributed more or less homogeneously throughout the entire nervous parenchyma. Microglial cells moving through the nervous parenchyma are ameboid microglia, which apparently differentiate into ramified microglia after reaching their definitive locations. The factors that control the invasion of the nervous parenchyma, migration within the developing CNS, and differentiation of microglial cells are still not understood, although extracellular matrix elements and soluble molecules have been suggested (180). Microglial cells within the developing CNS are involved in clearing cellular debris and withdrawing misdirected or transitory axons. Recently, with the use of serial analysis of gene expression (SAGE) to systematically analyze transcripts in a microglial cell line, more than 10,000 SAGE tags were sequenced and shown to represent 6,013 unique transcripts. Among the diverse transcripts were cytokines such as endothelial monocyte-activating polypeptide I (EMAP I), adhesion molecules such as CD9, CD53, CD107a, CD147, CD162, and mast cell high-affinity IgE receptor. In addition, transcripts that were characteristic of hematopoietic cells or mesodermal structures such as E3 protein, A1, EN-7, B94, and were detected. Further, the profile contained a transcript, Hn1, that is important in hematopoietic cells and neurologic development (181). These data strongly suggest the probable neural differentiation of microglia from the hematopoietic system in development. However, due to the difficulties of exactly characterizing microglia and differentiating these cells from other macrophage marker-carrying cells in the CNS, the antigen-presenting capability of these cells is somewhat controversial. Some part of this controversy is driven by the fact that, if microglia are mesodermal originated cells, then they should be very similar to blood-borne macrophages. Further, the CNS contains at least two populations of macrophages: the resident microglia of brain parenchyma and the CNS perivascular macrophages in the perivascular spaces, the leptomeninges, and the choroid plexus. These cells are continuously, slowly, recirculating between the blood and the CNS, carrying CNS or blood originated antigens to the perivascular space (173). Another complication in the discussion of this issue is that, in different neuropathologic diseases, infections, or during posttraumatic healing and inflammatory processes, a high number of macrophages can readily enter the CNS. These cells can also carry antigens or "pick-up" antigens in the brain parenchyma and function as central APCs and inflammatory effector cells in different situations.

It was also demonstrated that one class of microglial cells can be labeled early with only lectins, whereas another can be labeled with lectins and CD68 macrophage antibody. That may reflect a different origin of microglia in the early embryonic CNS compared with the fetal stages (182). This subdivision appears to be maintained in the adult brain as well. The microglia are characterized in part by their scarcity of MHC molecules and lack of constitutive antigen-presenting activity for naive CD4$^+$ T-cells. In contrast, some CNS macrophages constitutively express MHC molecules and present antigen to naive CD4$^+$ T-cells. Precursor cells were isolated from the CNS that, in the presence of colony-stimulating factor-1 (CSF-1), the macrophage growth factor, give rise to clones of cells that can be separated into two discrete subpopulations based on differences in cell density. The two cell populations give rise to progeny that differ in their content of cells constitutively expressing MHC class II and CD86 molecules and the ability to present antigen to naive CD4$^+$ T-cells (183). Probably the earliest marker used for microglia characterization was the binding of *Ricinus communis* agglutinin-1 (RCA-1) to these cells (184). With this marker, specific staining was observed in cell bodies and processes of microglia. Although endothelial cells and blood cells also reacted with RCA-1, they were easily distinguished morphologically from microglia. According to our current knowledge, astrocytes, oligodendrocytes, and neurons do not react with RCA-1 in the human brain. In Table 5.4 we attempt to summarize the most important characterization markers that differentiate microglia from macrophages or dendritic cells.

Despite the controversy regarding the origin of microglia cells, it is generally accepted that microglia are the most efficient APCs in the CNS. Microglia in vitro can express the essential molecules necessary for competent antigen presentation, such as MHC class II antigens

**TABLE 5.4**
*Characterization Markers That Differentiate Microglia from Macrophages or Dendritic Cells in the Central Nervous System*

|  | CD11B | CD11C | F4/80 | DEC205 | CD45 | MIDc8 (SEROTEC) | IBA1 | RCA-1 |
|---|---|---|---|---|---|---|---|---|
| Microglia | + | – | + | – | Low | – | + | + |
| Macrophage | + | –[1] | + | – | High | – | – | – |
| Dendritic cell | – | + | + | + | + | + | – | – |

[1]During inflammation.

(174,185–191). In addition, in vivo infusion and intracerebral injection of IFN-γ also leads to class II MHC upregulation on microglial cells (192–195). Class II expression on microglial cells is tightly regulated. It was demonstrated that IFN-γ–induced surface expression of MHC class II molecules on a microglial cell line can be inhibited by the cytokines TGF-β1, IL-4, and IL-10 but not IL-13 (196). In several nervous tissue diseases such as EAE, MS, dementia complex mediated by acquired immunodeficiency syndrome, and Alzheimer and Parkinson diseases, class II upregulation on microglial cells has also been found (197–201). These cells also can express costimulatory molecules such as B7, LFA-3, and ICAM-1 (202–204). Several laboratories have found that microglia are also fully competent APCs, able to stimulate naive CD4$^+$ T-cells and activate antigen-specific effector T-cell clones in an MHC class II–restricted manner. Interestingly, when microglial cells were compared with other CNS macrophages in antigen-presentation assays, these macrophages were found to be superior in their APC properties (176). These results indicate that, although microglial are presumed to be of hemopoietic origin, these cells are not as competent APCs as macrophages. As an answer to the apparent controversy, it was also proposed that microglia serve different functions under different inflammatory conditions, depending on the cytokine milieu and the type of cognate interaction they are involved in (205). Under some conditions, resting and IFN-γ–activated microglia cells cannot activate naive or MBP-specific CD4$^+$ T-cells in the presence of MBP and encephalomyelitic MBP Ac1-11 peptide. In addition, in the presence of Ac1-11 peptide, CD4$^+$ TCR-transgenic T-cells became anergized. Those investigators found that microglia became professional APCs only after a multistep activation process involving stimulation through cytokines and cognate signaling (205).

Interestingly, another study suggested that there is a differential capacity of macrophages and astrocytes to restimulate Th1 and Th2 responses and that this difference may contribute to the reactivation and regulation of local inflammatory processes during infectious and autoimmune diseases (206). IFN-γ–activated microglia cells expressed MHC class II, CD40, and ICAM-1 molecules and efficiently presented antigen to Th1 cells. Conversely, IFN-γ-treated astrocytes, which express MHC class II and ICAM-1, presented antigen less efficiently to Th1 cells but were as efficient as microglia in inducing IL-4 secretion by Th2 cells. Further, astrocytes are much less potent than microglia in presenting naturally processed OVA peptide to either T-cell subset, indicating inefficient antigen processing. These data suggest that microglia play a role in the activation of Th1 and Th2 cells, whereas astrocytes activate mainly Th2 responses in the CNS (206).

In summary, microglia cells are likely critical elements in the initiation of CNS immune responses by being able to present antigens and produce several inflammatory mediators in the brain parenchyma.

## Astrocytes as Immunocompetent Cells

Astrocytes are star-shaped cells that also belong to the glial cell family. The processes of astrocytes are often in contact with blood vessels (discussed in BBB and the Nature of Immunologic Privilege in the CNS). These cells provide physical and metabolic support to the neurons of the CNS. Astrocytes have also been suggested to be efficient APCs. These cells are the most numerous of glial cell types within the CNS, so their APC functions have been the subject of intensive studies. Astrocytes were the first CNS-originated cells to be demonstrated to upregulate MHC class II molecules with exposure to IFN-γ and IFN-γ with TNF-α (195,207–209). In addition, astrocytes can be activated by other proinflammatory stimuli such as IL-1β, LPS, or viral proteins to express adhesion molecules such as ICAM-1, VCAM-1, and CD62E (E-selectin) (203, 210–214). The expression of costimulatory molecules on astrocytes also has been controversial. Some investigators did not detect B7-1 (CD80) or B7-2 (CD86) costimulatory molecules on unstimulated or activated astrocytes (215,216), whereas others found B7 costimulatory molecule expression on astrocytes (217–219). Not surprisingly, the antigen-presentation properties of astrocytes have been debated. On one hand, the Th2-inducing capacity of astrocytes and their ability to produce anti-inflammatory mediators was suggested (220,221); on the other hand, apoptotic cell death of autoreactive T-cells resulting from their interaction with astrocytes has also been demonstrated (222). Some of these results may be due to the difficulties of purifying astrocytes, resulting in microglial contamination in these cultures. This hypothesis is supported by the fact that, although highly enriched in vitro cultures of astrocytes lacking microglia cannot present antigen immediately ex vivo to blood-derived CD4$^+$ T-cells in mixed lymphocyte cultures in situ with the cooperative help of microglia-derived cytokines or accessory surface molecules, astrocytes may function as CNS APCs (223). More detailed studies to characterize the antigen-presenting properties of astrocytes will need to performed to resolve these issues. Nevertheless, it is undeniable that astrocytes play an important role in regulating immune responses in the CNS by producing a plethora of proinflammatory cytokines such as TNF-α, IL-1, IL-6, macrophage CSF, and granulocyte–macrophage CSF (224–236).

## CONCLUSION

In this chapter we evaluated the current view of immunologic privilege in the CNS and concluded that there is a highly regulated communication between the immune and the nervous systems and that this bidirectional communication is augmented under pathologic conditions. The primary element maintaining the immunologic privileged status of the CNS is the BBB, which actively participates in immune responses via expression of adhesion molecules, cytokine, and chemokine production and interactions with effector T-cells at the BBB. The unique microenvironment of the CNS also actively participates in the development of immune responses in the nervous tissue. The profound influence of resident and invading APCs on the modulation of an immune response in the nervous tissue is also crucial for regulating immunity in the CNS. The balance of suppressor factors that can prevent or limit the initiation of inflammatory responses in the CNS against proinflammatory mediators that alter this balance is fundamental for immunity in the CNS. As a result of an overwhelming invasion of activated lymphocytes and invading APCs into the CNS, a predominantly proinflammatory local environment will form in the nervous tissue, facilitating inflammation in the nervous tissue. Understanding the mechanism of immuno-privilege in the CNS will provide the basis for better therapeutic interventions for immune-mediated CNS diseases such as MS.

## References

1. Barker CF, Billingham RE. Immunologicly privileged sites. *Adv Immunol* 1977; 25:1–54.
2. Carson MJ, Sutcliffe JG. Balancing function vs. self defense: The CNS as an active regulator of immune responses. *J Neurosci Res* 1999; 55:1–8.
3. Hickey WF. Migration of hematogenous cells through the blood–brain barrier and the initiation of CNS inflammation. *Brain Pathol* 1991; 1:97–105.
4. Hickey WF, Hsu BL, Kimura H. T-lymphocyte entry into the central nervous system. *J Neurosci Res* 1991; 28:254-260.
5. Brabb T, von Dassow P, Ordonez N, et al. In situ tolerance within the central nervous system as a mechanism for preventing autoimmunity. *J Exp Med* 2000; 192:871–880.
6. Kida S, Pantazis A, Weller RO. CSF drains directly from the subarachnoid space into nasal lymphatics in the rat. Anatomy, histology and immunologic significance. *Neuropathol Appl Neurobiol* 1993; 19:480–488.
7. Kida S, Weller RO, Zhang ET, Phillips MJ, Iannotti F. Anatomic pathways for lymphatic drainage of the brain and their pathologic significance. *Neuropathol Appl Neurobiol* 1995; 21:181–184.
8. Weller RO, Kida S, Zhang ET. Pathways of fluid drainage from the brain—morphological aspects and immunologic significance in rat and man. *Brain Pathol* 1992; 2:277–284.
9. Cserr HF, Harling-Berg CJ, Knopf PM. Drainage of brain extracellular fluid into blood and deep cervical lymph and its immunologic significance. *Brain Pathol* 1992; 2:269–276.
10. Harling-Berg C, Knopf PM, Merriam J, Cserr HF. Role of cervical lymph nodes in the systemic humoral immune response to human serum albumin microinfused into rat cerebrospinal fluid. *J Neuroimmunol* 1989; 25:185–193.
11. Harling-Berg CJ, Park TJ, Knopf PM. Role of the cervical lymphatics in the Th2-type hierarchy of CNS immune regulation. *J Neuroimmunol* 1999; 101:111–127.
12. Knopf PM, Cserr HF, Nolan SC, Wu TY, Harling-Berg CJ. Physiology and immunology of lymphatic drainage of interstitial and cerebrospinal fluid from the brain. *Neuropathol Appl Neurobiol* 1995; 21:175–180.
13. Qing Z, Sewell D, Sandor M, Fabry Z. Antigen-specific T-cell trafficking into the central nervous system. *J Neuroimmunol* 2000; 105:169–178.
14. Ehrlich P. *Das Sauerstoff-Bedurfnis des Organismus: eine Farbenanalytische studie.* Berlin: Hirchwald; 1885.
15. Ehrlich P. *Uber Beziehunger von chemisher constitution, Vertheilung, und pharmakologisher Wirlung.* New York: John Wiley & Sons; 1906: 567–595.
16. Goldman E. *Vital Faubung am Zentralnervensystem.* Abh Preuss Akad Wiss Phys-Math K1, 1913; 1–60.
17. Reese TS, Karnovsky MJ. Fine structural localization of a blood–brain barrier to exogenous peroxidase. *J Cell Biol* 1967; 34:207–217.
18. Rubin LL, Staddon JM. The cell biology of the blood–brain barrier. *Annu Rev Neurosci* 1999; 22:11–28.
19. Joo F. Endothelial cells of the brain and other organ systems: Some similarities and differences. *Prog Neurobiol* 1996; 48:255–273.
20. Risau W, Wolburg H. Development of the blood-brain barrier. *Trends Neurosci* 1990; 13:174–178.
21. Staddon JM, Rubin LL. Cell adhesion, cell junctions and the blood–brain barrier. *Curr Opin Neurobiol* 1996; 6:622–627.
22. DeBault KE, Cancilla PA. *Some properties of isolated endothelial cells in culture.* New York: Plenum Publishing Corporation, 1980; 69–74.
23. DeBault LE, Cancilla PA. g-Glutamyl transpeptidase in isolated brain endothelial cells: Induction by glial cells *in vitro. Science.* 1980; 207:652–655.
24. Schinkel AH, Smit JJ, van Tellingen O, et al. Disruption of the mouse mdr1a P-glycoprotein gene leads to a deficiency in the blood–brain barrier and to increased sensitivity to drugs. *Cell* 1994; 77:491–502.
25. Maher F, Vannucci SJ, Simpson IA. Glucose transporter proteins in brain. *FASEB J* 1994; 8:1003–1011.

26. Simpson IA, Vannucci SJ, Maher F. Glucose transporters in mammalian brain. *Biochem Soc Trans* 1994; 22:671–675.

27. Seulberger H, Lottspeich F, Risau W. The inducible blood–brain barrier specific molecule HT7 is a novel immunoglobulin-like cell surface glycoprotein. *EMBO J* 1990; 9:2151–2158.

28. Schlosshauer B, Bauch H, Frank R. Neurothelin: Amino acid sequence, cell surface dynamics and actin colocalization. *Eur J Cell Biol* 1995; 68:159–166.

29. Seulberger H, Unger CM, Risau W. HT7, neurothelin, basigin, gp42 and OX-47—many names for one developmentally regulated immuno-globulin–like surface glycoprotein on blood–brain barrier endothelium, epithelial tissue barriers and neurons. *Neurosci Lett* 1992; 140:93–97.

30. Jefferies WA, Brandon MR, Hunt SV, et al. Transferrin receptor on endothelium of brain capillaries. *Nature* 1984; 312:162–163.

31. Breier G, Breviario F, Caveda L, et al. Molecular cloning and expression of murine vascular endothelial-cadherin in early stage development of cardiovascular system. *Blood* 1996; 87:630–641.

32. Hallmann R, Mayer DN, Berg EL, Broermann R, Butcher EC. Novel mouse endothelial cell surface marker is suppressed during differentiation of the blood brain barrier. *Dev Dyn* 1995; 202:325–332.

33. Raine CS, Cannella B, Duijvestijn AM, Cross AH. Homing to central nervous system vasculature by antigen-specific lymphocytes. II. Lymphocyte/endothelial cell adhesion during the initial stages of autoimmune demyelination. *Lab Invest* 1990; 63:476–489.

34. Dobbie MS, Hurst RD, Clark JB. An immortalized *in vitro* model of the blood–brain barrier: Glutathione levels and sensitivity to oxidative stress. *Biochem Soc Trans* 1998; 26:S354.

35. Dobbie MS, Hurst RD, Klein NJ, Surtees RA. Upregulation of intercellular adhesion molecule-1 expression on human endothelial cells by tumour necrosis factor-alpha in an *in vitro* model of the blood–brain barrier. *Brain Res* 1999; 830:330–336.

36. Duvar S, Suzuki M, Muruganandam A, Yu RK. Glycosphingolipid composition of a new immortalized human cerebromicrovascular endothelial cell line. *J Neurochem* 2000; 75:1970–1976.

37. Hurst RD, Fritz IB. Properties of an immortalised vascular endothelial/glioma cell co- culture model of the blood–brain barrier. *J Cell Physiol* 1996; 167:81–88.

38. Kuchler-Bopp S, Delaunoy JP, Artault JC, Zaepfel M, Dietrich JB. Astrocytes induce several blood–brain barrier properties in non-neural endothelial cells. *Neuroreport* 1999; 10:1347–1353.

39. Lechardeur D, Schwartz B, Paulin D, Scherman D. Induction of blood-brain barrier differentiation in a rat brain-derived endothelial cell line. *Exp Cell Res* 1995; 220:161–170.

40. Muruganandam A, Herx LM, Monette R, Durkin JP, Stanimirovic DB. Development of immortalized human cerebromicrovascular endothelial cell line as an *in vitro* model of the human blood–brain barrier. *FASEB J* 1997; 11:1187–1197.

41. RayChaudhury A, Frazier WA, D'Amore PA. Comparison of normal and tumorigenic endothelial cells: Differences in thrombospondin production and responses to transforming growth factor- beta. *J Cell Sci* 1994; 107:39–46.

42. Fabry Z, Waldschmidt MM, Hendrickson D, et al. Adhesion molecules on murine brain microvascular endothelial cells: Expression and regulation of ICAM-1 and Lgp 55. *J Neuroimmunol* 1992; 36:1–11.

43. Waldschmidt, M.M., Fabry, Z., Keiner, J., Love-Homan, L. and Hart, M.N., Adhesion of splenocytes to brain microvascular endothelium in the BALB/c and SJL/j mouse systems, *J Neuroimmunol*, 35 (1991) 191-200.

44. Ponzio NM, Chapman-Alexander JM, Thorbecke GJ. Transfer of memory cells into antigen-pretreated hosts. I. Functional detection of migration sites for antigen-specific B cells. *Cell Immunol* 1977; 34:79–92.

45. Williams KC, Dooley NP, Ulvestad E, et al. Antigen presentation by human fetal astrocytes with the cooperative effect of microglia or the microglial-derived cytokine IL-1. *J Neurosci* 1995; 15:1869–1878.

46. Brankin B, Hart MN, Cosby SL, Fabry Z, Allen IV. Adhesion molecule expression and lymphocyte adhesion to cerebral endothelium: Effects of measles virus and herpes simplex 1 virus. *J Neuroimmunol* 1995; 56:1–8.

47. Brayton J, Qing Z, Hart MN, VanGilder JC, Fabry Z. Influence of adhesion molecule expression by human brain microvessel endothelium on cancer cell adhesion. *J Neuroimmunol* 1998; 89:104–112.

48. Fabry Z, Topham DJ, Fee D. TGF-beta 2 decreases migration of lymphocytes *in vitro* and homing of cells into the central nervous system *in vivo*. *J Immunol* 1995; 155:325–332.

49. Reyes TM, Fabry Z, Coe CL. Brain endothelial cell production of a neuroprotective cytokine, interleukin-6, in response to noxious stimuli. *Brain Res* 1999; 851:215–220.

50. Kniesel U, Wolburg H. Tight junctions of the blood-brain barrier. *Cell Mol Neurobiol* 2000; 20:57–76.

51. Wolburg H, Neuhaus J, Kniesel U, et al. Modulation of tight junction structure in blood-brain barrier endothelial cells. Effects of tissue culture, second messengers and cocultured astrocytes. *J Cell Sci* 1994; 107:1347–1357.

52. Janzer RC, Raff MC. Astrocytes induce blood-brain barrier properties in endothelial cells. *Nature* 1987; 325:253–257.

53. Stewart PA, Wiley MJ. Developing nervous tissue induces formation of blood–brain barrier characteristics in invading endothelial cells:.A study using quail–chick transplantation chimeras. *Dev Biol* 1981; 84:183–192.

54. Janzer RC, Lobrinus JA, Darekar P, Juillerat L. Astrocytes secrete a factor inducing the expression of HT7-protein and neurothelin in endothelial cells of chorioallantoic vessels. *Adv Exp Med Biol* 1993; 331:217–221.

55. Allt G, Lawrenson JG. Is the pial microvessel a good model for blood-brain barrier studies? *Brain Res Brain Res Rev* 1997; 24:67–76.

56. Cohen Z, Molinatti G, Hamel E. Astroglial and vascular interactions of noradrenaline terminals in the rat cerebral cortex. *J Cereb Blood Flow Metab* 1997; 17:894–904.

57. Igarashi Y, Utsumi, H, Chiba H, et al. Glial cell line-derived neurotrophic factor induces barrier function of endothelial cells forming the blood–brain barrier. *Biochem Biophys Res Commun* 1999; 261:108–112.

58. Rubin LL, Hall DE, Porter S, et al. A cell culture model of the blood-brain barrier. *J Cell Biol* 1991; 115:1725–1735.

59. Albrecht U, Seulberger H, Schwarz H, Risau W. Correlation of blood–brain barrier function and HT7 protein distribution in chick brain circumventricular organs. *Brain Res* 1990; 535:49–61.

60. Petrov T, Howarth AG, Krukoff TL, Stevenson BR. Distribution of the tight junction-associated protein ZO-1 in circumventricular organs of the CNS. *Brain Res Mol Brain Res* 1994; 21:235–246.

61. Bard F, Cannon,C, Barbour R, et al. Peripherally administered antibodies against amyloid beta-peptide enter the central nervous system and reduce pathology in a mouse model of Alzheimer disease. *Nat Med* 2000; 6:916–919.

62. Hill JO, Aguirre KM. CD4+ T-cell–dependent acquired state of immunity that protects the brain against *Cryptococcus neoformans*. *J Immunol* 1994; 152:2344–2350.

63. Tunkel AR, Wispelwey B, Scheld WM. Pathogenesis and pathophysiology of meningitis. *Infect Dis Clin North Am* 1990; 4:555–581.

64. Dallasta LM, Pisarov LA, Esplen JE, et al. Blood-brain barrier tight junction disruption in human immunodeficiency virus-1 encephalitis. *Am J Pathol* 1999; 155:1915–1927.

65. Luabeya MK, Dallasta LM, Achim CL, Pauza CD, Hamilton RL. Blood–brain barrier disruption in simian immunodeficiency virus encephalitis. *Neuropathol Appl Neurobiol* 2000; 26:454–462.

66. Abbott NJ. Inflammatory mediators and modulation of blood–brain barrier permeability. *Cell Mol Neurobiol* 2000; 20:131–147.

67. Proescholdt MA, Heiss JD, Walbridge S, et al. Vascular endothelial growth factor (VEGF) modulates vascular permeability and inflammation in rat brain. *J Neuropathol Exp Neurol* 1999; 58:613–627.

68. Butcher EC. Leukocyte-endothelial cell recognition: Three (or more) steps to specificity and diversity. *Cell* 1991; 67:1033–1036.

69. Campbell JJ, Butcher EC. Chemokines in tissue-specific and microenvironment-specific lymphocyte homing. *Curr Opin Immunol* 2000; 12:336–341.

70. Rowley DA, Gowans JL, Atkins RC, Ford WL, Smith ME. The specific selection of recirculating lymphocytes by antigen in normal and preimmunized rats. *J Exp Med* 1972; 136:499–513.

71. Sprent J, Tough DF. Lymphocyte life-span and memory. *Science* 1994; 265:1395–1400.

72. Ottaway CA, Parrott DM. Regional blood flow and its relationship to lymphocyte and lymphoblast traffic during a primary immune reaction. *J Exp Med* 1979; 150:218–230.

73. Ponzio NM, Chapman-Alexander JM, Thorbecke GJ. Transfer of memory cells into antigen-pretreated hosts. I. Functional detection of migration sites for antigen-specific B cells. *Cell Immunol* 1977; 34:79–92.

74. Cserr HF, DePasquale M. Harling-Berg CJ, Park JT, Knopf PM. Afferent and efferent arms of the humoral immune response to CSF-administered albumins in a rat model with normal blood–brain barrier permeability. *J Neuroimmunol* 1992; 41:195–202.

75. Cserr HF, Knopf PM. Cervical lymphatics, the blood-brain barrier and the immunoreactivity of the brain: A new view. *Immunol Today* 1992; 13:507–512.

76. Gordon LB, Knopf PM, Cserr HF. Ovalbumin is more immunogenic when introduced into brain or cerebrospinal fluid than into extracerebral sites. *J Neuroimmunol* 1992; 40:81–87.

77. Harling-Berg CJ, Knopf PM, Cserr HF. Myelin basic protein infused into cerebrospinal fluid suppresses experimental autoimmune encephalomyelitis. *J Neuroimmunol* 1991; 35:45–51.

78. Dianzani U, Malavasi F. Lymphocyte adhesion to endothelium. *Crit Rev Immunol* 1995; 15:167–200.

79. Asherson GL, Zembala M. Anatomic location of cells which mediate contact sensitivity in the lympho nodes and bone marrow. *Nat New Biol* 1973; 244:176–177.

80. Buysmann S, Van Diepen FNJ, Van Kooyk Y, Ten Berge RJM. The influence of OKT3 on expression of lymphocyte adhesion molecules *in vitro*. *Transplant Proc* 1994; 26:3249–3250.

81. Issekutz TB. Effect of antigen challenge on lymph node lymphocyte adhesion to vascular endothelial cells and the role of VLA-4 in the rat. *Cell Immunol* 1991; 138:300–312.

82. Issekutz TB. Inhibition of *in vivo* lymphocyte migration to inflammation and homing to lymphoid tissues by the TA-2 monoclonal antibody. A likely role for VLA-4 *in vivo*. *J Immunol* 1991; 147:4178–4184.

83. Issekutz TB, Issekutz AC. T lymphocyte migration to arthritic joints and dermal inflammation in the rat: differing migration patterns and the involvement of VLA-4. *Clin Immunol Immunopathol* 1991; 61:436–447.

84. Jenkins MK, Khoruts A, Ingulli E, et al. *in vivo* activation of antigen-specific cd4 T-cells. *Annu Rev Immunol* 2001; 19:23–45.

85. Reinhardt RL, Khoruts A, Merica R, Zell T, Jenkins MK. Visualizing the generation of memory CD4 T-cells in the whole body. *Nature* 2001; 410:101–105.

86. Chao CC, Sandor M, Dailey MO. Expression and regulation of adhesion molecules by gamma delta T-cells from lymphoid tissues and intestinal epithelium. *Eur J Immunol* 1994; 24:3180–3187.

87. Gordon EJ, Myers KJ, Dougherty JP, Rosen H, Ron Y. Both Anti-Cd11a (Lfa-I) and Anti-Cd11b (Mac-1) therapy delay the onset and diminish the severity of experimental autoimmune encephalomyelitis. *J Neuroimmunol* 1995; 62:153–160.

88. Pober JS, Cotran RS. Immunologic interactions of T lymphocytes with vascular endothelium. *Adv Immunol* 1991; 50:261–302.

89. Shimizu Y, Newman W, Gopal T, et al. Four molecular pathways of T-cell adhesion to endothelial cells: Roles of LFA-1, VCAM-1, and ELAM-1 and changes in pathway hierarchy under different activation conditions. *J Cell Biol* 1991; 113:1203–1212.

90. Butcher EC, Williams M, Youngman K, Rott L, Briskin M. Lymphocyte trafficking and regional immunity. *Adv Immunol* 1999; 72:209–253.

91. Ludowyk PA, Willenborg DO, Parish CR. Selective localisation of neuro-specific T lymphocytes in the central nervous system. *J Neuroimmunol* 1992; 37:237–250.

92. Wekerle H, Engelhardt B, Risau W, Meyermann R. Interaction of T lymphocytes with cerebral endothelial cells *in vitro*. *Brain Pathol* 1991; 1:107–114.

93. Baron JL, Madri JA, Ruddle NH, Hashim G, Janeway CA, Jr. Surface expression of alpha 4 integrin by CD4 T-cells is required for their entry into brain parenchyma. *J Exp Med* 1993; 177:57–68.

94. Baron JL, Reich EP, Visinti I, Janeway CA, Jr. The pathogenesis of adoptive murine autoimmune diabetes requires an interaction between alpha 4-integrins and vascular cell adhesion molecule-1. *J Clin Invest* 1994; 93:1700–1708.

95. Romanic AM, Graesser D, Baron JL, et al. T-cell adhesion to endothelial cells and extracellular matrix is modulated upon transendothelial cell migration. *Lab Invest* 1997; 76:11–23.

96. Flugel A, Berkowicz T, Ritter T, et al. Migratory activity and functional changes of green fluorescent effector cells before and during experimental autoimmune encephalomyelitis. *Immunity* 2001; 14:547–560.

97. Miller RJ, Meucci O. AIDS and the brain: Is there a chemokine connection? *Trends Neurosci* 1999; 22:471–479.

98. Edens HA, Parkos CA. Modulation of epithelial and endothelial paracellular permeability by leukocytes. *Adv Drug Deliv Rev* 2000; 41:315–328.

99. Hart MN, Fabry Z, Love-Homan L, et al. Brain microvascular smooth muscle and endothelial cells produce granulocyte macrophage colony-stimulating factor and support colony formation of granulocyte–macrophage-like cells. *Am J Pathol* 1992; 141:421–427.

100. Hart MN, Fabry Z, Waldschmidt M, Sandor M. Lymphocyte interacting adhesion molecules on brain microvascular cells. *Mole Immunol* 1990; 27:1355–1359.

101. Cannella B, Cross AH, Raine CS. Anti-adhesion molecule therapy in experimental autoimmune encephalomyelitis. *J Neuroimmunol* 1993; 46:43–55.

102. Sobel RA, Mitchell ME, Fondren G. Intercellular adhesion molecule-1 (ICAM-1) in cellular immune reactions in the human central nervous system. *Am J Pathol* 1990; 136:1309–1316.

103. Wilcox CE, Ward AM, Evans A, et al. Endothelial cell expression of the intercellular adhesion molecule-1 (ICAM-1) in the central nervous system of guinea pigs during acute and chronic relapsing experimental allergic encephalomyelitis. *J Neuroimmunol* 1990; 30:43–51.

104. Kuchroo VK, Martin CA, Greer JM, et al. Cytokines and adhesion molecules contribute to the ability of myelin proteolipid protein-specific T-cell clones to mediate experimental allergic encephalomyelitis. *J Immunol* 1993; 151:4371–4382.

105. Willenborg DO, Simmons RD, Tamatani T, Miyasaka M. ICAM-1-dependent pathway is not critically involved in the inflammatory process of autoimmune encephalomyelitis or in cytokine-induced inflammation of the central nervous system. *J Neuroimmunol* 1993; 45:147–154.

106. Austrup F, Vestweber D, Borges E, et al. LP- and E-selectin mediate recruitment of T-helper-1 but not T-helper-2 cells into inflamed tissues. *Nature* 1997; 385:81–83.

107. Engelhardt B, Vestweber D, Hallmann R, Schulz M. E- and P-selectin are not involved in the recruitment of inflammatory cells across the blood-brain barrier in experimental autoimmune encephalomyelitis. *Blood* 1997; 90:4459–4472.

108. Newman PJ. Switched at birth: A new family for PECAM-1. *J Clin Invest* 1999; 103:5–9.

109. Newton-Nash DK, Newman PJ. A new role for platelet-endothelial cell adhesion molecule-1 (CD31): Inhibition of TCR-mediated signal transduction. *J Immunol* 1999: 163:682–688.

110. Williams KC, Zhao RW, Ueno K, Hickey WF. Pecam-1 (Cd31) expression In the central nervous system and its role in experimental allergic encephalomyelitis in the rat. *J Neurosci Res* 1996; 45:747–757.

111. Wong D, Prameya R, Dorovini-Zis K. *in vitro* adhesion and migration of T lymphocytes across monolayers of human brain microvessel endothelial cells: regulation by ICAM-1, VCAM-1, E-selectin and PECAM-1. *J Neuropathol Exp Neurol* 1999; 58:138–152.

112. Qing Z, Sandor M, Radvany Z, et al. Inhibition of antigen specific T-cell trafficking into the central nervous system via blocking PECAM-1/CD31 molcule. *J Neuropathol Exp Neurol.* 2001; in press.

113. Seabrook TJ, Johnston M, Hay JB. Cerebral spinal fluid lymphocytes are part of the normal recirculating lymphocyte pool. *J Neuroimmunol* 1998; 91:100–107.

114. Mobley J, Evans G, Dailey MO, Perlman S. Immune response to a murine coronavirus: Identification of a homing receptor-negative CD4+ T-cell subset that responds to viral glycoproteins. *Virology* 1992; 187:443–452.

115. Mobley JL, Rigby SM, Dailey MO. Regulation of adhesion molecule expression by CD8 T-cells *in vivo*. II. Expression of L-selectin (CD62L) by memory cytolytic T-cells responding to minor histocompatibility antigens. *J Immunol* 1994; 153:5443–5452.

116. Engelhardt B, Conley FK, Kilshaw PJ, Butcher EC. Lymphocytes infiltrating the CNS during inflammation display a distinctive phenotype and bind to VCAM-1 but not to MAdCAM-1. *Int Immunol* 1995; 7:481–491.

117. Bauer J, Bradl M, Hickley WF. T-cell apoptosis in inflammatory brain lesions: Destruction of T-cells does not depend on antigen recognition (see comments). *Am J Pathol* 1998; 153:715–724.

118. Mosmann TR, Cherwinski H, Bond MW, Giedlin MA, Coffman RL. Two types of murine helper T-cell clone. I. Definition according to profiles of lymphokine activities and secreted proteins. *J Immunol* 1986l 136:2348–2352.

119. Abbas AK, Williams ME, Burstein HJ, et al. Activation and functions of CD4+ T-cell subsets, Immunol Rev 1991; 123:5–22.

120. Merrill JE. Proinflammatory and antiinflammatory cytokines in multiple sclerosis and central nervous system acquired immunodeficiency syndrome. *J Immunother* 1992; 12:167–170.

121. Merrill JE, Graves MC, Mulder DG. Autoimmune disease and the nervous system. Biochemical, molecular, and clinical update. *West J Med* 1992; 156:639–646.

122. Merrill JE, Kono DH, Clayton J, et al. Inflammatory leukocytes and cytokines in the peptide-induced disease of experimental allergic encephalomyelitis in SJL and B10.PL mice (published erratum appears in *Proc Natl Acad Sci USA* 1992; 89:10562). *Proc Natl Acad Sci USA* 1992; 89:574–578.

123. Khoury SJ, Hancock WW, Weiner HL. Oral tolerance to myelin basic protein and natural recovery from experimental autoimmune encephalomyelitis are associated with downregulation of inflammatory cytokines and differential upregulation of transforming growth factor beta, interleukin 4, and prostaglandin E expression in the brain. *J Exp Med* 1992; 176:1355–1364.

124. Khoruts A, Miller SD, Jenkins MK. Neuroantigen-specific Th2 cells are inefficient suppressors of experimental autoimmune encephalomyelitis induced by effector Th1 cells. *J Immunol* 1995; 155:5011–5017.

125. Mondino A, Khoruts A, Jenkins MK. The anatomy of T-cell activation and tolerance. *Proc Natl Acad Sci USA* 1996; 93:2245–2252.

126. Goverman J, Woods A, Larson L, et al. Transgenic mice that express a myelin basic protein-specific T-cell receptor develop spontaneous autoimmunity. *Cell* 1993; 72:551–560.

127. Lafaille JJ, Nagashima K, Katsuki M, Tonegawa S. High incidence of spontaneous autoimmune encephalomyelitis in immunodeficient anti-myelin basic protein T-cell receptor transgenic mice. *Cell* 1994; 78:399–408.

128. Kaye J, Hedrick SM. Analysis of specificity for antigen, Mls, and allogenic MHC by transfer of T-cell receptor alpha- and beta-chain genes. *Nature* 1988; 336:580–583.

129. Kaye J, Hsu ML, Sauron ME, et al. Selective development of CD4+ T-cells in transgenic mice expressing a class II MHC-restricted antigen receptor. *Nature* 1989; 341:746–749.

130. Dittel BN, Visintin I, Merchant RM, Janeway CA, Jr. Presentation of the self antigen myelin basic protein by dendritic cells leads to experimental autoimmune encephalomyelitis. *J Immunol* 1999; 163:32–39.

131. Fischer HG, Bielinsky AK. Antigen presentation function of brain-derived dendriform cells depends on astrocyte help. *Int Immunol* 1999; 11:1265–1274.

132. Fischer HG, Bonifas U, Reichmann G. Phenotype and functions of brain dendritic cells emerging during chronic infection of mice with Toxoplasma gondii. *J Immunol* 2000; 164:4826–4834.

133. Brodsky FM, Guagliardi LE. The cell biology of antigen processing and presentation. *Annu Rev Immunol* 1991; 9:707–744.

134. Kourilsky P, Claverie JM. *MHC–Antigen Interaction: What Does the T-cell Receptor See?* San Diego: Academic Press, 1989; 107–194.

135. Townsend A, Bodmer H. Antigen recognition by class I-restricted T lymphocytes. *Annu Rev Immunol* 1989; 7:601–624.

136. Unanue ER. Antigen-presenting function of the macrophage. *Annu Rev Immnol* 1984; 2:395–428.

137. Allison JP, L LL. Structure, function and serology of the T-cell antigen receptor complex. *Ann Rev Immunol* 1987; 5:503–540.

138. Allison JP, Havran WL. The immunobiology of T-cells with invariant gd antigen receptors. *Ann Rev Immunol* 1991; 19:679–705.

139. Raulet DH. The structure, function and molecular genetics of the gd T-cell receptor. *Ann Rev Immunol* 1989; 7:175–207.

140. Wilson RK, Lai E, Concannon R, Barth RK, Hood LE. Structure, organization and polymorphism of murine and human T-cell receptor a and b chain families. *Immunol Rev* 1988; 101:149–172.

141. Kappler JW, Wade T, White J. A T-cell receptor Vb segment that imparts eactivity to a class II major histocompatibility complex product. *Cell* 1987; 49:263–271.

142. Rudensky AY, Maric M, Eastman S, et al. Intracellular assembly and transport of endogenous peptide-MHC class II complexes. *Immunity* 1994; 1:585–594.

143. Jenkins, M.K., The ups and downs of T-cell costimulation. *Immunity* 1 (1994) 443-6.

144. Jenkins MK, Schwartz RH. Antigen presentation by chemically modified splenocytes induces antigen-specific T-cell unresponsiveness *in vitro* and *in vivo*. *J Exp Med* 1987; 165:302–319.

145. Chambers CA, Allison JP. Costimulatory regulation of T-cell function. *Curr Opin Cell Biol* 1999; 11:203–210.

146. Kobata T, Azuma M, Yagita H, Okumura K. Role of costimulatory molecules in autoimmunity. *Rev Immunogenet* 2000; 2:74–80.

147. Mak TW. Insights into the ontogeny and activation of T-cells. *Clin Chem* 1994; 40:2128–2131.

148. Sharpe AH. Analysis of lymphocyte costimulation *in vivo* using transgenic and 'knockout' mice. *Curr Opin Immunol* 1995; 7:389–395.

149. Slavik JM, Hutchcroft JE, Bierer BE. CD28/CTLA-4 and CD80/CD86 families: Signaling and function. *Immunol Res* 1999; 19:1–24.

150. Wingren AG, Parra E, Varga M, et al. T-cell activation pathways: B7, LFA-3, and ICAM-1 shape unique T-cell profiles. *Crit Rev Immunol* 1995; 15:235–253.

151. Allison JP. CD28-B7 interactions in T-cell activation. *Curr Opin Immunol* 1994; 6:414–419.

152. June CH, Bluestone JA, Nadler LM, Thompson CB. The B7 and CD28 receptor families. *Immunol Today* 1994; 15:321–331.

153. June CH, Vandenberghe P, Thompson CB. The CD28 and CTLA-4 receptor family. *Chem Immunol* 1994; 59:62–90.

154. Lenschow DJ, Walunas TL, Bluestone JA. CD28/B7 system of T-cell costimulation (review). *Ann Rev Immunol* 1996; 14:233–258.

155. Gimmi CD, Freeman GJ, Gribben JG, et al. B-cell surface antigen B7 provides a costimulatory signal that induces T-cells to proliferate and secrete interleukin 2. *Proc Natl Acad Sci USA* 1991; 88:6575–6579.

156. Freeman GJ, Gray GS, Gimmi CD, et al. Structure, expression, and T-cell costimulatory activity of the murine homologue of the human B lymphocyte activation antigen B7. *J Exp Med* 1991; 174:625–631.

157. Walunas TL, Lenschow DJ, Bakker CY. CTLA-4 can function as a negative regulator of T-cell activation. *Immunity* 1994; 1:405–413.

158. Karandikar NJ, Vanderlugt CL, Walunas TL, Miller SD, Bluestone JA. Ctla-4—a Negative Regulator Of Autoimmune Disease. *J Exp Med* 1996; 184:783–788.

159. Perkins D, Wang ZM, Donovan C, et al. Regulation Of Ctla-4 Expression During T-cell Activation. *J Immunol* 1996; 156:4154–4159.

160. Walunas TL, Bakker CY, Bluestone JA. Ctla-4 Ligation Blocks Cd28-Dependent T-cell Activation. *J Exp Med* 1996; 183:2541–2550.

161. McIntosh KR, Linsley PS, Drachman DB. Immunosuppression and induction of anergy by Ctla4ig *in vitro*—effects on cellular and antibody responses of lymphocytes from rats with experimental autoimmune myasthenia gravis. *Cell Immunol* 1995; 166:103–112.

162. Khoury SJ, Akalin E, Chandraker A, et al. Cd28-B7 Costimulatory Blockade By Ctla4ig Prevents Actively Induced Experimental Autoimmune Encephalomyelitis and Inhibits Th1 But Spares Th2 Cytokines In the Central Nervous System. *J Immunol* 1995; 155:4521–4524.

163. Jemison LM, Williams SK, Lublin FD, Knobler RL, Korngold R. Interferon-gamma–inducible endothelial cell class II major histocompatibility complex expression correlates with strain- and site-specific susceptibility to experimental allergic encephalomyelitis. *J Neuroimmunol* 1993; 47:15–22.

164. Prat A, Biernacki K, Becher B, Antel JP. B7 expression and antigen presentation by human brain endothelial cells: requirement for proinflammatory cytokines. *J Neuropathol Exp Neurol* 2000; 59:129–136.

165. McCarron RM, Spatz M, Kempski O, et al. Interaction between myelin basic protein-sensitized T lymphocytes and murine cerebral vascular endothelial cells. *J Immunol* 1986; 137: 3428–3435.

166. Pryce G, Male D, Sedgwick J. Antigen presentation in brain: Brain endothelial cells are poor stimulators of T-cell proliferation. *Immunology* 1989; 66:207–212.

167. Rollins SA, Kennedy SP, Chodera AJ, et al. Evidence that activation of human T-cells by porcine endothelium involves direct recognition of porcine SLA and costimulation by porcine ligands for LFA-1 and CD2. *Transplantation*. 1994; 57:1709–1716.

168. Vallee I, Guillaumin JM, Thibault G, et al. Human T lymphocyte proliferative response to resting porcine endothelial cells results from an HLA-restricted, IL-10-sensitive, indirect presentation pathway but also depends on endothelial-specific costimulatory factors. *J Immunol* 1998; 161:1652–1658.

169. Bourdoulous S, Beraud E, Le Page C, et al. Anergy induction in encephalitogenic T-cells by brain microvessel endothelial cells is inhibited by interleukin-1. *Eur J Immunol* 1995; 25:1176–1183.

170. Fabry Z, Waldschmidt MM, Moore SA, Hart MN. Antigen presentation by brain microvessel smooth muscle and endothelium. *J Neuroimmunol* 1990; 28:63–71.

171. Karasin A, Macvilay S, Hart MN, Fabry Z. Murine endothelia do not express MHC class II I-Ealpha subunit and differentially regulate I-Aalpha expression along the vascular tree. *Endothelium* 1998; 6:83–93.

172. Fabry Z, Sandor M, Gajewski TF, et al. Differential activation of Th1 and Th2 CD4+ cells by murine brain microvessel endothelial cells and smooth muscle/pericytes. *J Immunol* 1993; 151:38–47.

173. Hickey WF, Kimura H. Perivascular microglial cells of the CNS are bone marrow-derived and present antigen *in vivo*. *Science* 1988; 239:290–292.

174. Bo L, Mork S, Kong PA, et al. Detection of MHC class II-antigens on macrophages and microglia, but not on astrocytes and endothelia in active multiple sclerosis lesions. *J Neuroimmunol* 1994; 51:135–146.

175. Ulvestad E, Williams K, Bo L, et al. HLA class II molecules (HLA-DR, -DP, -DQ) on cells in the human CNS studied in situ and *in vitro*. *Immunology*. 1994; 82:535–541.

176. Ford AL, Goodsall AL, Hickey WF, Sedgwick JD. Normal adult ramified microglia separated from other central nervous system macrophages by flow cytometric sorting. Phenotypic differences defined and direct ex vivo antigen presentation to myelin basic protein- reactive CD4+ T-cells compared. *J Immunol* 1995; 154:4309–4321.

177. Tran EH, Hoekstra K, van Rooijen N, Dijkstra CD, Owens T. Immune invasion of the central nervous system parenchyma and experimental allergic encephalomyelitis, but not leukocyte extravasation from blood, are prevented in macrophage-depleted mice. *J Immunol* 1998; 161:3767–3775.

178. Ling EA, Wong WC. The origin and nature of ramified and amoeboid microglia: A historical review and current concepts. *Glia* 1993; 7:9–18.

179. Cuadros MA, Navascues J. The origin and differentiation of microglial cells during development. *Prog Neurobiol* 1998; 56:173–189.

180. Tanaka J, Maeda N. Microglial ramification requires nondiffusible factors derived from astrocytes. *Exp Neurol* 1996; 137:367–375.

181. Tang W, Lai YH, Han XD, et al. Murine Hn1 on chromosome 11 is expressed in hemopoietic and brain tissues. *Mamm Genome* 1997; 8:695–696.

182. Andjelkovic AV, Nikolic B, Pachter JS, Zecevic N. Macrophages/microglial cells in human central nervous system during development: An immunohistochemical study. *Brain Res* 1998; 814:13–25.

183. Walker WS. Separate precursor cells for macrophages and microglia in mouse brain: Immunophenotypic and immunoregulatory properties of the progeny. *J Neuroimmunol* 1999; 94:127–133.

184. Mannoji H, Yeger H, Becker LE. A specific histochemical marker (lectin *Ricinus communis* agglutinin-i) for normal human microglia, and application to routine histopathology. *Acta Neuropathol* 1986; 71:341–343.

185. Jiang H, Milo R, Swoveland P, et al. Interferon beta-1b reduces interferon gamma–induced antigen-presenting capacity of human glial and B cells. *J Neuroimmunol* 1995; 61:17–25.

186. Perry VH. A revised view of the central nervous system microenvironment and major histocompatibility complex class II antigen presentation. *J Neuroimmunol* 1998; 90:113–121.

187. Tomimoto H, Akiguchi I, Akiyama H, Kimura J, Yanagihara T. T-cell infiltration and expression of MHC class II antigen by macrophages and microglia in a heterogeneous group in leukoencephalopathy. *Am J Pathol* 1993; 143:579–586.

188. Tran CT, Wolz P, Egensperger R, et al. Differential expression of MHC class II molecules by microglia and neoplastic astroglia: Relevance for the escape of astrocytoma cells from immune surveillance. *Neuropathol Appl Neurobiol* 1998; 24:293–301.

189. Walker WS, Gatewood J, Olivas E, Askew D, Havenith CE. Mouse microglial cell lines differing in constitutive and interferon- gamma-inducible antigen-presenting activities for naive and memory CD4+ and CD8+ T-cells. *J Neuroimmunol* 1995; 63:163–174.

190. Wucherpfennig KW. Autoimmunity in the central nervous system: Mechanisms of antigen presentation and recognition. *Clin Immunol Immunopathol* 1994; 72:293–306.

191. Xu J, Ling EA. Upregulation and induction of surface antigens with special reference to MHC class II expression in microglia in postnatal rat brain following intravenous or intraperitoneal injections of lipopolysaccharide. *J Anat* 1994; 184:285–296.

192. Steiniger B, Falk P, Van der Meide PH. Interferon-gamma *in vivo*. Induction and loss of class II MHC antigens and immature myelomonocytic cells in rat organs. *Eur J Immunol* 1988; 18:661–669.

193. Steiniger B, van der Meide PH, Falk P, Klempnauer J. Induction of class II MHC antigen expression in rat organs after systemic application of recombinant gamma interferon. *Adv Exp Med Biol* 1988; 237:795–799.

194. Vass K, Lassmann H. Intrathecal application of interferon gamma. Progressive appearance of MHC antigens within the rat nervous system. *Am J Pathol* 1990; 137:789–800.

195. Wong GH, Bartlett PF, Clark-Lewis I, Battye F, Schrader JW. Inducible expression of H-2 and Ia antigens on brain cells. *Nature* 1984; 310:688–691.

196. O'Keefe GM, Nguyen VT, Benveniste EN. Class II transactivator and class II MHC gene expression in microglia: Modulation by the cytokines TGF-beta, IL-4, IL-13 and IL-10. *Eur J Immunol* 1999; 29:1275–1285.

197. Achim CL, Morey MK, Wiley CA. Expression of major histocompatibility complex and HIV antigens within the brains of AIDS patients. *AIDS* 1991; 5:535–541.

198. Achim CL, Wiley CA. Expression of major histocompatibility complex antigens in the brains of patients with progressive multifocal leukoencephalopathy. *J Neuropathol Exp Neurol* 1992; 51:257–263.

199. Dickson DW, Lee SC, Mattiace LA, Yen SH, Brosnan C. Microglia and cytokines in neurological disease, with special reference to AIDS and Alzheimer's disease. *Glia* 1993; 7:75–83.

200. Hofman FM, von Hanwehr RI, Dinarello CA, et al. Immunoregulatory molecules and IL 2 receptors identified in multiple sclerosis brain. *J Immunol* 1986; 136:3239–3245.

201. McGeer PL, Kawamata T, Walker DG, et al. Microglia in degenerative neurological disease. *Glia* 1993; 7:84–92.

202. De Simone R, Giampaolo A, Giometto B, et al. The costimulatory molecule B7 is expressed on human microglia in culture and in multiple sclerosis acute lesions. *J Neuropathol Exp Neurol* 1995; 54:175–187.

203. Shrikant P, Weber E, Jilling T, Benveniste EN. Intercellular adhesion molecule-1 gene expression by glial cells. Differential mechanisms of inhibition by IL-10 and IL-6. *J Immunol* 1995; 155:1489–1501.

204. Williams K, Ulvestad E, Antel JP. B7/BB-1 antigen expression on adult human microglia studied *in vitro* and in situ. *Eur J Immunol* 1994; 24:3031–3037.

205. Matyszak MK, Denis-Donini S, Citterio S, et al. Microglia induce myelin basic protein-specific T-cell anergy or T-cell activation, according to their state of activation. *Eur J Immunol* 1999; 29:3063–3076.

206. Aloisi F, Ria,F, Penna G, Adorini L. Microglia are more efficient than astrocytes in antigen processing and in Th1 but not Th2 cell activation. *J Immunol* 1998; 160:4671–4680.

207. Fontana A, Fierz W, Wekerle H. Astrocytes present myelin basic protein to encephalitogenic T-cell lines. *Nature* 1984; 307:273–276.

208. Hirsch MR, Wietzerbin J, Pierres M, Goridis C. Expression of Ia antigens by cultured astrocytes treated with gamma-interferon. *Neurosci Lett* 1983; 41:199–204.

209. Vidovic M, Sparacio SM, Elovitz M, Benveniste EN. Induction and regulation of class II major histocompatibility complex mRNA expression in astrocytes by interferon-gamma and tumor necrosis factor-alpha. *J Neuroimmunol* 1990; 30:189–200.

210. Aloisi F, Borsellino G, Samoggia P, et al. Astrocyte cultures from human embryonic brain: Characterization and modulation of surface molecules by inflammatory cytokines. *J Neurosci Res* 1992; 32:494–506.

211. Benveniste EN, Huneycutt BS, Shrikant P, Ballestas ME. Second messenger systems in the regulation of cytokines and adhesion molecules in the central nervous system. *Brain Behav Immunol* 1995; 9:304–314.

212. Frohman EM, Frohman TC, Dustin ML, et al. The induction of intercellular adhesion molecule 1 (ICAM-1) expression on human fetal astrocytes by interferon-gamma, tumor necrosis factor alpha, lymphotoxin, and interleukin-1: Relevance to intracerebral antigen presentation. *J Neuroimmunol* 1989; 23:117–124.

213. Hurwitz AA, Lyman WD, Guida MP, Calderon TM, Berman JW. Tumor necrosis factor alpha induces adhesion molecule expression on human fetal astrocytes. *J Exp Med* 1992; 176:1631–1636.

214. Rosenman SJ, Shrikant P, Dubb L, Benveniste EN, Ransohoff RM. Cytokine-induced expression of vascular cell adhesion molecule-1 (VCAM- 1) by astrocytes and astrocytoma cell lines. *J Immunol* 1995; 154:1888–1899.

215. Cross AH, Ku G. Astrocytes and central nervous system endothelial cells do not express B7-1 (CD80) or B7-2 (CD86) immunoreactivity during experimental autoimmune encephalomyelitis. *J Neuroimmunol* 2000; 110:76–82.

216. Satoh J, Lee YB, Kim SU. T-cell costimulatory molecules B7-1 (CD80) and B7-2 (CD86) are expressed in human microglia but not in astrocytes in culture. *Brain Res* 1995; 704:92–96.

217. Cornet A, Bettelli E, Oukka M, et al. Role of astrocytes in antigen presentation and naive T-cell activation. *J Neuroimmunol* 2000; 106:69–77.

218. Nikcevich KM, Gordon KB, Tan L, et al. IFN-gamma-activated primary murine astrocytes express B7 costimulatory molecules and prime naive antigen-specific T-cells. *J Immunol* 1997; 158:614–621.

219. Soos JM, Ashley TA, Morrow J, Patarroyo JC, Szente BE, Zamvil SS. Differential expression of B7 co-stimulatory molecules by astrocytes correlates with T-cell activation and cytokine production. *Int Immunol* 1999; 11:1169–1179.

220. Aloisi F, Ria F, Columba-Cabezas S, et al. Relative efficiency of microglia, astrocytes, dendritic cells and B cells in naive CD4+ T-cell priming and Th1/Th2 cell restimulation. *Eur J Immunol* 1999; 29:2705–2714.

221. Aloisi F, Serafini B, Adorini L. Glia–T-cell dialogue. *J Neuroimmunol* 2000; 107:111–117.

222. Gold R, Schmied M, Tontsch U, et al. ntigen presentation by astrocytes primes rat T lymphocytes for apoptotic cell death. A model for T-cell apoptosis *in vivo*. *Brain* 1996; 119:651–659.

223. Williams KC, Dooley NP, Ulvestad E, et al. Antigen presentation by human fetal astrocytes with the cooperative effect of microglia or the microglial-derived cytokine IL-1. *J Neurosci* 1995; 15:1869–1878.

224. Baldwin GC, Benveniste EN, Chung GY, Gasson JC, Golde DW. Identification and characterization of a high-affinity granulocyte-macrophage colony-stimulating factor receptor on primary rat oligodendrocytes. *Blood* 1993; 82:3279–3282.

225. Benveniste EN. Lymphokines and monokines in the neuroendocrine system. *Prog Allergy* 1988; 43:84–120.

226. Benveniste EN. Inflammatory cytokines within the central nervous system: Sources, function, and mechanism of action. *Am J Physiol* 1992; 263:C1–C16.

227. Benveniste EN. Cytokine circuits in brain. Implications for AIDS dementia complex. *Res Publ Assoc Res Nerv Ment Dis* 1994; 72:71–88.

228. Benveniste EN. Cytokine actions in the central nervous system. *Cytokine Growth Factor Rev* 1998; 9:259–275.

229. Benveniste EN, Sparacio SM, Norris JG, Grenett HE, Fuller GM. Induction and regulation of interleukin-6 gene expression in rat astrocytes. *J Neuroimmunol* 1990; 30:201–212.

230. Bethea JR, Gillespie GY, Benveniste EN. Interleukin-1 beta induction of TNF-alpha gene expression: Involvement of protein kinase C. *J Cell Physiol* 1992; 152:264–273.

231. Bethea JR, Gillespie GY, Chung IY, Benveniste EN. Tumor necrosis factor production and receptor expression by a human malignant glioma cell line, D54-MG. *J Neuroimmunol* 1990; 30:1–13.

232. Merrill JE, Benveniste EN. Cytokines in inflammatory brain lesions: helpful and harmful. *Trends Neurosci* 1996; 19:331–338.

233. Norris JG, Benveniste EN. Interleukin-6 production by astrocytes: Induction by the neurotransmitter norepinephrine. *J Neuroimmunol* 1993; 45:137–145.

234. Oh JW, Schwiebert LM, Benveniste EN. Cytokine regulation of CC and CXC chemokine expression by human astrocytes. *J Neurovirol* 1999; 5:82–94.

235. Van Wagoner NJ, Benveniste EN. Interleukin-6 expression and regulation in astrocytes. *J Neuroimmunol* 1999; 100:124–139.

236. Van Wagoner NJ, Oh JW, Repovic P, Benveniste EN. Interleukin-6 (IL-6) production by astrocytes: Autocrine regulation by IL-6 and the soluble IL-6 receptor. *J Neurosci* 1999; 19:5236–5244.

237. de Vries HE, Blom-Roosemalen MC, van Oosten M, et al. The influence of cytokines on the integrity of the blood–brain barrier *in vitro*. *J Neuroimmunol* 1996; 64:37–43.

238. Gloor SM, Weber A, Adachi N, Frei K. Interleukin-1 modulates protein tyrosine phosphatase activity and permeability of brain endothelial cells. *Biochem Biophys Res Commun* 1997; 239:804–809.

239. Sharief MK, Ciardi M, Thompson EJ. Blood–brain barrier damage in patients with bacterial meningitis: Association with tumor necrosis factor-alpha but not interleukin-1 beta. *J Infect Dis* 1992; 166:350–358.

240. Yang GY, Gong C, Qin Z, Liu XH, Lorris Betz A. Tumor necrosis factor alpha expression produces increased blood–brain barrier permeability following temporary focal cerebral ischemia in mice. *Brain Res Mol Brain Res* 1999; 69:135–143.

# 6 Experimental Autoimmune Encephalomyelitis

*LaChelle R. Arredondo*
*Amy E. Lovett-Racke*
*Michael K. Racke, M.D.*

Multiple sclerosis (MS) is a neurologic disease characterized by inflammation and demyelination within the central nervous system (CNS). Genetic and environmental factors are thought to predispose individuals for the development of MS. The precise etiology of MS remains elusive, although the inflammatory nature of the lesions in the CNS strongly suggests an immunopathologic mechanism of disease.

Experimental autoimmune encephalomyelitis (EAE) is a well-characterized animal disease used extensively as a model system to study basic immune function. In particular, EAE parallels MS in many ways and has thus become a useful tool in MS research. Like MS, EAE is an inflammatory, demyelinating disease of the CNS whose development and course varies according to several genetic and environmental determinants. Unlike MS, the etiology of EAE has been clearly defined as an autoimmune disease caused by myelin-specific CD4$^+$ T-cells, initially by Pettinelli and McFarlin (1) and subsequently by numerous laboratories. These CD4$^+$ T helper (Th) lymphocytes are of the type 1 phenotype, as defined by the specific pattern of cytokine production, where the T-cells secrete lymphotoxin (LT), interferon-gamma (IFNγ), and interleukin-2 (IL-2). The Th1 cells are crucial to the induction and development of EAE, but not to the exclusion of other types of immune cells. Throughout the course of disease, other immune cells, including Th2 cells, CD8$^+$

T-cells, macrophages, B cells, and possibly natural killer (NK) cells, are also involved in the pathogenesis of EAE. Research in several laboratories has led to valuable information about the roles of these various immune cells in organ-specific immune responses. These findings have led to an increased understanding of the basic mechanisms of autoimmunity, in particular inflammatory demyelination in the CNS.

## EAE: A CD4$^+$ T-CELL–MEDIATED DEMYELINATING DISEASE

In the late 1800s and early 1900s, a disease called post-vaccinal encephalomyelitis (PVE) occurred in a number of people receiving the rabies virus vaccine. An inactivated form of the virus was inoculated and grown in the spinal cords of rabbits. The vaccine itself consisted of a homogenate of the infected spinal cords, which contained the virus. Initially, the encephalomyelitis was attributed to the rabies virus in the vaccine; however, later studies found that factors in the spinal cord independent of the virus were responsible for PVE. In those studies, monkeys receiving normal spinal cord homogenate and monkeys receiving infected spinal cord homogenate developed a demyelinating disease soon after the vaccination. Those studies and many more in the years that followed led to the development of the experimental system known today as experimental autoimmune encephalomyelitis.

The ability to induce EAE by administration of spinal cord homogenate led researchers to suspect myelin as a major encephalitogenic component of the homogenate. Studies using myelin basic protein (MBP) to induce EAE confirmed the primary role of myelin antigens in the disease process (2,3). Since those studies, EAE has been induced using several myelin components, including MBP, proteolipid protein (PLP), myelin oligodendrocyte protein (MOG), and encephalitogenic peptides derived from these proteins (Table 6.1).

Although myelin and its components could induce disease, the precise mechanism of demyelination was not known until the 1970s and 1980s. In 1977, Panitch and McFarlin reported the induction of EAE in naive Lewis rats after the transfer of splenocytes from syngeneic donors previously immunized with MBP (4). Induction of the disease was enhanced if the sensitized cells were incubated in concanavalin A (ConA) or MBP before transfer. In 1981, Pettinelli and McFarlin extended this research to mice, showing that lymph node cells from MBP-sensitized SJL/J mice were capable of transferring disease into naive syngeneic recipients (1). The direct transfer of EAE in mice had been described by Bernard and colleagues (5). These authors described a complex protocol that included the use of spinal cord homogenate and *Bordetella pertussis* toxin in the initial immunization and large numbers of cells in the transfer and irradiation of the recipients (5). This report also implicated T-cells in disease mediation, because anti-Thy 1.2 antibodies prevented the induction of EAE. By eliminating specific populations of the lymph node cells with the use of several monoclonal antibodies, Pettinelli and McFarlin determined that $CD4^+$ T (Lyt $1^+ 2^-$ T) cells were responsible for mediating disease.

Neuropathology of the active lesion in the CNS of mice with relapsing EAE shows a severe inflammatory response, primary demyelination with moderate remyelination, and some axonal loss (6). These lesions become more gliotic and depleted of axons, but less severely demyelinated as the disease becomes chronic (7). The mode of disease induction affects lesion pathology in mice

with EAE. After induction of EAE via immunization with CNS antigens in adjuvant, lesions exhibit more severe gliosis and axonal loss, but scattered demyelination (6). After induction of EAE via adoptive transfer of MBP-specific lymphocytes, lesions exhibit more demyelination, more remyelination, and less axonal loss (6,7). In the mouse models of EAE, these lesions are present primarily in the spinal cord, irrespective of the mode of disease induction (8). They do differ from the lesions observed in MS patients, as they are limited in size and differ in distribution. Within the lesion itself, similarities between MS and EAE are apparent, including the primary features of axonal demyelination and remyelination (9).

The clinical course of EAE varies among the many different animal models. In a recently developed marmoset model, animals developed a relapsing–remitting form of EAE, characterized by inflammation and demyelination in the CNS and moderate neurologic dysfunction, features very reminiscent of MS (10). Although this new marmoset model is intriguing, current researchers primarily use rodent models of EAE because of the quality of reagents, the wealth of genetic information, and the diversity of molecular biology techniques available. Among the rodent models, the clinical course of EAE is quite diverse. In the Lewis rat and several mouse strains, EAE manifests as an acute, monophasic disease that appears to be self-limiting. Recovery from the monophasic disease is associated with increased apoptosis of T-cells in the inflammatory lesion (11,12). In other strains of mice, in particular SJL, EAE develops as a relapsing–remitting disease with greater clinical and pathologic similarity to MS. These animal models provide a method for investigating the mechanisms of immune-mediated pathogenesis in the CNS.

## MHC RESTRICTION AND DISEASE SUSCEPTIBILITY

Susceptibility to EAE varies between different strains in both the mouse and rat. Initially, susceptibility to EAE was linked primarily to the major histocompatability complex (MHC) class II genetic locus (13,14). In mice,

---

### TABLE 6.1
### Commonly Used Myelin Peptides Used to Induce Experimental Autoimmune Encephalomyelitis

| Peptide | Predominant mouse strains when used | Encephalitogenic sequence |
|---|---|---|
| MBP Ac1-11 | PL/J, B10.PL | ASQKRPSQRSK |
| MBP 89-101 | SJL | FKNIVTPRTPPP |
| PLP 139-151 | SJL | HSLGKWLGHPDKF |
| MOG 35-55 | B6 | MEVGWYRSPFSRVVHLYRNGK |

MBP, myelin basic protein; MOG, myelin oligodendrocyte glycoprotein; PLP, proteolipid protein.

strains expressing the H-2 u, s, q, and k loci were generally considered susceptible to MBP-induced EAE, whereas strains expressing the H-2 b and d loci were considered resistant. Molecular studies have shown that MHC components expressed by these alleles differ in their binding affinities to particular peptides. Differences in binding affinity regulate the interaction between the antigen-presenting cell (APC) and the T-cell and contribute to the effector response of the T-cell. Although most encephalitogenic regions of MBP correspond to peptides with high MHC-binding affinities, other nonencephalitogenic regions of MBP also have peptides with high MHC-binding affinities (15). One exception to this general observation is the low binding affinity of the immunodominant N-terminal epitope of MBP and the H-2u MHC. In another study, moderate to strong binding affinities were essential for development of immune responses, but immunogenicity was not sufficient for encephalitogenicity (16). These and other findings suggest that variables other than MHC affinity are also involved in determining the susceptibility to EAE (15–18). Another variable that contributes to the susceptibility to develop EAE is the antigen used to induce disease. MBP and PLP are the most prominent protein constituents of myelin and are most commonly used as encephalitogenic antigens. Several strains of mice and rats are highly susceptible to disease induced by immunization with either MBP or PLP or by transfer of MBP- or PLP-specific T-cells (14,19). Although it is primarily a T-cell–mediated disease, EAE can exhibit a strong antibody component that may be involved in demyelination of the CNS of affected mice (20–22). This antibody component often involves the production of autoantibodies against MOG, another constituent of myelin (23). Recent studies have demonstrated that strains resistant to disease induction using MBP or PLP are quite susceptible to disease induction using MOG (24–27). Thus, even though C57/BL6 mice are considered to be highly resistant to MBP-induced EAE, they are quite susceptible to MOG-induced EAE. In addition, 129 mice, which are also H-2b, are quite susceptible to MBP-induced EAE. It is clear that the genetic background affecting EAE susceptibility is much more complicated than just MHC haplotype.

In addition to the use of different antigens, novel modes of disease induction have weakened the distinction between susceptibility and resistance considerably. Typically, susceptible strains of mice develop EAE after a single immunization with MBP or PLP in complete Freund adjuvant (CFA), followed by injections of pertussis toxin (13,14). Other more typically MBP-resistant strains do not develop EAE under these conditions but will develop EAE after performing an adoptive transfer step (where the draining lymph node cells are stimulated with MBP in vitro), followed by immunization with MBP in CFA (28). After this mode of induction, these typically resistant strains develop consistent and severe disease similar to that seen in the traditionally susceptible strains. This suggests that resistance to EAE is a relative state and that, under appropriate conditions, most mouse strains can be induced to develop EAE, regardless of MHC haplotype.

## T-CELL RECEPTOR SPECIFICITY AND USAGE

When considering the various components of the trimolecular complex, T-cell receptor (TCR) usage in EAE has received a great deal of attention. The antigen-specific TCR is a heterodimeric transmembrane glycoprotein comprised of $\alpha$ and $\beta$ chains encoded in the germline in distinct regions, including variable (V), diversity (D; for the $\beta$ chain only), joining (J), and constant (C) regions. Numerous genes exist for each region. Functional TCR chains are formed during T-cell development by gene rearrangements that splice together components of the V and J (V-D-J for the $\beta$ chain) regions and by posttranscriptional RNA splicing that adds the C region (29,30). TCR diversity originates from the random use of these V-D-J genes, variation between the junctional sites between the V-D-J genes, and the variable association of the $\alpha$ and $\beta$ chains.

Early studies in B10.PL and PL mice found that the V$\alpha$ and V$\beta$ chains of T-cells specific for the Ac1-9 peptide of MBP were highly restricted. Most of these T-cells express TCR carrying the V$\beta$8.2 chain, with the remainder carrying the V$\beta$13 chain. The Va chains expressed by these T-cells are restricted to expression of V$\alpha$2.3, V$\alpha$4.2, or V$\alpha$4.3 TCR V$\alpha$ chains. Further, the junctional sites, or CDR3 region of the TCR, which have been associated with peptide binding, are quite similar among these T-cells (31,32,35). Identification of the preference of MBP Ac1-11–specific T-cells for these particular V genes led to the development of B10.PL TCR transgenic mice expressing the V$\alpha$2.3 and V$\beta$8.2 genes (36). These transgenic mice are crossed to create V$\alpha$2.3, V$\beta$8.2 TCR transgenic mice, which are highly susceptible to EAE induction and occasionally develop spontaneous EAE. TCR usage is less restricted in SJL mice immunized with MBP peptide 89-101 but do show a preference for V$\beta$17 and V$\alpha$1.1 (37). Further, the TCRs from the SJL T-cell clones exhibit a conserved a-chain rearrangement between V$\alpha$1.1 and J$\alpha$BBM142 in the third hypervariable complementary determining region-3 (CDR3) region. Another study in the SJL mouse suggested that V$\beta$4 usage is increased in T-cells recognizing MBP (38). Similarly, TCR usage is quite heterogeneous in the SJL mouse when it comes to recognition of the immunodominant epitope of PLP 139-151 (39).

The CDR3 region of the variable chain confers antigenic specificity to the TCR. These regions are often fairly conserved in TCRs that recognize a common peptide bound to the same MHC molecule. In Lewis rats immunized with MBP to induce EAE, several different T-cell clones specific for peptide 68-88 of MBP expressed TCR comprised of the Vβ8.2 chain (40). Most of these Vβ8.2 chains shared two conserved amino acids in the CDR3 region, which were not observed in Vβ8.2 TCR of T-cells from adjuvant-immunized Lewis rats. In addition, the CDR3 motifs identified in the α-chain rearrangement between Vα1.1 and JαBBM142 in the TCRs of MBP 89-101–specific T-cells from SJL mice also were expressed by other encephalitogenic clones, including MBP-specific clones from PL mice (37). These data support the idea that CDR3 regions are fairly conserved between TCRs that recognize peptides from myelin antigens.

Recent evidence has suggested that the TCR β-chain usage during EAE in Lewis rats may not be as restricted as indicated by earlier studies (41). Vβ3.3 TCRs were identified in T-cell lines established from lymphocytes of Vβ8.2-depleted Lewis rats. The proportion of the Vβ3.3$^+$ T-cells increased after immunization with MBP, suggesting that they proliferated in response to the antigen. Further, Vβ3.3$^+$ T-cells were identified in spinal cord lesions of Lewis rats with EAE. Notably, Vβ3.3$^+$ TCRs used a CDR3 motif that is very similar to the motif used in the CDR3 region of Vβ8.2 TCRs identified by Gold and colleagues, implicating conserved CDR3 elements in both Vβ8.2 and Vβ3.3 TCR reactive to MBP (40). These data indicate that, although the TCR β-chain usage may be more heterogeneous than previously suggested, conserved elements within the CDR3 region of the TCR chains play an important role in MBP recognition.

Implication of the Vα2.3 and Vβ8.2 TCRs in the recognition of the immunodominant epitope of MBP by the H-2u MHC of B10.PL mice led to the development of mice transgenic for these TCR (36,42). In the mouse developed by Goverman (36), the α2.3- and Vβ8.2-rearranged TCR genes were used to generate transgenic lines that were bred together to generate mice expressing the complete transgenic Vα2.3;Vβ8.2 TCR. T-cells from these transgenic mice are reactive to MBP presented in the context of the H-2u MHC. These transgenic mice are highly susceptible to induction of EAE by MBP in CFA with pertussis toxin and by pertussis toxin or CFA alone. Further, transgenic mice maintained in normal animal facilities occasionally develop spontaneous EAE, whereas those maintained in specific pathogen-free (SPF) facilities do so at a much lower frequency, implicating an environmental agent in the development of spontaneous EAE. These MBP-specific TCR transgenic mice have been used extensively in EAE studies, many of which are discussed in this review.

The rearranged α and β genes of a different I-Au–restricted, MBP Ac1-9–specific CD4$^+$ T-cell clone were used to generate another TCR transgenic line of mice (42). These transgenic mice were crossed with recombinase activating gene 1 (RAG-1)-deficient mice to render them incapable of rearranging TCR and antibody genes to produce mature lymphocytes of their own. Thus, only T-cells expressing the transgenic TCR were present in these mice. Those crosses produced TCR transgenic H-2u mice that were homozygous for the RAG-1 mutation (T/R$^-$ mice) and littermates that carried a normal RAG-1 gene (T/R$^+$ mice). Spontaneous EAE developed in all of the T/R mice but in only some of the T/R$^+$ mice in SPF facilities. The clinical course of spontaneous EAE was variable in onset and rate of progression, with no signs of remission. Development of spontaneous EAE was associated with inflammation in the brain and spinal cord, as is typically observed in EAE. Because spontaneous EAE occurred in all of the T/R$^-$ mice but in only some of the T/R$^+$ mice, the investigators argued that nontransgenic lymphocytes in the T/R$^+$ mice confer some protection from disease initiation. Potential mechanisms for these protective effects include bystander suppression and immune deviation, concepts that are discussed later in this review.

Recently, additional transgenic mice expressing myelin-specific TCR were introduced (43) that recognize the immunodominant epitope of PLP 139-151. Initially, two different transgenic lines were established using the TCRs from two separate T-cell clones. The first TCR (5B6) contained the Vα4 and Vβ6 chains, and the second TCR (4E3) contained the Vα11 and Vβ16 chains. T-cells from mice from each of these transgenic lines proliferated vigorously and produced IL-2 and IFN-γ with stimulation with PLP 139-151. Those transgenic mice were highly susceptible to induction of EAE with PLP 139-151 in CFA and by pertussis toxin or CFA alone, similar to the MBP-specific TCR transgenic mice. Interestingly, both PLP 139-151–specific TCR transgenic lines were more prone to develop spontaneous EAE than the MBP-specific TCR transgenic mice, even in SPF facilities. Further, one of the transgenic lines was so susceptible to spontaneous EAE that it could not be maintained on the SJL background, but only on the normally resistant B10.S background. Because those animals were housed in SPF facilities, their development of spontaneous EAE might not have been due to an environmental agent. Additional studies using these transgenic mice may provide valuable information about the roles of PLP and PLP-specific T-cells in the development of EAE.

The limited heterogeneity of TCR V genes expressed by encephalitogenic MBP-specific T-cells in EAE enabled selective immunotherapy targeted against these TCR. Antibodies directed against MBP-specific TCR could prevent and ameliorate the clinical signs of EAE after adoptive transfer of MBP-specific T-cells or active immunization with MBP (31,34,44). In our own studies, using a monoclonal antibody to deplete donor (PL × SJL) F1 mice of Vβ8-expressing T-cells did not reduce the incidence of EAE induction, although the onset of disease was delayed (45). This demonstrates that, in severe disease, therapy directed against a predominant, specific Vβ TCR family may attenuate, but not fully prevent, disease onset or relapse. Using an alternative strategy, vaccination with whole inactivated encephalitogenic T-cells or synthetic peptides corresponding to determinants of the β chain of the TCR that are conserved among encephalitogenic T-cells conferred resistance to the induction of EAE in rats (46–48).

More recent studies have focused on the use of altered peptide ligands (APLs), encephalitogenic peptides with changes in the TCR contact residues, which results in partial activation, antagonism, or anergy of the encephalitogenic T-cell (49,50). One study showed that single amino acid changes at different positions in the MBP 87-99 peptide generate APLs capable of blocking the development of EAE by 2 different mechanisms (51). One APL was capable of inducing apoptosis of antigen-specific T-cells, and another caused the secretion of IL-4 rather than of IFN-γ by the antigen-specific cells. Several additional studies have reported the protection conferred by recognition of an APL. In one study, induction of EAE by immunization with several different antigens, including the 178-191 peptide of PLP, the 92-106 peptide of MOG, and MBP, was blocked by the administration of an APL of the 139-151 peptide of PLP (52). In a similar study, induction of EAE by transfer of T-cells specific for two epitopes of MBP could be blocked by the administration of an APL of 1 MBP epitope (53). In the latter study, the protective effect of the APL was blocked by the administration of anti–IL-4, suggesting that the induction of Th2 cells suppresses EAE. Transforming growth factor-β (TGF-β) has also been implicated as an effector of APL activity because anti–TGF-β partly eliminates the protection conferred by an APL of PLP 139-151 (54). In addition, cytokines, including IL-4, IL-13, and TGF-β, derived from APL-specific Th2 cells, decrease the encephalitogenic potential of antigen-specific splenocytes, if administered during in vitro stimulation (55).

Application of APL therapy has been complicated by recent studies showing that the in vitro effects of an APL do not absolutely predict the in vivo effects, presumably due to the diversity of the T-cell repertoire in vivo (56–58). Several APLs with changes in the MHC:TCR contact residue at position 6 of the Ac1-9 peptide of MBP, the immunodominant epitope for encephalitogenic T-cells from mice of the H-2u MHC haplotype, were found to be highly antagonistic to encephalitogenic T-cells in vitro and were assayed for their suppressive effects in vivo (56,57). These APLs not only failed to protect wild-type mice of the H-2u MHC haplotype from EAE induced by immunization with the Ac1-9 peptide, but they actually induced disease. The investigators attributed the encephalitogenicity of the APLs to the polyclonal nature of the T-cell repertoire in the wild-type mice, which is further supported by the fact that transgenic mice expressing the Ac1-9–specific TCR did not develop disease with

immunization with the APLs. In contrast, subsequent studies targeting another MHC:TCR contact residue identified APLs with limited antagonist activity in vitro but significant suppressive activity in vivo (58). Taken together, these studies indicate that the effects of an APL on T-cells in vitro is not indicative of its effects on the diverse repertoire of T-cells in vivo. Although the therapeutic application of APL in autoimmune disorders is intriguing, selection of appropriate analog peptides may be quite difficult, particularly when such a therapy is considered in humans.

## T-CELL COSTIMULATION

In addition to the TCR recognition of antigen bound by MHC class II on the surface of the APC, a second signal is required for proper activation of the T-cell. The second signal, termed *costimulation*, involves recognition of accessory molecules on the APC and the T-cell (Figure 6.1). Although several receptor–ligand pairs can provide costimulation, the signal provided by the interaction of B7 molecules on the APC and T-cell surface proteins cluster determinant 28 (CD28) and CTLA-4 appears to be the predominant one for T-cell activation. Costimulation provided by B7:CD28 signaling is important in the initiation of the autoimmune response in EAE. Further, costimulation provided by B7-1 is important in disease development, and B7-2 may play an important regulatory role. The interaction between B7 and CTLA-4 appears to play a critical role in downregulating the immune response in EAE.

The T-cell surface protein CD28 appears to be critical for IL-2 production because T-cells from a CD28-deficient mouse could not produce IL-2 upon stimulation with the mitogenic lectin ConA (59). Signaling through CD28 involves the B7 family of cells surface receptors. Two members of the B7 family of CD28 ligands have been defined, B7-1 (CD80) and B7-2 (CD86) (60–64). These molecules are only moderately homologous, but each can provide costimulation to T-cells for proliferation and IL-2 production. This complementary activity is probably responsible for the immunocompetence of the B7-1–deficient mouse (61). B7-1 and B7-2 are expressed differentially on various APCs. Further, the kinetics of expression and binding of B7-1 and B7-2 differ (65–67). B7-2 is expressed on monocytes constitutively, whereas B7-1 can be induced on these APCs with IFN-γ. Both B7 molecules are expressed on B-cell populations after an activation stimulus, with B7-2 being expressed within 6 hours and B7-1 expression peaking after 48 hours. Expressions of B7-1 and B7-2 also have been observed on T-cells themselves (68,69). Interestingly, B7-2 expressed on T-cells appears incapable of interacting with CD28 but is capable of interacting with CTLA-4, implying that B7 mole-

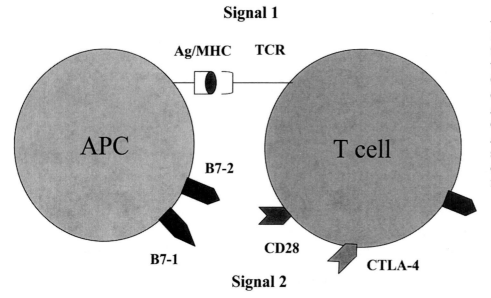

**Signal 1**

**FIGURE 6.1**

Diagrammatic representation of the 2-signal model of T-cell activation. The ligands for CD28, CTLA-4, B7-1, and B7-2 are expressed predominantly on APCs, although they can also be expressed on T-cells themselves. Ag, antigen; APC, antigen-presenting cell; MHC, major histocompatibility complex; TCR, T-cell receptor.

cules expressed on T-cells may directly contribute to the regulation of an immune response (70). In fact, our group showed that T-cells appear to be the main cell type expressing B7 molecules in the CNS during various stages of EAE (71).

T-cells also express CTLA-4, a surface molecule similar to CD28 that is also capable of engaging the B7 family of molecules. Originally, CTLA-4, in combination with CD28, was believed to provide a positive signal through binding the B7 family of molecules (72). Recent studies in several laboratories have indicated that CTLA-4–mediated signaling of the B7 family of molecules provides a negative or regulatory signal for T-cell activity (73–75). Studies using mice deficient in CTLA-4 further support the hypothesis that CTLA-4 mediates a regulatory signal because these mice develop a severe lymphoproliferative disorder (76,77). These studies suggest that B7-mediated costimulation provides regulatory activating signals for immune responses driven by T-cell activity.

B7 signaling through CD28 and/or CTLA-4 offers several avenues for regulatory intervention in an immune response mediated by T-cell function. Studies using CTLA-4Ig, a soluble fusion protein capable of preventing the interaction between B7 and CD28 or CTLA-4, have revealed a great deal about signaling through these molecules (78). For example, administration of CTLA-4Ig prevents rat cardiac allograft rejection and pancreatic islet cell xenograft rejection in mice (79–81). In both instances, the mechanism of suppression appears to involve the induction of antigen-specific tolerance.

Costimulation provided by the B7:CD28/CTLA-4 pathway is important for the development of autoimmunity. Our laboratory examined the role of this pathway in the induction of EAE (71,82–86) In the adoptive transfer model of EAE, administration of CTLA-4Ig or anti-

CD28 F(ab) inhibits the proliferation and IL-2 production of MBP-specific lymph node cells during activation in vitro, resulting in reduced clinical disease at subsequent transfer. B7-mediated costimulation is an important factor in determining encephalitogenicity. It is important to note that, once activated autoreactive cells are injected into naive recipients, CTLA-4Ig intervention does not alter the course of disease, which is consistent with the concept that activated T-cells do not require costimulation to perform their effector function. However, wild-type cells injected into mice deficient in both B7-1 and B7-2 are resistant to disease (87,88).

In models of EAE induced by active immunization, several intriguing observations have been made. Disease induced by immunization with MBP followed by pertussis toxin (PT) injection was inhibited with a single injection of CTLA-4Ig (84). In another model, which used a two-immunization schedule without subsequent PT injection, disease was inhibited after administration of a single injection of CTLA-4Ig EAE (82). However, in that model, disease was actually enhanced after administration of multiple doses of CTLA-4Ig. These paradoxical results suggest that B7 costimulation may provide a regulatory role during an immune response.

We and others have found that B7-1 provides an important stimulus for the development of encephalitogenic T-cells (74–82,84,89,90). Kuchroo and colleagues reported that B7-1 costimulation results in the development of Th1 cells, and B7-2 costimulation results in the development of Th2 cells (89). Although our laboratory was unable to demonstrate this dichotomy for B7-mediated stimulation, we did observe that anti-B7-1 administration protects against EAE, whereas anti-B7-2 administration exacerbates EAE. Studies using mice deficient in either B7-1 or B7-2 demonstrated that both molecules make significant contributions to the production of both IFN-γ and IL-4, although neither molecule plays an obligatory role in the production of either cytokine (91). Interestingly, in the autoimmune diabetes that develops in the nonobese diabetic (NOD) mouse, the effect of treatment using antibodies against B7 molecules is reversed (92). Anti–B7-1 administration exacerbates diabetes, whereas anti–B7-2 protects against diabetes.

Recently, a new model of acute EAE was developed in NOD mice with a peptide from PLP$_{56-70}$ (88). That model was used to investigate the potential roles of CD28, B7-1, and B7-2 in the pathogenesis of EAE. In that model, treatment with CTLA-4Ig or a combination of anti–B7-1 and anti–B7-2 monoclonal antibodies (mAbs) significantly delayed disease onset and reduced disease severity in wild-type NOD mice compared with control immunoglobulin (Ig)–treated animals. Treatment with anti–B7-1 or anti–B7-2 alone did not significantly alter clinical disease when compared with treatment with a control hamster Ig. To further examine the roles of these costimulatory molecules in this EAE model, B7-1–, B7-2–, and CD28–deficient mice were backcrossed onto the NOD strain. Disease was absent in CD28-deficient NOD mice and significantly reduced in B7-2–deficient NOD mice as compared with wild-type NOD animals, although these animals produced normal or enhanced levels of IFN-γ and tumor necrosis factor-α (TNF-α) in response to antigen in vitro. B7-1–deficient NOD mice developed clinical EAE similar to that in wild-type NOD mice, despite developing enhanced antigen-specific T-cell responses in vitro. Taken together, these data indicate that B7/CD28 signaling is critical for EAE induction in the NOD strain and in traditional EAE strains. Autoimmune target tissue-specific upregulation of B7-1 may function by binding to CTLA-4 with greater affinity than B7-2 and downregulating T-cell responses (75,93–95). These results suggest that B7-1 plays a dual role in EAE by interacting with CD28 and CTLA-4 to regulate disease.

Previous work has shown that naive T-cells, which have not encountered antigen since exiting the thymus, depend on costimulation, whereas memory T-cells, which have encountered antigen at least once, do not. For example, MHC–peptide complexes stimulated primed TCR transgenic T-cells, but only poorly stimulated naive TCR transgenic T-cells (96). Providing costimulation through CD28 enhanced the stimulation of the naive TCR transgenic T-cells by the MHC–peptide complexes. Memory T-cells depended considerably less on costimulation than did naive T-cells (97,98). In fact, our laboratory found that antigenic stimulation of MBP-specific lymphocytes makes them much less dependent on B7-mediated costimulation at subsequent antigenic stimulation (99,100). These data may explain the lack of effect of costimulatory blockade in ongoing EAE, where the encephalitogenic cells have already seen antigen and are no longer

costimulation dependent. These findings suggest that the blockade of costimulation has limited therapeutic use in ongoing autoimmune diseases due to the presence of memory, autoreactive T-cells. However, the lack of inflammation in the CNS of B7-1/B7-2–deficient mice suggests that costimulation is important for inflammatory cells to invade the CNS.

## CYTOKINES

EAE is characterized by a delayed hypersensitivity reaction resulting from inflammatory cell infiltration into the CNS. Although the infiltrate consists of a variety of immune cells, including T-cells and macrophages, initial formation of the lesion has been associated with neuroantigen-specific autoimmune T-cells (101). In this scenario, antigen-specific cells recognize one or more myelin antigens at the blood–brain barrier (BBB). It is thought that the most likely site of immune recognition is the perivascular monocyte (102). These cells are activated and release a variety of cytokines and chemokines that alter adhesion molecule expression on surrounding cells, including endothelial cells, and attract myelin-specific and nonspecific immune cells (Figure 6.2). The alteration of adhesion molecule expression allows infiltration of the activated T-cell and the numerous nonspecific cells swarming to the site into the CNS, thereby establishing the inflammatory lesion and initiating the demyelination process. T-cells associated with the delayed hypersensitivity reaction are classified as Th1 CD4$^+$ T-cells, a phenotype distinguished by the production of proinflammatory cytokines including IFN-γ, TNF-β/LT, and IL-2. In contrast, regulation of the inflammatory lesion has been correlated with the activity of Th2 CD4$^+$ T-cells, a phenotype distinguished by the production of regulatory cytokines including IL-4, IL-5, IL-10, and IL-13. The contributions of these subsets of CD4$^+$ T-cells is discussed below in relation to the activity of the cytokines and chemokines these cells produce. In addition, the effects of these cytokines are summarized in Table 6.2.

Expression of the cytokines associated with the Th1 phenotye has been correlated with disease activity (103–110). Many of these cytokines are secreted by CNS antigen-specific encephalitogenic Th1 clones in vitro (111–113). Both mRNA and protein expression of inflammatory cytokines occur in the CNS during the course of EAE, with detectable levels at the preclinical stage, significantly higher levels at the acute stage, and diminished levels at the recovery or remission stage. Similar results for mRNA expression in the CNS have been observed in our own studies and are used as markers for disease activity (114,115).

Information about the activity of these cytokines during EAE has been obtained by the exogenous application

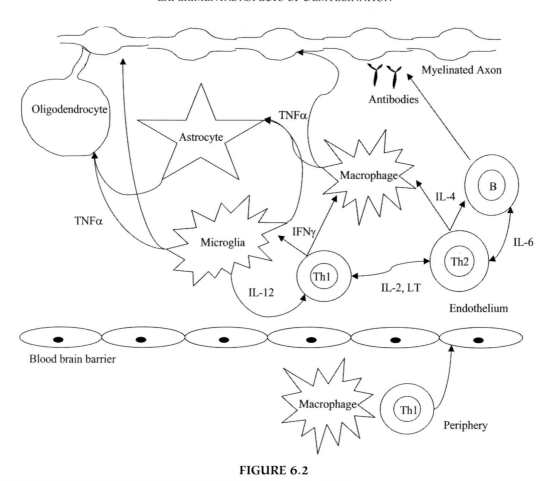

**FIGURE 6.2**

Diagrammatic representation of some of the potential cytokine circuits in experimental autoimmune encephalomyelitis. In this condition, myelin-specific CD4+, T$_h$1 cells are activated in the periphery before crossing the blood–brain barrier. Once across the blood–brain barrier, resident CNS microglia are thought to be the initial APCs. As other inflammatory cells are recruited into the CNS, these T$_h$1 cells interact with many different cell types. B, B cell; IFN-γ, interferon-γ; IL, interleukin; LT, lymphotoxin; T$_h$, T-helper cell; TNF-γ, tumor necrosis factor-γ.

**TABLE 6.2**
*Effects of Various Cytokines on the Disease Course of EAE[1]*

| CYTOKINE | EFFECT ON DISEASE SEVERITY | EFFECT WITH NEUTRALIZATION | EAE IN GENE-DEFICIENT OR TRANSGENIC MICE |
|---|---|---|---|
| IFN-γ | Reduced (116–118) | Exacerbated (116,117,119) | Exacerbated in IFN-γ-/− (120–122) |
| TNF-α | Exacerbated (129–131) | Reduced (132–133) | Conflicting (136–140) |
| IL-2 | Exacerbated (143–144) | Reduced (119) | Not reported |
| IL-4 | Reduced (114,149,169,170) | | Exacerbated or no effect in IL-4−/− (175,176) |
| IL-6 | Not reported | Reduced (148) | Conflicting (151–153) |
| IL-10 | Conflicting (149,182) | Exacerbated (149,182) | Exacerbated in IL-10 −/− (183) |
| IL-12 | Exacerbated (155–156) | Reduced (157–159) | |
| TGFβ | Reduced (186–187) | Exacerbated (164,188) | Exacerbated in mice where TGF-β expressed in CNS (192) |

[1]References cited are those noted in the text that describe the effect of these cytokines on the clinical course of EAE. CNS, central nervous system; EAE, experimental autoimmune encephalomyelitis; IFN-γ, interferon-γ; IL, interleukin; TGF-β, transforming growth factor-β; TNF-α, tumor necrosis factor-α.

of these cytokines and inhibitors of these cytokines and through the use of targeted gene knockouts in mice. In contrast to its anticipated role in pathogenesis, in vivo administration of IFN-γ actually decreased the severity of EAE in both mice and rats (116–118). In addition, these and other studies have shown an increase in severity of EAE in mice after anti-IFN-γ administration (116,117,119). Studies using knockout mice correlate well with the reports using anti-IFN-γ antibodies. EAE can be induced successfully in homozygous IFN-γ −/− and homozygous IFN-γR −/− mice, which corroborates the reports using anti–IFN-γ antibodies (120–122). In the IFN-γ -/- and IFN-γR -/- mice, the disease course is normal or more severe when compared with heterozygous littermates or wild-type controls. Taken together, these data indicate that IFN-γ is not required for the induction or perpetuation of EAE. Although it is traditionally characterized as a proinflammatory cytokine, IFN-γ clearly has multiple effects on immune function. It should be noted that MS patients treated by IFN-γ injection experienced exacerbation of the disease (123), suggesting that the role of IFN-γ in inflammatory diseases of the CNS is complex and may change with progression of the disease over time.

TNF-α and LT-α (TNF-β) are proinflammatory cytokines produced during the course of EAE in vivo and by encephalitogenic T-cells in vitro. Administration of TNF-α in vivo contributed to the development of clinical EAE and associated demyelination (129–131). Neutralizing antibody against TNF-α successfully prevented the transfer of disease by MBP-activated T-cells in SJL/J mice (132,133). In fact, little or no inflammation or demyelination was observed in the CNS tissue from mice treated with the antibodies. In addition, soluble TNF-α receptors (sTNF-R) were successful in treating EAE (134,135).

Experiments using TNF knockout mice also have produced conflicting results, which are largely attributed to the H-2b MHC restriction of the strain used in gene-targeting procedures. Mice with the MHC class II H-2b haplotype are relatively resistant to EAE induction with MBP. EAE has been successfully induced in these strains by using MOG as the antigen, although the disease course differs as it is often monophasic and chronic. TNF-α knockout mice appeared to be more resistant to disease induction, as shown by delayed disease onset (136,137). However, Liu and colleagues reported that TNF-deficient mice are more susceptible to MOG-induced disease, as shown by the development of extensive inflammation and demyelination (138), which was reduced by treatment with exogenous TNF-α. These differences may be due to disparity in experimental design and technique. To further explore and clarify the role of TNF-α in EAE, different groups backcrossed the TNF-deficient strain with the classic EAE-susceptible strain SJL/J (139,140). In initial experiments, both TNF-α and LT were targeted and disease was induced using mouse spinal cord homogenate

or PLP peptide 139-151 (139). These studies suggested that the antigen used affects disease susceptibility in these gene-targeted mice; however, the controls in those studies were not littermates but SJL wild-type mice, which possess an MHC different from that of the experimental mice. In a more recent study, MBP was used to induce EAE in TNF-α–deficient mice and the more appropriate congenic SJL.H-2b control. Disease onset, incidence, and severity were comparable between SJL.H-2b and SJL/J (H-2s) mice challenged with MBP. In TNF-α–deficient SJL.H2-b mice, although disease incidence and severity was comparable, onset was significantly delayed after challenge with MBP. The proliferative response of MBP-specific T-cells was not affected by TNF-α deficiency; however, the cytokine profile of those T-cells was not examined, so the overall role of TNF-α in MBP-specific T-cell responses cannot be determined. Thus, discrepancies in experimental design and results complicate interpretation of the TNF-deficiency studies, although TNF-α clearly has a role in the development and progression of clinical EAE in wild-type mice.

Interestingly, LT-α–deficient mice backcrossed onto the C57BL/6 strain were characterized by dramatic splenic disorganization, no peripheral lymph nodes, and resistance to induction of EAE by immunization with the MOG peptide, although these mice displayed an antibody response and a T-cell proliferative response to MOG (141). LT-α–deficient mice were susceptible to EAE when MOG-specific T-cells were passively transferred into them, implicating T-cell production of LT-α as a critical factor in the development of EAE pathogenesis. In a more recent report, radiation bone marrow chimeras were generated to explore the effects of LT-α–deficiency in mice with normal peripheral lymphoid systems (137). The transfer of LT-α–deficient hematopoietic cells into lethally irradiated C57BL/6 recipients did not alter the susceptibility of the recipient to induction of EAE by immunization with the MOG peptide after reconstitution of the immune system, suggesting that LT-α is not a direct mediator of pathogenesis.

IL-2 is a critical factor for the survival and expansion of T-cells, and anergy induction of T-cells is strongly associated with the repression of IL-2 gene expression (142). IL-2 is expressed with Th1-associated cytokines during the pathogenesis of EAE. Administration of IL-2 intensified EAE induced by adoptive transfer (143,144), suggesting that continued expansion of encephalitogenic T-cells can exacerbate EAE. Anti-IL-2 antibody had only a marginal effect in the active induction of EAE but drastically reduced the clinical signs of passive EAE, even when mixed with a disease-enhancing dose of anti-IFN-γ (119). Treatment of Lewis rats with monoclonal anti–IL-2 receptor (IL-2R) antibody conferred protection against the adoptive transfer of EAE by MBP-specific T-cells but not against active induction of EAE by immunization with MBP in CFA (145). This discrepancy may be due to variations in IL-2R expression on lymphocytes in vivo compared with those activated in vitro. In addition, IL-2 plays a major role in antigen-induced programmed cell death (PCD). T-cells proceeding through the cell cycle under the influence of IL-2 are highly susceptible to PCD induced by high doses of antigen, whereas resting cells are much less susceptible (146). This mechanism, which requires repeated antigen encounters at close intervals, provides a self-limiting negative feedback loop to regulate T-cell proliferation and function during an immune response. During EAE, encephalitogenic T-cells are susceptible to this mechanism (146). In other studies, coadministration of exogenous IL-2 with high doses of MBP reproducibly worsened EAE, although MBP-specific T-cells were deleted in numbers comparable to high doses of MBP alone (144). This finding implies that the endogenous IL-2 produced by activated T-cells is sufficient for resultant PCD, whereas the addition of exogenous IL-2 may stimulate other cells capable of contributing to inflammation and demyelination. The activation of other inflammatory cells by IL-2 is capable of worsening disease and emphasizes the complex and pleiotropic nature of IL-2.

IL-6 is a pleiotropic cytokine expressed by resident CNS cells and by infiltrating lymphocytes during the course of EAE (147). Studies of the role of IL-6 in the pathogenesis of EAE have produced conflicting results. Although Gijbels and colleagues reported that administration of anti-IL-6 antibody successfully suppresses EAE, the mechanism of action of the antibody does not appear to be neutralizing, because the levels of IL-6 in the blood and spinal fluid of animals receiving antibody were substantially higher than those in control animals (148). In contrast, Willenborg and colleagues did not observe any effect on EAE in mice treated with anti–IL-6 antibody (149). They did report that transgenic expression of IL-6 in the CNS of mice effectively suppresses the disease. In a related study, the administration of recombinant IL-6 suppressed the demyelination associated with a viral model of MS, Theiler murine encephalomyelitis (TMEV) (150). These studies suggest that increased levels of circulating IL-6 prevent the development of EAE.

Three recent reports addressing the role of IL-6 in EAE using IL-6–deficient mice produced some contradictory results (151–153). In all cases, the IL-6–deficient mice (B6.129) were completely resistant to EAE induced by an immunodominant peptide (encompassing residues 38–50) of MOG, whereas wild-type IL-6–competent littermates were highly susceptible to disease. Treatment with IL-6 during the preclinical phase restored the induction of EAE in those IL-6–deficient mice, which exhibit a normal disease course. In adoptive transfer experiments, MOG-specific T-cells derived from IL-6–deficient mice and activated in vitro did not transfer disease to IL-6–defi-

cient or wild-type recipients (152,153). When wild-type MOG-specific T-cells were transferred into IL-6–deficient recipients, Mendel and colleagues found only mild or no disease in the recipients. In direct contrast, Okuda and colleagues found typical disease under the same conditions. In both studies, administration of recombinant IL-6 had no effect on the observed course of EAE. In IL-6–deficient mice exhibiting little or no disease, a concomitant absence of inflammation in the CNS was also observed (151,152). In IL-6–deficient mice exhibiting EAE, inflammation in the CNS was observed (153).

During in vitro analysis of IL-6–deficient splenocytes, Samoilova and colleagues observed a decrease in cytokine production and proliferation in response to antigen but vigorous cytokine production and proliferation in response to the mitogen ConA (151). In contrast, Mendel and colleagues observed antigen-specific proliferation of lymph node cells from IL-6–deficient mice and wild-type littermates (152). Okuda and colleagues reported increased production of the Th2 cytokines IL-4 and IL-10 and decreased production of Th1 cytokines IFN-$\gamma$ and IL-2 in the IL-6–deficient lymphcytes compared with the wild-type lymphocytes in response to antigen (153). All three groups agreed that IL-6 regulates T-cell function and is crucial to the induction phase of EAE. Samoilova and colleagues contended that IL-6 is involved in the activation and differentiation of autoreactive T-cells as an important mediator in the costimulation pathway. Mendel and colleagues also supported a role for IL-6 in the costimulation pathway, but as an indirect mediator. They also contended that IL-6 is involved in the immune infiltration and inflammatory lesion development in the CNS. Okuda and colleagues argued that IL-6 contributes to the induction phase of EAE by modulating the Th1/Th2 phenotype of the autoreactive T-cells. In all cases, the investigators supported the investigation of IL-6 as a therapeutic target relevant to inflammation in the CNS and various autoimmune disorders.

Immunohistochemistry demonstrates that TNF-$\alpha$ and IL-12, which are produced by macrophages, contribute to the pathogenesis of EAE. IL-12 is a cytokine crucial to the differentiation of naive CD4$^+$ T-cells into Th1 cells and is expressed in the CNS of mice during the onset of EAE (110,154). Inclusion of IL-12 during in vitro priming of MBP-specific T-cells exacerbates EAE after adoptive transfer, and administration of IL-12 in vivo accelerates the onset of, exacerbates, and prolongs clinical EAE in mice and rats (155,156). Administration of neutralizing IL-12 antibody decreased the severity of EAE (157–159). IL-12 is a powerful stimulus for the proliferation and IFN-$\gamma$ production by Th1 cells, both of which contribute to the pathogenesis of EAE. However, in vivo administration of neutralizing anti–IFN-$\gamma$ did not decrease the effects of IL-12 during in vitro priming of encephalitogenic T-cells (155). Further, administration of anti–IL-12 completely prevented the induction of EAE in IFN-γ–deficient mice, suggesting that IL-12 plays a role in pathogenesis independent of IFN-γ (160). One alternative role for IL-12 in the pathogenesis of EAE may involve the autocrine induction of nitric oxide (NO) synthesis in macrophages, because mice treated with IL-12 exhibited increased infiltration of macrophages staining positively for inducible NO synthase (iNOS) in CNS lesions (161). Oligodendrocyte cytotoxicity and astrocyte reactive gliosis can be due to the actions of NO (162). Further, NO inhibitors can ameliorate the clinical course of EAE (163). Therefore, in addition to inducing encephalitogenic T-cells to produce IFN-γ, IL-12 may contribute to the pathogenesis of EAE by inducing activated macrophages to produce NO, which leads to oligodendrocyte cytotoxicity and astrocyte gliosis.

Conversely, expression of the cytokines associated with the Th2 phenotype, including IL-4, IL-10, and TGF-β, has been linked to recovery or remission of disease (104,164,165). IL-4 drives the differentiation of naive CD4$^+$ T-cells to Th2 cells and may play a regulatory role in EAE because its expression is prominent in the CNS during the remission phases of EAE in SJL mice (105,128,166). Adoptive transfer of MBP-specific Th2 cells that secrete IL-4 cannot transfer EAE into immunocompetent recipients (111–114,167,168). Our laboratory and others have shown that in vivo administration of IL-4 reduces the severity of EAE (114,149,169,170). Despite the antagonistic effects of IL-4 and Th2 cells on EAE, cotransfer of IL-4–secreting Th2 cells with encephalitogenic Th1 cells does not consistently reduce the clinical signs of EAE (171,172). Several procedures reported to reduce the pathogenesis of EAE rely heavily on the production of IL-4. These procedures include induction of myelin-specific oral tolerance (166,173), use of altered peptide ligands (53), administration of retinoic acid (174), and induction of tolerance using intraperitoneal administration of high-dose antigen (85).The pathogenesis of EAE in IL-4–deficient mice depends on the genetic strain of the mouse. Liblau and colleagues reported that PL/J mice deficient for IL-4 develop EAE, with normal disease course and pathology (175). Falcone and colleagues reported that C57BL/6 and BALB/c mice deficient in IL-4 develop EAE, with a more severe disease course and enhanced infiltration of inflammatory cells into the CNS compared with wild-type littermate controls (176). In all three strains, IL-4–deficient mice are capable of entering the recovery phase of disease, indicating that IL-4 is not the only factor capable of regulating EAE pathogenesis. IL-10 may be a prime candidate for contributing to recovery from EAE because increased levels of IL-10 mRNA in the CNS of IL-4–deficient C57BL/6 mice was observed during their recovery.

IL-10 is expressed by Th2 cells and by macrophages, astrocytes, and microglia (109,177). IL-10 can suppress cytokine production by Th1 cells and inhibit NO production and antigen presentation by macrophages (178–180). Recently, strict classification of IL-10 as a Th2 cytokine has been challenged because it can be induced by IL-12 during a Th1 response, presumably as part of a negative feedback loop designed to limit macrophage activity (181). IL-10 mRNA expression correlated with the onset of remission when EAE was induced by adoptive transfer or active immunization (104,110,127). Conversely, others demonstrated that IL-10 mRNA is expressed before disease onset and consistently throughout the course of EAE in SJL/J mice after induction with PLP peptide 139-151 or TMEV. (161).

In vivo administration of IL-10 as a therapeutic agent during EAE has produced different effects. After immunization with mouse spinal cord homogenate, SJL/J mice treated with a recombinant *Vaccinia* virus expressing IL-10 displayed reduced disease severity (149). After adoptive transfer of myelin-specific T-cells, SJL/J mice treated with IL-10 displayed normal to moderately increased disease severity (182). In addition, treatment with anti–IL-10 antibody had similar effects on EAE induced by adoptive transfer in SJL/J mice, with the mice displaying normal to increased disease severity. Recent reports using transgenic and knockout techniques strongly suggest that IL-10 is an important regulator of EAE pathogenesis. IL-10–deficient mice on the C57BL/6 genetic background are more susceptible and develop more severe EAE than wild-type C57BL/6 mice after immunization with the encephalitogenic MOG peptide (183). Further, Bettelli et al. reported that transgenic (FVB x SJL)F1 mice overexpressing IL-10 in T-cells are completely resistant to induction of EAE after immunization with PLP despite a normal T-cell proliferative response to the antigen. Another group used transfected T-cells expressing IL-10 under the control of an antigen-inducible IL-2 promoter region to deliver IL-10 to the CNS (184). With adoptive transfer of these transgenic T-cell clones, antigen-inducible expression of IL-10 leads to the inhibition of onset of EAE and is able to treat EAE, even after the onset of neurologic signs. A third group generated transgenic mice expressing human IL-10 under the control of an MHC class II promoter on the BALB/c background (185). These human IL-10 transgenic mice were completely resistant to EAE induced by intradermal immunization with mouse spinal cord homogenate, whereas littermate control mice were highly susceptible to disease. The human IL-10 transgenic BALB/c mice also were crossed to SJL/J mice to generate (SJL/J x BALB/c)F1 transgenic mice for a more conventional model system. A low incidence of EAE and reduced disease severity was observed in the human IL-10 transgenic F1 mice, whereas nontransgenic littermates were highly susceptible to EAE induction. Although proliferative activity of T-cells from these IL-10 transgenic mice was not reported, cytokine profiles showed that myelin-reactive Th1 cells are generated in response to immunization. Presumably, in vivo expression of IL-10 by T-cells or APCs suppresses the effector function of Th1 cells. These studies support IL-10 as a potential therapeutic agent in cell-mediated autoimmune diseases.

TGF-β is a pleiotropic cytokine produced by T-cells, macrophages, and many other cell types. We observed the expression of TGF-β in the CNS of mice during acute and chronic phases of EAE (164). In vitro administration of TGF-β inhibited the activation and proliferation of myelin-specific lymph node cells and reduced their capacity to transfer EAE (186). In addition, in vivo administration of TGF-β improved clinical and pathologic signs of EAE, even when given after disease onset (186,187). Further, in vivo administration of anti–TGF-β at disease onset exacerbated the clinical course of EAE and caused more extensive pathologic lesions (164,188). These findings show that TGF-β is another important regulator of EAE pathogenesis.

However, there have been several paradoxical observations regarding the role of TGF-β in the regulation of EAE. For example, culturing MBP-specific lymph node cells in the presence of MBP and TGF-β inhibited their ability to proliferate and transfer EAE (186). Interestingly, lymph node cells initially stimulated in the presence of MBP and TGF-β easily transferred disease with subsequent antigen stimulation, suggesting that exposure to TGF-β does not result in the differentiation of the cells into a nonencephalitogenic phenotype. In addition, certain T-cell lines cultured in the presence of TGF-β actually had enhanced encephalitogenic potential (189). Thus, exposure of encephalitogenic T-cells to TGF-β does not eliminate their encephalitogenic potential, particularly if the T-cells have been activated.

Notably, in several EAE models, including studies performed in our laboratory, systemic administration of TGF-β inhibited clinical disease (186,187,190). Systemic administration of TGF-β also inhibited the signs of experimental arthritis, indicating that the regulatory phenomenon observed is not specific to the CNS (191). From this discussion, one can surmise that TGF-β seems to mediate a suppressive effect in a number of autoimmune disease models, including EAE. The recent observation that TGF-β expressed under the glial fibrillary acidic protein promoter actually exacerbated rather than suppressed disease is intriguing (192). This suggests that local expression of TGF-β in the CNS is not sufficient to suppress clinical signs of EAE and may participate in perpetuation of the disease. Determining whether TGF-β expression mediates its protective effects in the CNS or whether this takes place in the peripheral lymphoid organs will be an important future pursuit.

Several nontraditional cytokines or growth factors have been implicated in EAE, particularly as potential therapeutic agents. For example, nerve growth factor (NGF), although traditionally characterized as a neurotrophic factor, may also play an important role in the immune response. NGF is expressed by activated immune cells and this expression is functionally regulated (193–195). Further, NGF can modulate the activity of immune cells through its receptor tyrosine receptor kinase-A (196–199). The expression of NGF is elevated in rats with EAE, suggesting that it plays a role in the pathogenesis of the disease (200). In a recent paper, anti-NGF antibody administration exacerbated the clinical and histologic signs of EAE in Lewis rats (201). In our own studies, administration of NGF ameliorated the clinical signs of EAE in mice after adoptive transfer or active induction (313). Thus, NGF likely plays a role in the pathogenesis of EAE and may be an intriguing candidate for therapeutic intervention in immune-mediated demyelination in the CNS.

Another approach to the treatment of inflammatory demyelination involves the administration of a growth factor that promotes remyelination. One such agent, insulin-like growth factor (IGF-1), is a potent inducer of oligodendrocyte development and myelin production (202–206). Administration of IGF-1 reduced the severity of EAE in Lewis rats, a model in which the course of disease is monophasic (207–209). Recent studies in our laboratory using IGF-1 alone or in a more stable complex with its major serum-binding protein, IGFBP3, addressed its effects in a relapsing mouse model of EAE (210). Treatment with the IGF-1/IGFBP3 complex delayed disease onset, presumably due to the inhibition of inflammatory cells infiltrating the CNS. Intercellular adhesion molecule-1 (ICAM-1) expression in the CNS was reduced after treatment, indicating that the permeability of the BBB is decreased by IGF-1/IGFBP3 treatment. Although delayed, mice that received the IGF-1/IGFBP3 complex eventually developed severe EAE. In fact, the dose correlated directly with severity, indicating that IGF-1/IGFBP3 is capable of potentiating an immune response. Because lymphocytes express receptors for IGF-1, antigen-specific proliferation and cytokine production by T-cells were assayed with clinical outcome. IGF-1 alone and the IGF-1/IGFBP3 complex enhanced proliferation of MBP-specific lymph node cells in vitro but did not alter their cytokine production, their surface molecule expression, or their ability to transfer disease. These findings suggest that the delay in disease onset after IGF-1/IGFBP3 administration is not due to changes in the encephalitogenic T-cells themselves but rather to slowed inflammatory cell extravasation across the BBB. Eventually the T-cells do invade the CNS and cause severe EAE, possibly because they have expanded in response to IGF-1/IGFBP3. Although IGF-1 treatment appeared to be effective in preventing EAE in the rat model and slowed the development of EAE in the mouse model, IGF-1 also appeared capable of exacerbating the disease. Thus, the differences between the monophasic rat and relapsing mouse models of EAE must be taken into account when evaluating potential therapies.

Administration of glial growth factor-2 (GGF-2), another signal that promotes proliferation and survival of the oligodendrocyte, effectively delayed onset, decreased severity, and reduced relapses in mice with EAE (211,212). In addition, treated mice exhibited more remyelination in CNS lesions than did nontreated mice, implicating GGF-2 as a promising therapeutic agent with pleiotropic effects. In another study, platelet-derived growth factor (PDGF), which induces the proliferation and development of oligodendrocytes, was delivered by the transfer of autoreactive transgenic Th2 cells, leading to the amelioration of ongoing EAE induced by immunization with PLP 139-151 (213). These and other nontraditional cytokines hold promise as therapeutic agents capable of repairing previous damage and preventing further damage incurred during inflammatory responses in the CNS.

## IMMUNE DEVIATION

Many early studies implicated Th1 cells in the pathogenesis of EAE. Encephalitogenic MBP-specific T-cell lines secreted cytokines associated with the Th1 phenotype (111). Transfer of MBP-specific T-cells predominantly expressing Th1 cytokines induced EAE in naive mice, whereas transfer of MBP-specific T-cells expressing predominantly Th2 cytokines did not transfer EAE into naive mice (114,214,215). Further, not all Th2 cells are incapable of inducing EAE. Th1 and Th2 cells transgenic for an MBP-specific TCR can mediate EAE at transfer into immunodeficient mice under extremely artificial conditions (215).

To modify the pathogenesis of EAE, researchers coinjected Th2 cells with encephalitogenic Th1 cells into naive SJL mice (171). Coinjection of Th2 cells with Th1 cells in a 2:1 ratio did not prevent the induction of EAE. Further, when the Th2:Th1 ratio was 10:1, those investigators reported extensive eosinophilia rather than the typical lymphocytic infiltrate in the CNS. Coinjection of Th2 cells with encephalitogenic Th1 cells did not prevent disease; however, injection of Th2 cells before active immunization with myelin antigen did prevent disease (216). Taken together, these data indicate that Th2 cells cannot prevent EAE by inhibiting the function of activated Th1 cells, but Th2 cells can prevent EAE by altering the activation of Th1 cells and shifting the resultant responder population to a Th2 phenotype.

Several experiments have focused on altering the phenotypic balance of Th cells from the encephalitogenic Th1-dominant response to the protective Th2-dominant response, a phenomenon termed *immune deviation*. Administration of IL-4 during EAE induction was suc-

cessful in ameliorating disease by diminishing demyelination and decreasing inflammation in the CNS (114). Administration of IL-4 after EAE induction resulted in only mild therapeutic effects, confirming earlier findings that Th2-associated effects were unable to inhibit ongoing Th1 responses. Other regimens that successfully altered the Th response and inhibited EAE include the modulation of costimulatory signals, the use of altered peptide ligands, and the administration of retinoids (52,174,217).

Although immune deviation is a promising method for therapeutic intervention in Th1-associated autoimmune diseases, recent studies using mice deficient in various Th1-associated cytokines indicated that a complete switch from a Th1 response to a Th2 response might not be optimal for limiting disease progression. In mice deficient in IFN-γ, IFN-γ receptor, and TNF-α, EAE could still be induced and, in some cases, was more severe than in wild-type mice (120–122,138,139). These findings suggest that Th1-associated cytokines play a regulatory role in the pathogenesis of EAE and may possess self-limiting regulatory activity or induce regulatory activity in surrounding cells. In either case, decreasing the Th1 response in ongoing disease may have unexpected negative consequences for therapeutic applications.

## CHEMOKINES

Several laboratories have described the expression patterns of various chemokines and their receptors during the pathogenesis of EAE, which appear dependent on the animal model and the mode of disease induction examined (218). In general, C-C and C-X-C chemokines, including monocyte chemoattractant protein-1 (MCP-1), RANTES, macrophage inflammatory protein-1α (MIP-1α), TCA-3, and interferon-inducible protein-10 (IP-10), are associated with the initial acute attack and subsequent relapses. The chemokine receptors, CCR1, CCR2, and CCR5, are highly expressed in the CNS during EAE (225).

The role of particular chemokines during the clinical course of EAE has been examined with the use of neutralizing antibodies. Anti–MIP-α, not anti–MCP-1 or anti-RANTES, decreased inflammation in the CNS and prevented the development of clinical EAE, indicating that MIP-1α is critical to the induction of disease (226). Interestingly, anti–MCP-1 administration reduced the severity of clinical disease during relapses, implicating MCP-1 as an important mediator of relapses during the clinical course of EAE (227). Vβ8.2 TCR transgenic mice, which are protected from EAE after injection with Vβ8.2 recombinant protein, had decreased inflammation in the CNS and significantly reduced expression of several chemokines, including RANTES, MIP-1α, IP-10, and MCP-1 (225). In addition, the CNS expression of several chemokine receptors, including CCR1, CCR2, and CCR5, also was reduced after TCR vaccination.

Because encephalitogenic T-cells increase expression of chemokines with antigen stimulation in vitro, they may use chemokines to mediate inflammation in the CNS (113,224). In 1 theory, activated myelin-specific T-cells enter the CNS and respond to antigen by increasing their production of chemokines, thereby directly recruiting macrophages and additional T-cells into the CNS. Alternatively, encephalitogenic T-cells may enter the CNS and indirectly recruit additional inflammatory cells by inducing resident CNS cells to produce chemokines. Astrocytes, microglia, pericytes, endothelial cells, and smooth muscle cells can produce chemokines under the appropriate conditions in vitro (228–231). Recent studies have indicated that encephalitogenic T-cells actually contribute to chemokine production by direct and indirect routes. First, chemokine mRNA is not detectable without infiltrating inflammatory cells, suggesting these cells are responsible for the initial production of chemokines (220). Second, astrocytes express RANTES, IP-10, MIP-1α, and MCP-1 after the migration of MBP-specific T-cells into the CNS, presumably due to the effects of TNF-α and IFN-γ released by the infiltrating T-cells (232). Activation of astrocytes and possibly other resident CNS cells could be responsible for additional chemokine expression and further recruitment of inflammatory cells into the CNS.

In addition to their chemotactic functions, chemokines also have been implicated in T-cell activation (233–237). MIP-α and RANTES promote T-cell activation independent of antigen or in synergism with other factors. Further, RANTES induced tyrosine phosphorylation of multiple proteins in T-cells, including focal adhesion kinase, zeta associated protein (ZAP)-70, and paxillin (239). Thus, RANTES may influence the generation of T-cell focal adhesions and subsequent T-cell activation, although these functions have not been investigated with regard to EAE.

Chemokine activity is critical for the recruitment of inflammatory cells into the CNS. Therefore, they are promising targets for therapeutic intervention in diseases characterized by inflammation in the CNS. Blocking the activity of MIP-α successfully prevented the induction of EAE (226). Further, and perhaps more important for application in human diseases such as MS, blocking the activity of MCP-1 successfully ameliorated relapses associated with ongoing EAE (227). Further examination of the roles of chemokines in the induction and progression of EAE will provide additional information about the pathogenesis of inflammation in the CNS.

## TOLERANCE

Autoimmunity develops when the immune system no longer demonstrates tolerance for an autoantigen. Under-

standing the mechanisms that restore tolerance to CNS autoantigens is a critical focus in EAE and MS research.

At stimulation with antigen, T-cells undergo activation, anergy, or death via apoptosis (240–242). T-cells actively engaged in the cell cycle, as directed by IL-2, are highly susceptible to apoptosis induced by high doses of antigen, whereas resting cells are not. This mechanism serves as a negative feedback loop, limiting T-cell proliferation and cytokine production during an immune response (146,241,243,244). Apoptosis induced in this manner requires repeated antigen stimulation through the TCR and may involve several downstream factors, including the Fas antigen, IFN-γ, growth cytokines, TNF-α, and cytolytic mechanisms. Induction of apoptosis of antigen-specific T-cells by repeated antigen stimulation is one mechanism for restoring tolerance to a specific autoantigen. In fact, the use of the encephalitogenic antigen is a well-documented treatment for EAE (248–250). The mechanism for the immune suppression was not well-defined in those early reports but has been examined closely in recent work by our laboratory and others.

Synthetic peptides of MBP induced anergy of autoreactive T-cells, which reduced the severity of EAE (251). Our laboratory found that high-dose intravenous antigen therapy eliminates MBP-specific, autoreactive T-cells, which attenuates the immune response and the clinical signs of EAE (144,146). Recently, we investigated the mechanism of tolerance in Vβ8.2 TCR transgenic mice, which exhibit a much higher MBP-specific T-cell precursor frequency than wild-type mice (85,86). These mice are highly susceptible to induction of disease by immunization with MBP or the Ac1-11 peptide of MBP in CFA and do not require subsequent injections of PT for the development of EAE. Lymphocytes from naive Vβ8.2 transgenic mice proliferated in response to MBP in a standard 4-day proliferation assay, thereby providing a consistent readout for our studies examining T-cell activation. After intravenous injection of the Ac1-11 peptide of MBP, splenocytes were anergized, as shown by decreased MBP-specific proliferation and IL-2 production (86). Administration of anti–CTLA-4 at the time of tolerization potentiated these effects. Interestingly, intravenous administration of antigen, in a single dose with or without concomitant anti–CTLA-4 injection, did not prevent EAE at subsequent immunization, suggesting that, although most MBP-specific T-cells are anergized, a population of T-cells remains unaffected and can mediate EAE. After intraperitoneal administration of the Ac1-11 peptide of MBP, splenocytes exhibited a Th2 phenotype, which was potentiated by the administration of anti–CTLA-4 at the time of tolerization (85). Tolerance in lymph node cells from the same mice was partly blocked by CTLA-4, as shown by slight a restoration of the proliferative response to MBP. In contrast to intravenous administration of antigen, intraperitoneal administration of antigen, in a single dose with or without concomitant anti-CTLA-4 injection, inhibited EAE at subsequent immunization, presumably due to the switch from an antigen-specific Th1 response to an antigen-specific Th2 response. In a primate model of EAE, intraperitioneal administration of antigen dramatically enhanced disease (252). It should be noted that the tolerization protocol applied in those studies was quite different from the protocol we used in mice. The primates were immunized with rMOG in adjuvant and then given 300 μg rMOG intraperitioneal on days 7 through 18 as the tolerization protocol. The monkeys were protected from disease during intraperitioneal treatment but developed severe EAE after treatment stopped.

Oral administration of guinea pig MBP diminished the development of EAE at immunization with guinea pig MBP in CFA (253–255). Upon further examination of the tolerized animals, histopathologic signs of disease were reduced and MBP-specific lymphocyte proliferation was profoundly suppressed (253). Additional studies focusing on high-dose oral tolerance suggested that MBP-specific T-cells are anergized or deleted by the oral administration of MBP (256,257). As demonstrated by Weiner and colleagues, low-dose oral tolerance stimulates the production of regulatory T-cells capable of transferring tolerance from MBP-fed donors to naive recipients (258–260). The active mechanism of low-dose oral tolerance appears to be a cytokine-mediated immune deviation away from a predominant Th1 response toward a predominant Th2 and Th3 (TGF-β–producing) response (166,216,261). The active suppression of low-dose oral tolerance also may suppress unrelated immune responses, a phenomenon termed *bystander suppression*. The concept of bystander suppression was encouraged by the demonstration that the oral administration of MBP could suppress PLP-induced EAE in SJL mice (262). This finding suggested that regulatory cells generated in the gut could migrate to the CNS and prevent the encephalitogenic response to PLP. The effectiveness of some APLs also has been attributed to bystander suppression mediated by the production of regulatory cytokines such as IL-4, IL-13, and TGF-β, in the CNS. As discussed previously, inhibition of adoptively transferred EAE by an APL of an MBP peptide depends on the activity of IL-4 because the administration of anti–IL-4 reverses the inhibition (53). Similarly, anti–TGF-β partly eliminates the protection conferred by an APL of PLP 139-151 (54). Many of these studies imply, but do not definitively show, that bystander suppression occurs in the CNS. Recent evidence has shown that bystander suppression also may occur in the peripheral lymphoid system. SJL mice immunized with keyhole limpet hemocyanin (KLH) in IFA developed KLH-specific Th2 cells that mediated suppression of EAE induced by immunization with MBP and KLH (172).

The MBP-specific T-cells produced in that system were of the Th2 phenotype but primed in the periphery rather than in the CNS.

Recent data suggested that MBP and PLP exist as parts of molecules expressed in lymphoid tissue (263,264). Further, immunogenic forms of MBP can be expressed in lymphoid tissues during the disease process (265). These myelin components in the lymphoid tissues may play a role in bystander suppression. Lymphoid tissues provide the ideal environment for efficiently converting the phenotype of a large number of T-cells. Although the CNS contains localized sites of inflammation, it is much less conducive as an organ for extensive immune regulatory activity.

## EPITOPE SPREADING

The relapsing–remitting nature of some models of EAE has been an intriguing focus of research in recent years, and understanding the mechanism behind the remission and subsequent relapses would provide potential avenues for inducing permanent disease remission and preventing further relapses. Recent studies have implicated Fas (CD95/APO-1) and its ligand (FasL/CD95L) in the apoptotic clearance of infiltrating T-cells from the CNS, a phenomenon associated with remission of clinical EAE (266–271). Adoptive transfer of MBP-specific T-cells into *gld* (generalized lymphoproliferative disease) mice, which are deficient in FasL, induced a similar but not identical onset of EAE compared with that induced in wild-type mice (270,271). The severity of EAE in *gld* mice is highly variable compared with the severity in wild-type mice. In addition, these mice developed a chronic clinical course, whereas their wild-type counterparts recovered from the acute phase of clinical EAE. The CNS from these chronic *gld* mice displayed extensive CD4$^+$ T-cell infiltration throughout disease, presumably due to the lack of apoptotic elimination that occurs in wild-type mice. Thus, FasL appears to function in the regulation of acute disease and contributes to the onset of remission by eliminating the infiltrating CD4$^+$ T-cells, which express Fas.

In EAE, disease is induced by immunization with a component of myelin or by transfer of myelin-reactive T-cells. The initial acute attack is dominated by an immune response to the particular myelin antigen used to induce disease; however, subsequent attacks are often mediated by immune responses to additional myelin antigens. For example, after immunization of the SJL/J mouse with the peptide 139-151 of PLP in CFA, a relapsing–remitting model of EAE develops. In this model, T-cells isolated from the periphery during the initial acute attack are specific for the peptide PLP 139-151. As disease progresses, T-cells isolated from the periphery during subsequent acute attacks are specific for other myelin antigens, including peptides from other regions of PLP (intramolecular) and from other myelin proteins such as MBP (intermolecular). This phenomenon, termed *epitope spreading*, is an enticing candidate for interventional therapies in ongoing disease.

Intramolecular epitope spreading was first described by McCarron and colleagues after examining the responses to MBP in the (PL × SJL) F1 mouse (272). In that study, after disease induced by the N-terminal epitope of EAE, responses were noted to the $H-2^S$–restricted epitope. Intermolecular epitope spreading in EAE was first described by Perry and colleagues (273). Although EAE was induced by the adoptive transfer of lymphoctyes activated by the 87-99 peptide of MBP, lymphocytes reactive to a peptide of PLP also were isolated from diseased mice but not from healthy or control mice. T lymphocytes developed responses to PLP 139-151 after the initial acute attack resulting from the transfer of lymphocytes specific for the 84-104 peptide of MBP. Evidence for intramolecular epitope spreading was observed after the adoptive transfer of lymphocytes activated by the 139-151 peptide of PLP-caused EAE and resulted in the production of lymphocytes not only responsive to the 178-191 epitope of PLP but also capable of inducing EAE after their transfer into naive mice. Miller and colleagues also showed that epitope spreading occurs in TMEV-induced demyelinating disease (TMEV-IDD), a viral disease model in which virus-specific lymphocytes mediate the initial myelin damage with lymphocytes responsive to several myelin epitopes developing as disease progresses (274–276).

Epitope spreading is costimulation dependent, relying on the presence of B7-1 molecules for this phenomenon to occur. Administration of anti-B7-1 F(ab) fragments prevented clinical relapses, ameliorated CNS pathology, and blocked epitope spreading, whereas anti–B7-2 F(ab) fragments had no effect on disease (90). In contrast, the administration of anti–B7-1 mAb, which may actually cause signaling through B7-1, exacerbated clinical relapses, enhanced CNS pathology, and promoted epitope spreading (277). Because costimulation mediated through the CD28:B7 pathway is required for the activation of naive T lymphocytes, it follows that activation of lymphocytes specific for endogenous myelin epitopes also would be dependent on costimulation. One of the attractive features of using costimulatory blockade as a means to block epitope spreading is that one would not require knowledge of the encephalitogenic epitopes for such a strategy to be effective.

## THEILER MURINE ENCEPHALOMYELITIS VIRUS-INDUCED DEMYELINATING DISEASE

TMEV-IDD is another mouse model of MS. Like EAE, susceptibility to TMEV is determined by MHC and non-MHC genes (278–281). TMEV-IDD is initiated by a TMEV-specific $CD4^+$ T-cell attack on virally infected cells of the CNS (282). TMEV persists as a chronic productive infection in CNS white matter macrophages. The persistent infection leads to chronic activation of myelin-reactive $CD4^+$ T-cells via epitope spreading (274). TMEV infection is associated with inflammatory demyelinating lesions of the spinal cord similar to those in EAE and MS (283,284). Depletion or tolerance of T lymphocytes abrogates the disease (285).

As in EAE, the $CD4^+$ T-cells responsible for TMEV-IDD appear to be of a Th1 phenotype. Lymph node cells of TMEV-infected mice produce Th1-associated cytokines and antibodies, including IL-2, TNF-$\alpha$, IFN-$\gamma$, and $IgG_{2a}$, but not Th2-associated cytokines (286,287). In addition, TMEV-infected mice mount a delayed type hypersensitivity (DTH) reaction to portions of the virus, with an immunodominant epitope identified in the VP2 nucleocapsid (288,289). Treatment of SJL mice with TMEV-coupled ethyl carbodiimide–treated splenocytes before or after infection with live TMEV induced tolerance, successfully preventing the development of disease, including inflammation and demyelination in the CNS (285). Tolerance induction conferred a reduction in DTH and T-cell proliferative responses to viral antigen and a significant reduction in the absolute numbers of mononuclear cells infiltrating the CNS. Treatment with TMEV-coupled splenocytes failed to prevent the development of EAE, demonstrating the specificity of in vivo tolerance induction. Although TMEV immunopathogenesis initially targets the viral infection in the CNS, subsequent demyelination in the CNS also appears to be immunopathogenic, presumably due to epitope spreading from viral to endogenous myelin antigens.

Microglia, resident APCs of the CNS, isolated directly from the CNS of TMEV-infected SJL mice present epitopes of PLP to T-cell lines (275). These experiments demonstrate that, with viral infection of the CNS, myelin antigens can be processed and presented by resident microglial cells to activate naive T-cells. Only CNS APCs isolated from TMEV-infected mice with previous myelin damage were able to endogenously present the PLP epitopes to specific Th1 lines. Localized virus-induced myelin damage activates CNS-resident APCs to process and present endogenous autoantigen epitopes to autoantigen-specific T-cells, which may provide a mechanism by which epitope spreading may occur.

TMEV is an important model for examining the effects of virus-induced inflammation and demyelination in the CNS because a possible etiologic mechanism for the development of MS is viral infection. Although no single virus has been implicated, the possibility remains that one or more viruses may have the capacity to induce CNS demyelination. Although molecular mimicry initially was thought to be the mechanism of viral induction of CNS demyelination, the data discussed above suggest that activation of CNS APCs by a viral infection such as TMEV can lead to the activation of autoreactive T-cells and perpetuation of an inflammatory, demyelinating process without involving molecular mimicry.

## MOLECULAR MIMICRY

Several lines of evidence implicate environmental factors, particularly viruses, in the development of autoimmunity. First, monozygotic twins are highly discordant for several autoimmune disorders, including MS, indicating that genetic factors are not always sufficient to induce disease (290). Second, viral infections are associated with exacerbations in several autoimmune diseases (291–294). Third, epidemiologic studies have linked viruses with several human autoimmune diseases, including MS (293–296). Fourth, viral infections increase development of spontaneous autoimmune disease in several animal models (297). Fifth, in several transgenic models in which mice express an autoimmune gene or an antigen-specific recognition molecule (TCR or antibody), spontaneous autoimmunity occurs only in standard animal facilities, not in pathogen-free animal facilities (36,298). Taken together, these data strongly implicate pathogenic participation in the development of autoimmunity.

A popular theory contends that pathogen-induced autoimmunity can be attributed to molecular mimicry, a phenomenon in which activated T-cells that are specific for a viral antigen are so similar to a host antigen that the T-cells attack the host antigen (299). Research in several laboratories has identified many different microbial products that activate T-cells cross-reactive to endogenous autoantigens. These microbes include bacteria (300–302), viruses (303–308), and yeast (301). In a specific example, T-cells isolated from the cerebrospinal fluid of MS patients could be activated by a viral determinant and a host myelin protein (305). Several additional studies have suggested that molecular mimicry is more than an epiphenomenon (309,310).

Initially, the homology necessary for molecular mimicry between microbial peptide and endogenous peptide was thought to be sequence oriented. Several viral peptides homologous to the encephalitogenic epitope of the MBP were identified in computer-assisted searches (311). In support of the molecular mimicry theory, the hepatitis B virus polymerase (HBVP), which is most similar to MBP of those identified, induces pathology similar to that induced by the MBP peptide itself (299). In addition, HBVP elicits a cellular and humoral immune response against MBP. Although sequence homology is a useful tool for identifying potential cross-reactive epitopes, recent studies have identified another tool for detecting these epitopes. Crucial motifs corresponding to contact

residues between the peptide–MHC complex and the TCR provide a structural determinant with which to search for and detect potential cross-reactive epitopes. By using such motifs for MBP-specific T-cells, several pathogenic peptides capable of inducing EAE were identified (306,312). Another group using peptide spot synthesis for global amino acid replacements of the Ac1-11 peptide of MBP identified additional pathogenic peptides capable of activating T-cells specific for MBP Ac1-11 peptide (302). Several of these peptides can induce EAE in mice transgenic for an MBP Ac1-11-specific TCR. The identification of multiple pathogenic peptides with the use of different methods provides further support for the molecular mimicry theory.

Although evidence supports molecular mimicry as a mechanism by which pathogens may induce the development of autoimmunity, it is not the only mechanism. As discussed previously, virus-induced, T-cell–mediated myelin damage is capable of activating CNS-resident APCs to process and present endogenous autoantigen epitopes to autoantigen-specific T-cells, thus activating them and leading to an autoimmune state (275). Another mechanism might involve viral induction of inflammatory cells to increase the production of cytokines and chemokines, which augments the recruitment and activation of additional inflammatory cells, some of which might be autoantigen specific. In a more direct route, viruses might preferentially infect and destroy one lymphocyte subset, thereby disrupting the normal balance of the immune system and inducing an autoimmune state. Any or all of these mechanisms, including molecular mimicry, may be responsible for the active role pathogens likely play in the development of autoimmunity.

## CONCLUSION

In this review we have commented on many of the aspects currently being examined in the EAE model. The use of the EAE model has led to the development of several experimental strategies for the treatment of patients with MS. In fact, a primary immunomodulatory agent used in the treatment of MS, copolymer-1 (Copaxone®), was developed almost exclusively from studies showing efficacy in the EAE model. We anticipate that many of the strategies discussed in this review will move into the clinical arena and the results of these new therapeutic trials in MS are eagerly anticipated.

### Acknowledgments

This work was supported by grants from the National Institutes of Health, National Multiple Sclerosis Society, and the Yellow Rose Foundation to MKR. L.R.A. was supported in part by a fellowship from the Spinal Cord Research Foundation. The authors thank Nancy Monson, Ph.D., for critical reading of the manuscript. This work is dedicated to the memory of Dale E. McFarlin, M.D., one of the pioneers in the study of EAE.

# References

1. Pettinelli C B, McFarlin DE. Adoptive transfer of experimental allergic encephalomyelitis in SJL/J mice after *in vitro* activation of lymph node cells by myelin basic protein: requirement for Lyt 1+ 2- T lymphocytes. *J Immunol* 1981; 127(4):1420–1423.

2. Bernard CC, Carnegie PR. Experimental autoimmune encephalomyelitis in mice: immunologic response to mouse spinal cord and myelin basic proteins. *J Immunol* 1975; 114(5):1537–1540.

3. Yasuda T, Tsumita T, Nagai Y, Mitsuzawa E, Ohtani S. Experimental allergic encephalomyelitis (EAE) in mice. I. Induction of EAE with mouse spinal cord homogenate and myelin basic protein. *Jpn J Exp Med* 1975; 45(5):423–427.

4. Panitch HS, McFarlin DE. Experimental allergic encephalomyelitis: enhancement of cell-mediated transfer by concanavalin A. *J Immunol* 1977; 119(3):1134–1137.

5. Bernard CC, Leydon J, Mackay IR. T-cell Necessity in the pathogenesis of experimental autoimmune encephalomyelitis in mice. *Eur J Immunol* 1976; 6(9):655–660.

6. Brown A, McFarlin DE, Raine,CS. Chronologic neuropathology of relapsing experimental allergic encephalomyelitis in the mouse. *Lab Invest* 1982; 46(2):171–185.

7. Cross AH, McCarron R, McFarlin DE, Raine CS. Adoptively transferred acute and chronic relapsing autoimmune encephalomyelitis in the PL/J mouse and observations on altered pathology by intercurrent virus infection. *Lab Invest* 1987; 57(5):499–512.

8. Raine CS, Barnett LB, Brown A, Behar T, McFarlin DE. Neuropathology of experimental allergic encephalomyelitis in inbred strains of mice. *Lab Invest* 1980; 43(2):150–157.

9. Raine CS. The Dale E. McFarlin memorial lecture: The immunology of the multiple sclerosis lesion. *Ann Neurol* 1994; 36 (suppl):S61–S72.

10. Genain CP, Hauser SL. Creation of a model for multiple sclerosis in *Callithrix jacchus* marmosets [see comments]. *J Mol Med* 1997; 75(3):187–197.

11. McCombe PA, Nickson I, Tabi Z, Pender MP. Apoptosis of V beta 8.2+ T lymphocytes in the spinal cord during recovery from experimental autoimmune encephalomyelitis induced in Lewis rats by inoculation with myelin basic protein. *J Neurol Sci* 1996; 139(1):1–6.

12. Gold R, Hartung HP, Lassmann H. T-cell apoptosis in autoimmune diseases: Termination of inflammation in the nervous system and other sites with specialized immune-defense mechanisms. *Trends Neurosci* 1997; 20(9):399–404.

13. Fritz RB, Skeen MJ, Chou CH, Garcia M, Egorov IK. Major histocompatibility complex-linked control of the murine immune response to myelin basic protein. *J Immunol* 1985; 134(4):2328–2332.

14. Fritz RB, McFarlin DE. Encephalitogenic epitopes of myelin basic protein. *Chem Immunol* 1989; 46:101–125.

15. Wall M, Southwood S, Sidney J, et al. High affinity for class II molecules as a necessary but not sufficient characteristic of encephalitogenic determinants. *Int Immunol* 1992; 4(7):773–777.

16. Greer JM, Sobel RA, Sette A, et al. Immunogenic and encephalitogenic epitope clusters of myelin proteolipid protein. *J Immunol* 1996; 156(1):371–379.

17. Baker D, Rosenwasser OA, O'Neill JK, Turk JL. Genetic analysis of experimental allergic encephalomyelitis in mice. *J Immunol* 1995; 155(8):4046–4051.

18. Sundvall M, Jirholt J, Yang HT, et al. Identification of murine loci associated with susceptibility to chronic experimental autoimmune encephalomyelitis. *Nat Genet* 1995; 10(3):313–317.

19. Martin R, McFarland HF, McFarlin DE. Immunological aspects of demyelinating diseases. *Annu Rev Immunol* 1992; 10:153–187.

20. Linington C, Webb M, Woodhams PL. A novel myelin-associated glycoprotein defined by a mouse monoclonal antibody. *J Neuroimmunol* 1984; 6(6):387–396.

21. Smith ME, deJong LJ. Antibody to myelin constituents: a possible factor in induction of cell- mediated demyelination. *Neurochem Res* 1987; 12(2):167–172.

22. Schluesener HJ, Sobel RA, Linington C, Weiner HL. A monoclonal antibody against a myelin oligodendrocyte glycoprotein induces relapses and demyelination in central nervous system autoimmune disease. *J Immunol* 1987; 139(12):4016–4021.

23. Wekerle H. Remembering MOG: Autoantibody mediated demyelination in multiple sclerosis? [news; comment]. *Nat Med* 1999; 5(2):153–154.

24. Amor S, Groome N, Linington C, et al. Identification of epitopes of myelin oligodendrocyte glycoprotein for the induction of experimental allergic encephalomyelitis in SJL and Biozzi AB/H mice. *J Immunol* 1994; 153(10):4349–4356.

25. Adelmann M, Wood J, Benzel I, et al. The N-terminal domain of the myelin oligodendrocyte glycoprotein (MOG) induces acute demyelinating experimental autoimmune encephalomyelitis in the Lewis rat. *J Neuroimmunol* 1995; 63(1):17–27.

26. Mendel I, Kerlero R, Ben Nun A. A myelin oligodendrocyte glycoprotein peptide induces typical chronic experimental autoimmune encephalomyelitis in H-2b mice: Fine specificity and T-cell receptor V beta expression of encephalitogenic T-cells. *Eur J Immunol* 1995; 25(7):1951–1959.

27. Stefferl A, Linington C, Holsboer F, Reul JM. Susceptibility and resistance to experimental allergic encephalomyelitis: Relationship with hypothalamic–pituitary–adrenocortical axis responsiveness in the rat. *Endocrinology* 1999; 140(11):4932–4938.

28. Shaw MK, Kim C, Ho KL, Lisak RP, Tse HY. A combination of adoptive transfer and antigenic challenge induces consistent murine experimental autoimmune encephalomyelitis in C57BL/6 mice and other reputed resistant strains. *J Neuroimmunol* 1992; 39(1-2):139–149.

29. Kronenberg M, Goverman J, Haars R, et al. Rearrangement and transcription of the beta-chain genes of the T-cell antigen receptor in different types of murine lymphocytes. *Nature* 1985; 313(6004):647–653.

30. Wilson A, Held W, MacDonald HR. two waves of recombinase gene expression in developing thymocytes. *J Exp Med* 1994; 179(4):1355–1360.

31. Acha-Orbea H, Mitchell DJ, Timmermann L, et al. Limited heterogeneity of T-cell receptors from lymphocytes mediating autoimmune encephalomyelitis allows specific immune intervention. *Cell* 1988; 54(2):263–273.

32. Urban JL, Kumar V, Kono DH, et al. Restricted use of T-cell receptor V genes in murine autoimmune encephalomyelitis raises possibilities for antibody therapy [see comments]. *Cell* 1988; 54(4):577–592.

33. Zamvil SS, Mitchell DJ, Lee NE, et al. Predominant expression of a T-cell receptor V beta gene subfamily in autoimmune encephalomyelitis [published erratum in *J Exp Med* 1988; 168(1):455]. *J Exp Med* 1988; 167(5):1586–1596.

34. Zamvil SS, SteinmanL. The T lymphocyte in experimental allergic encephalomyelitis. *Annu Rev Immunol* 1990; 8:579–621.

35. Burns FR, Li XB, Shen N, et al. Both rat and mouse T-cell receptors specific for the encephalitogenic determinant of myelin basic protein use similar V alpha and V beta chain genes even though the major histocompatibility complex and encephalitogenic determinants being recognized are different. *J Exp Med* 1989; 169(1):27–39.

36. Goverman J, Woods A, Larson L, et al. Transgenic mice that express a myelin basic protein–specific T-cell receptor develop spontaneous autoimmunity. *Cell* 1993; 72(4):551–560.

37. Yamamura T, Kondo T, Sakanaka S, et al. Analysis of T-cell antigen receptors of myelin basic protein specific T-cells in SJL/J mice demonstrates an alpha chain CDR3 motif associated with encephalitogenic T-cells. *Int Immunol* 1994; 6(7):947–954.

38. Padula SJ, Lingenheld EG, Stabach PR, et al. Identification of encephalitogenic V beta-4–bearing T-cells in SJL mice. Further evidence for the V region disease hypothesis? *J Immunol* 1991; 146(3):879–883.

39. Kuchroo VK, Sobel RA, Laning JC, et al. Experimental allergic encephalomyelitis mediated by cloned T-cells specific for a synthetic peptide of myelin proteolipid protein. Fine specificity and

T-cell receptor V beta usage. *J Immunol* 1992; 148(12):3
776–3782.

40. Gold DP, Offner H, Sun D, et al. Analysis of T-cell receptor beta chains in Lewis rats with experimental allergic encephalomyelitis: conserved complementarity determining region 3. *J Exp Med* 1991; 174(6):1467–1476.

41. Chan A, Gold R, Giegerich G, et al. Usage of Vbeta3.3 T-cell receptor by myelin basic protein–specific encephalitogenic T-cell lines in the Lewis rat. *J Neurosci Res* 1999; 58(2):214–225.

42. Lafaille JJ, Nagashima K, Katsuki M, Tonegawa S. High incidence of spontaneous autoimmune encephalomyelitis in immunodeficient anti–myelin basic protein T-cell receptor transgenic mice. *Cell* 1994; 78(3):399–408.

43. Waldner H, Whitters MJ, Sobel RA, Collins M, Kuchroo VK. Fulminant spontaneous autoimmunity of the central nervous system in mice transgenic for the myelin proteolipid protein-specific T-cell receptor [in process citation]. *Proc Natl Acad Sci USA* 2000; 97(7):3412–3417.

44. Zaller DM, Osman G, Kanagawa O, Hood L. Prevention and treatment of murine experimental allergic encephalomyelitis with T-cell receptor V beta-specific antibodies. *J Exp Med* 1990; 171(6):1943–1955.

45. Racke MK, Quigley L, Cannella B, et al. Superantigen modulation of experimental allergic encephalomyelitis: activation of anergy determines outcome. *J Immunol* 1994; 152(4):2051–2059.

46. Ben Nun A, Wekerle H, Cohen IR. Vaccination against autoimmune encephalomyelitis with T-lymphocyte line cells reactive against myelin basic protein. *Nature* 1981; 292(5818):60–61.

47. Howell MD, Winters ST, Olee T, et al. Vaccination against experimental allergic encephalomyelitis with T-cell receptor peptides [published erratum appears in *Science* 1990; 247(4947):1167]. *Science* 1989; 246(4930):668–670.

48. Vandenbark AA, Hashim G, Offner H. Immunization with a synthetic T-cell receptor V-region peptide protects against experimental autoimmune encephalomyelitis. *Nature* 1989; 341(6242):541–544.

49. Karin, N., Mitchell, D. J., Brocke, S., Ling, N., and Steinman, L. Reversal of experimental autoimmune encephalomyelitis by a soluble peptide variant of a myelin basic protein epitope: T-cell receptor antagonism and reduction of interferon gamma and tumor necrosis factor alpha production. *J.Exp.Med* 1994;180(6):2227–2237.

50. Kuchroo VK, Greer JM, Kaul D, et al. A single TCR antagonist peptide inhibits experimental allergic encephalomyelitis mediated by a diverse T-cell repertoire. *J Immunol* 1994; 153(7):3326–3336.

51. Gaur A, Boehme SA, Chalmers D, et al. Amelioration of relapsing experimental autoimmune encephalomyelitis with altered myelin basic protein peptides involves different-cellular mechanisms. *J Neuroimmunol* 1997; 74:149–158.

52. Nicholson LB, Greer JM, Sobel RA, Lees MB, Kuchroo VK. An altered peptide ligand mediates immune deviation and prevents autoimmune encephalomyelitis. *Immunity* 1995; 3(4):397–405.

53. Brocke S, Gijbels K, Allegretta M, et al. Treatment of experimental encephalomyelitis with a peptide analogue of myelin basic protein [published erratum appears in *Nature* 1998; 392(6676):630]. *Nature* 1996; 379(6563):343–346.

54. Santambrogio L, Lees MB, Sobel RA. Altered peptide ligand modulation of experimental allergic encephalomyelitis: immune responses within the CNS. *J Neuroimmunol* 1998; 81:1–13.

55. Young DA, Lowe LD, Booth SS, et al. IL-4, IL-10, IL-13, and TGF-beta from an altered peptide ligand- specific Th2 cell clone down-regulate adoptive transfer of experimental autoimmune encephalomyelitis [in process citation]. *J Immunol* 2000; 164(7):3563–3572.

56. Anderton SM, Wraith DC. Hierarchy in the ability of T-cell epitopes to induce peripheral tolerance to antigens from myelin. *Eur J Immunol* 1998; 28(4):1251–1261.

57. Anderton SM, Manickasingham SP, Burkhart C, et al. Fine specificity of the myelin-reactive T-cell repertoire: Implications for TCR antagonism in autoimmunity. *J Immunol* 1998; 161(7):3357–3364.

58. Anderton SM, Kissler S, Lamont AG, Wraith DC. Therapeutic potential of TCR antagonists is determined by their ability to modulate a diverse repertoire of autoreactive T-cells. *Eur J Immunol* 1999; 29(6):1850–1857.

59. Green JM, Noel PJ, Sperling AI, et al. Absence of B7-dependent responses in CD28-deficient mice. *Immunity* 1994; 1(6):501–508.

60. Freeman GJ, Borriello F, Hodes RJ, et al. Murine B7-2, an alternative CTLA4 counter-receptor that costimulates T-cell proliferation and interleukin 2 production. *J Exp Med* 1993; 178(6):2185–2192.

61. Freeman GJ, Borriello F, Hodes RJ, et al. Uncovering of functional alternative CTLA-4 counter-receptor in B7- deficient mice [see comments]. *Science* 1993; 262(5135):907–909.

62. Freeman GJ, Gribben JG, Boussiotis VA, et al. Cloning of B7-2: a CTLA-4 counter-receptor that costimulates human T-cell proliferation [see comments]. *Science* 1993; 262(5135):909–911.

63. Hathcock KS, Laszlo G, Dickler HB, et al. Identification of an alternative CTLA-4 ligand costimulatory for T-cell activation [see comments]. *Science* 1993; 262(5135):905–907.

64. Hathcock KS, Laszlo G, Pucillo C, Linsley P, Hodes RJ. Comparative analysis of B7-1 and B7-2 costimulatory ligands: Expression and function. *J Exp Med* 1994; 180(2):631–640.

65. Freedman AS, Freeman GJ, Rhynhart K, Nadler LM. Selective induction of B7/BB-1 on interferon-gamma stimulated monocytes: A potential mechanism for amplification of T-cell activation through the CD28 pathway. *Cell Immunol* 1991; 137(2):429–437.

66. Larsen CP, Ritchie SC, Hendrix R, et al. Regulation of immunostimulatory function and costimulatory molecule (B7-1 and B7-2) expression on murine dendritic cells. *J Immunol* 1994; 152(11):5208–5219.

67. Linsley PS, Greene JL, Brady W, et al. Human B7-1 (CD80) and B7-2 (CD86) bind with similar avidities but distinct kinetics to CD28 and CTLA-4 receptors [published erratum appears in Immunity 1995; 2:203]. *Immunity* 1994; 1(9):793–801.

68. Sansom D M, Hall ND. B7/BB1, the ligand for CD28, is expressed on repeatedly activated human T-cells *in vitro*. *Eur J Immunol* 1993; 23(1):295–298.

69. Azuma M, Yssel H, Phillips JH, Spits H, Lanier LL. Functional expression of B7/BB1 on activated T lymphocytes. *J Exp Med* 1993; 177(3):845–850.

70. Greenfield EA, Howard E, Paradis T, et al. B7.2 expressed by T-cells does not induce CD28-mediated costimulatory activity but retains CTLA4 binding: Implications for induction of antitumor immunity to T-cell tumors. *J Immunol* 1997; 158(5):2025–2034.

71. Cross AH, Lyons JA, San M, et al. T-cells are the main cell type expressing B7-1 and B7-2 in the central nervous system during acute, relapsing and chronic experimental autoimmune encephalomyelitis. *Eur J Immunol* 1999; 29(10):3140–3147.

72. Linsley PS, Greene JL, Tan P, et al. Coexpression and functional cooperation of CTLA-4 and CD28 on activated T lymphocytes. *J Exp Med* 1992; 176(6):1595–1604.

73. Walunas TL, Lenschow DJ, Bakker CY, et al. CTLA-4 can function as a negative regulator of T-cell activation. *Immunity* 1994; 1(5):405–413.

74. Perrin PJ, Maldonado JH, Davis TA, June CH, Racke MK. CTLA-4 blockade enhances clinical disease and cytokine production during experimental allergic encephalomyelitis. *J Immunol* 1996; 157(4):1333–1336.

75. Karandikar NJ, Vanderlugt CL, Walunas TL, Miller SD, Bluestone JA. CTLA-4: a negative regulator of autoimmune disease. *J Exp Med* 1996; 184(2):783–788.

76. Waterhouse P, Penninger JM, Timms E, et al. Lymphoproliferative disorders with early lethality in mice deficient in Ctla-4 [see comments]. *Science* 1995; 270(5238):985–988.

77. Tivol EA, Borriello F, Schweitzer AN, et al. Loss of CTLA-4 leads to massive lymphoproliferation and fatal multiorgan tissue destruction, revealing a critical negative regulatory role of CTLA-4. *Immunity* 1995; 3(5):541–547.

78. Gimmi CD, Gribben JG, Freeman GJ, Nadler LM. [Failing B7 costimulation engenders a peripheral clonal T-cell anergy in a human antigen-specific model]. *Schweiz Med Wochenschr* 1993; 123(47):2255–2256.

79. Lenschow DJ, Zeng Y, Thistlethwaite JR, et al. Long-term survival of xenogeneic pancreatic islet grafts induced by CTLA4Ig [see comments]. *Science* 1992; 257(5071):789–792.

80. Lin H, Bolling SF, Linsley PS, et al. Long-term acceptance of major histocompatibility complex mismatched cardiac allografts induced by CTLA4Ig plus donor-specific transfusion. *J Exp Med* 1993; 178(5):1801–1806.

81. Lin H, Rathmell JC, Gray GS, et al. Cytotoxic T lymphocyte antigen 4 (CTLA4) blockade accelerates the acute rejection of cardiac allografts in CD28-deficient mice: CTLA4 can function independently of CD28. *J Exp Med* 1998; 188(1):199–204.

82. Racke MK, Scott DE, Quigley L, et al. Distinct roles for B7-1 (CD-80) and B7-2 (CD-86) in the initiation of experimental allergic encephalomyelitis. *J Clin Invest* 1995; 96(5):2195–2203.

83. Perrin PJ, Scott D, June CH, Racke MK. B7-mediated costimulation can either provoke or prevent clinical manifestations of experimental allergic encephalomyelitis. *Immunol Res* 1995; 14(3):189–199.

84. Perrin PJ, Scott D, Quigley L, et al. Role of B7:CD28/CTLA-4 in the induction of chronic relapsing experimental allergic encephalomyelitis. *J Immunol* 1995; 154(3):1481–1490.

85. Ratts RB, Arredondo LR, Bittner P, et al. The role of CTLA-4 in tolerance induction and T-cell differentiation in experimental autoimmune encephalomyelitis: I.P. antigen administration. *Int Immunol* 1999; 11(12):1881–1888.

86. Ratts RB, Arredondo LR, Bittner P, et al. The role of CTLA-4 in tolerance induction and antigen administration cell differentiation in experimental autoimmune encephalomyelitis: I. V. antigen administration. *Int Immunol* 1999; 11(12):1889–1896.

87. Chang TT, Jabs C, Sobel,RA, Kuchroo VK, Sharpe AH. Studies in B7-deficient mice reveal a critical role for B7 costimulation in both induction and effector phases of experimental autoimmune encephalomyelitis. *J Exp Med* 1999; 190(5):733–740.

88. Girvin AM, Dal Canto MC, Rhee L, et al. A critical role for B7/CD28 costimulation in experimental autoimmune encephalomyelitis: A comparative study using costimulatory molecule-deficient mice and monoclonal antibody blockade. *J Immunol* 2000; 164(1):136–143.

89. Kuchroo VK, Das MP, Brown JA, et al. B7-1 and B7-2 costimulatory molecules activate differentially the Th1/Th2 developmental pathways: Application to autoimmune disease therapy. *Cell* 1995; 80(5):707–718.

90. Miller SD, Vanderlugt CL, Lenschow DJ, et al. Blockade of CD28/B7-1 interaction prevents epitope spreading and clinical relapses of murine EAE. *Immunity* 1995; 3(6):739–745.

91. Schweitzer AN, Borriello F, Wong RC, Abbas AK, Sharpe AH. Role of costimulators in T-cell differentiation: Studies using antigen-presenting cells lacking expression of CD80 or CD86. *J Immunol* 1997; 158(6):2713–2722.

92. Lenschow DJ, Ho SC, Sattar H, et al. Differential effects of anti-B7-1 and anti-B7-2 monoclonal antibody treatment on the development of diabetes in the nonobese diabetic mouse. *J Exp Med* 1995; 181:1145–1155.

93. Chambers CA, Allison JP. Co-stimulation in T-cell responses. *Curr Opin Immunol* 1997; 9(3):396–404.

94. Karandikar NJ, Vanderlugt CL, Eagar T, et al. Tissue-specific up-regulation of B7-1 expression and function during the course of murine relapsing experimental autoimmune encephalomyelitis. *J Immunol* 1998; 161(1):192–199.

95. Karandikar NJ, Vanderlugt CL, Bluestone JA, Miller SD. Targeting the B7/CD28:CTLA-4 costimulatory system in CNS autoimmune disease. *J Neuroimmunol* 1998; 89(1-2):10–18.

96. Sagerstrom CG, Kerr EM, Allison JP, Davis MM. Activation and differentiation requirements of primary T-cells in vitro. *Proc Natl Acad Sci USA* 1993; 90(19):8987–8991.

97. Damle NK, Klussman K, Linsley PS, Aruffo A. Differential costimulatory effects of adhesion molecules B7, ICAM-1, LFA-3, and VCAM-1 on resting and antigen-primed CD4+ T lymphocytes. *J Immunol* 1992; 148(7):1985–1992.

98. Croft M, Bradley LM, Swain SL. Naive versus memory CD4 T-cell response to antigen. Memory cells are less dependent on accessory cell costimulation and can respond to many antigen-presenting cell types including resting B cells. *J Immunol* 1994; 152(6):2675–2685.

99. Lovett-Racke AE, Trotter JL, Lauber J, et al. Decreased dependence of myelin basic protein–reactive T-cells on CD28-mediated costimulation in multiple sclerosis patients. A marker of activated/memory T-cells [published erratum appears in J Clin Invest 1998; 101(7):1542]. *J Clin Invest* 1998; 101(4):725–730.

100. Perrin PJ, Lovett-Racke A, Phillips SM, Racke MK. Differential requirements of naive and memory T-cells for CD28 costimulation in autoimmune pathogenesis. *Histol Histopathol* 1999; 14(4):1269–1276.

101. Cross AH, Cannella B, Brosnan CF, Raine CS. Homing to central nervous system vasculature by antigen-specific lymphocytes. I. Localization of 14C-labeled cells during acute, chronic, and relapsing experimental allergic encephalomyelitis. *Lab Invest* 1990; 63(2):162–170.

102. Hickey WF, Kimura H. Perivascular microglial cells of the CNS are bone marrow-derived and present antigen in vivo. *Science* 1988; 239(4837):290–292.

103. Baker D, O'Neill JK, Turk JL. Cytokines in the central nervous system of mice during chronic relapsing experimental allergic encephalomyelitis. *Cell Immunol* 1991; 134(2):505–510.

104. Kennedy MK, Torrance DS, Picha KS, Mohler KM. Analysis of cytokine MRNA expression in the central nervous system of mice with experimental autoimmune encephalomyelitis reveals that IL-10 mRNA expression correlates with recovery. *J Immunol* 1992; 149(7):2496–2505.

105. Merrill JE, Kono DH, Clayton J, et al. Inflammatory leukocytes and cytokines in the peptide-induced disease of experimental allergic encephalomyelitis in SJL and B10.PL mice [published erratum appears in *Proc Natl Acad Sci USA* 1992; 89(21):10562]. *Proc Natl Acad Sci USA* 1992; 89(2):574–578.

106. Stoll G, Muller S, Schmidt B, et al. Localization of interferon-gamma and Ia-antigen in T-cell line–mediated experimental autoimmune encephalomyelitis. *Am J Pathol* 1993; 142(6):1866–1875.

107. Weinberg AD, Wallin JJ, Jones RE, et al. Target organ-specific up-regulation of the MRC OX-40 marker and selective production of Th1 lymphokine MRNA by encephalitogenic T helper cells isolated from the spinal cord of rats with experimental autoimmune encephalomyelitis. *J Immunol* 1994; 152(9):4712–4721.

108. Renno T, Lin JY, Piccirillo C, Antel J, Owens T. Cytokine production by cells in cerebrospinal fluid during experimental allergic encephalomyelitis in SJL/J mice. *J Neuroimmunol* 1994; 49(1–2):1–7.

109. Renno T, Krakowski M, Piccirillo C, Lin JY, Owens T. TNF-alpha expression by resident microglia and infiltrating leukocytes in the central nervous system of mice with experimental allergic encephalomyelitis. Regulation by Th1 cytokines. *J Immunol* 1995; 154(2):944–953.

110. Issazadeh S, Ljungdahl A, Hojeberg B, Mustafa M, Olsson T. Cytokine production in the central nervous system of Lewis rats with experimental autoimmune encephalomyelitis: Dynamics of MRNA expression for interleukin-10, interleukin-12, cytolysin, tumor necrosis factor alpha and tumor necrosis factor beta. *J Neuroimmunol* 1995; 61(2):205–212.

111. Ando DG, Clayton J, Kono D, Urban JL, Sercarz EE. Encephalitogenic T-cells in the B10.PL model of experimental allergic encephalomyelitis (EAE) are of the Th-1 lymphokine subtype. *Cell Immunol* 1989; 124(1):132–143.

112. Baron JL, Madri JA, Ruddle NH, Hashim G, Janeway CA Jr. Surface expression of alpha 4 integrin by CD4 T-cells is required for their entry into brain parenchyma. *J Exp Med* 1993; 177(1):57–68.

113. Kuchroo VK, Martin CA, Greer JM, et al. Cytokines and adhesion molecules contribute to the ability of myelin proteolipid protein-specific T-cell clones to mediate experimental allergic encephalomyelitis. *J Immunol* 1993; 151(8):4371–4382.

114. Racke MK, Bonomo A, Scott DE, et al. Cytokine-induced immune deviation as a therapy for inflammatory autoimmune disease. *J Exp Med* 1994; 180(5):1961–1966.

115. Lovett-Racke AE, Bittner P, Cross AH, Carlino JA, Racke MK. Regulation of experimental autoimmune encephalomyelitis with insulin-like growth factor (IGF-1) and IGF-1/IGF-binding protein-3 complex (IGF-1/IGFBP3). *J Clin Invest* 1998; 101(8):1797–1804.

116. Billiau A, Heremans H, Vandekerckhove F, et al. Enhancement of experimental allergic encephalomyelitis in mice by antibodies against IFN-gamma. *J Immunol* 1988; 140(5):1506–1510.

117. Voorthuis JA, Uitdehaag BM, De Groot CJ, et al. Suppression of experimental allergic encephalomyelitis by intraventricular administration of interferon-gamma in Lewis rats. *Clin Exp Immunol* 1990; 81(2):183–188.

118. Lublin FD, Knobler RL, Kalman B, et al. Monoclonal anti-gamma interferon antibodies enhance experimental allergic encephalomyelitis. *Autoimmunity* 1993; 16(4):267–274.

119. Duong TT, St. Louis J, Gilbert JJ, Finkelman FD, Strejan GH. Effect of anti-interferon-gamma and anti–interleukin-2 mono-clonal antibody treatment on the development of actively and passively induced experimental allergic encephalomyelitis in the SJL/J mouse. *J Neuroimmunol* 1992; 36(2-3):105–115.

120. Ferber IA, Brocke S, Taylor-Edwards C, et al. Mice with a disrupted IFN-gamma gene are susceptible to the induction of experimental autoimmune encephalomyelitis (EAE). *J Immunol* 1996; 156(1):5–7.

121. Krakowski M, Owens T. Interferon-gamma confers resistance to experimental allergic encephalomyelitis. *Eur J Immunol* 1996; 26(7):1641–1646.

122. Willenborg DO, Fordham S, Bernard CC, Cowden WB, Ramshaw IA. IFN-gamma plays a critical down-regulatory role in the induction and effector phase of myelin oligodendrocyte gly-coprotein–induced autoimmune encephalomyelitis. *J Immunol* 1996; 157(8):3223–3227.

123. Panitch HS, Bever CT Jr. Clinical trials of interferons in multiple sclerosis. What have we learned? *J Neuroimmunol* 1993; 46(1-2):155–164.

124. Powell MB, Mitchell D, Lederman J, et al. Lymphotoxin and tumor necrosis factor-alpha production by myelin basic protein-specific T-cell clones correlates with encephalitogenicity. *Int Immunol* 1990; 2(6):539–544.

125. Held W, Meyermann R, Qin Y, Mueller C. Perforin and tumor necrosis factor alpha in the pathogenesis of experimental allergic encephalomyelitis: Comparison of autoantigen induced and trans-ferred disease in Lewis rats. *J Autoimmun* 1993; 6(3):311–322.

126. Voskuhl RR, Martin R, Bergman C, et al. T helper 1 (Th1) functional phenotype of human myelin basic protein–specific T lymphocytes. *Autoimmunity* 1993; 15(2):137–143.

127. Tanuma N, Kojima T, Shin T, et al. Competitive PCR quantification of pro- and anti-inflammatory cytokine mRNA in the central nervous system during autoimmune encephalomyelitis. *J Neuroimmunol* 1997; 73(1-2):197–206.

128. Begolka WS, Vanderlugt CL, Rahbe SM, Miller SD. Differential expression of inflammatory cytokines parallels progression of central nervous system pathology in two clinically distinct models of multiple sclerosis. *J Immunol* 1998; 161(8):4437–4446.

129. Kuroda Y, Shimamoto Y. Human tumor necrosis factor-alpha augments experimental allergic encephalomyelitis in rats. *J Neuroimmunol* 1991; 34(2-3):159–164.

130. Crisi GM, Santambrogio L, Hochwald GM, et al. Staphylococcal enterotoxin B and tumor-necrosis factor-alpha–induced relapses of experimental allergic encephalomyelitis: protection by transforming growth factor-beta and interleukin-10. *Eur J Immunol* 1995; 25(11):3035–3040.

131. Taupin V, Renno T, Bourbonniere L, et al. Increased severity of experimental autoimmune encephalomyelitis, chronic macrophage/microglial reactivity, and demyelination in trans-genic mice producing tumor necrosis factor-alpha in the central nervous system. *Eur J Immunol* 1997; 27(4):905–913.

132. Ruddle NH, Bergman CM, McGrath KM, et al. An antibody to lymphotoxin and tumor necrosis factor prevents transfer of experimental allergic encephalomyelitis. *J Exp Med* 1990; 172(4):1193–1200.

133. Selmaj K, Raine CS, Cross AH. Anti–tumor necrosis factor therapy abrogates autoimmune demyelination. *Ann Neurol* 1991; 30(5):694–700.

134. Selmaj K, Papierz W, Glabinski A, Kohno T. Prevention of chronic relapsing experimental autoimmune encephalomyelitis by soluble tumor necrosis factor receptor I. *J Neuroimmunol* 1995; 56(2):135–141.

135. Selmaj KW, Raine CS. Experimental autoimmune encephalo-myelitis: immunotherapy with anti–tumor necrosis factor anti-bodies and soluble tumor necrosis factor receptors. *Neurology* 1995; 45(suppl 6):S44–S49.

136. Korner H, Riminton DS, Strickland DH, et al. Critical points of tumor necrosis factor action in central nervous system autoimmune inflammation defined by gene targeting. *J Exp Med* 1997; 186(9):1585–1590.

137. Sean D, Korner H, Strickland DH, et al. Challenging cytokine redundancy: Inflammatory cell movement and clinical course of experimental autoimmune encephalomyelitis are normal in lymphotoxin-deficient, but not tumor necrosis factor–deficient, mice. *J Exp Med* 1998; 187(9):1517–1528.

138. Liu J, Marino MW, Wong G, et al. TNF is a potent anti-inflammatory cytokine in autoimmune-mediated demyelination. *Nat Med* 1998; 4(1):78–83.

139. Frei K, Eugster HP, Bopst M, et al. Tumor necrosis factor alpha and lymphotoxin alpha are not required for induction of acute experimental autoimmune encephalomyelitis. *J Exp Med* 1997; 185(12):2177–2182.

140. Kassiotis G, Pasparakis M, Kollias G, Probert L. TNF accelerates the onset but does not alter the incidence and severity of myelin basic protein–induced experimental autoimmune encephalomyelitis. *Eur J Immunol* 1999; 29(3):774–780.

141. Suen WE, Bergman CM, Hjelmstrom P, Ruddle NH. A critical role for lymphotoxin in experimental allergic encephalomyelitis. *J Exp Med* 1997; 186(8):1233–1240.

142. Telander DG, Malvey EN, Mueller DL. Evidence for repression of IL-2 gene activation in anergic T-cells. *J Immunol* 1999; 162(3):1460–1465.

143. Schluesener HJ, Lassmann H. Recombinant interleukin 2 (IL-2) promotes T-cell line-mediated neuroautoimmune disease. *J Neuroimmunol* 1986; 11(1):87–91.

144. Racke MK, Critchfield JM, Quigley L, et al. Intravenous antigen administration as a therapy for autoimmune demyelinating disease. *Ann Neurol* 1996; 39(1):46–56.

145. Engelhardt B, Diamantstein T, Wekerle H. Immunotherapy of experimental autoimmune encephalomyelitis (EAE): Differential effect of anti–IL-2 receptor antibody therapy on actively induced and T-line mediated EAE of the Lewis rat. *J Autoimmun* 1989; 2(1):61–73.

146. Critchfield JM, Racke MK, Zuniga-Pflucker JC, et al. T-cell deletion in high antigen dose therapy of autoimmune encephalomyelitis. *Science* 1994; 263(5150):1139–1143.

147. Gijbels K, Van Damme J, Proost P, Put W, et al. Interleukin 6 production in the central nervous system during experimental autoimmune encephalomyelitis. *Eur J Immunol* 1990; 20(1):233–235.

148. Gijbels K, Brocke S, Abrams JS, Steinman L. Administration of neutralizing antibodies to interleukin-6 (IL-6) reduces experimental autoimmune encephalomyelitis and is associated with elevated levels of IL-6 bioactivity in central nervous system and circulation. *Mol Med* 1995; 1(7):795–805.

149. Willenborg DO, Fordham SA, Cowden WB, Ramshaw IA. Cytokines and murine autoimmune encephalomyelitis: Inhibition or enhancement of disease with antibodies to select cytokines, or by delivery of exogenous cytokines using a recombinant *Vaccinia* virus system. *Scand J Immunol* 1995; 41(1):31–41.

150. Rodriguez M, Pavelko KD, McKinney CW, Leibowitz JL. Recombinant human IL-6 suppresses demyelination in a viral model of multiple sclerosis. *J Immunol* 1994; 153(8):3811–3821.

151. Samoilova EB, Horton JL, Hilliard B, Liu TS, Chen Y. IL-6-deficient mice are resistant to experimental autoimmune encephalomyelitis: Roles of IL-6 in the activation and differentiation of autoreactive T-cells. *J Immunol* 1998; 161(12):6480–6486.

152. Mendel I, Katz A, Kozak N, Ben Nun A, Revel M. Interleukin-6 functions in autoimmune encephalomyelitis: A study in gene-targeted mice. *Eur J Immunol* 1998; 28(5):1727–1737.

153. Okuda Y, Sakoda S, Fujimura H, et al. IL-6 plays a crucial role in the induction phase of myelin oligodendrocyte glucoprotein 35-55 induced experimental autoimmune encephalomyelitis. *J Neuroimmunol* 1999; 101(2):188–196.

154. Bright JJ, Musuro BF, Du C, Sriram S. Expression of IL-12 in CNS and lymphoid organs of mice with experimental allergic encephalitis. *J Neuroimmunol* 1998; 82(1):22–30.

155. Leonard JP, Waldburger KE, Goldman SJ. Prevention of experimental autoimmune encephalomyelitis by antibodies against interleukin 12. *J Exp Med* 1995; 181(1):381–386.

156. Smith T, Hewson AK, Kingsley CI, Leonard JP, Cuzner ML. Interleukin-12 induces relapse in experimental allergic encephalomyelitis in the Lewis rat. *Am J Pathol* 1997; 150(6):1909–1917.

157. Constantinescu CS, Wysocka M, Hilliard B, et al. Antibodies against IL-12 prevent superantigen-induced and spontaneous relapses of experimental autoimmune encephalomyelitis. *J Immunol* 1998; 161(9):5097–5104.

158. Heremans H, Dillen C, Groenen M, Matthys P, Billiau A. Role of endogenous interleukin-12 (IL-12) in induced and spontaneous relapses of experimental autoimmune encephalomyelitis in mice. *Eur Cytokine Netw* 1999; 10(2):171–180.

159. Ichikawa M, Koh CS, Inoue A, et al. Anti-IL-12 antibody prevents the development and progression of multiple sclerosis–like relapsing–remitting demyelinating disease in NOD mice induced with myelin oligodendrocyte glycoprotein peptide. *J Neuroimmunol* 2000; 102(1):56–66.

160. Segal BM, Dwyer BK, Shevach EM. An interleukin (IL)-10/IL-12 immunoregulatory circuit controls susceptibility to autoimmune disease. *J Exp Med* 1998; 187(4):537–546.

161. Begolka WS, Miller SD. Cytokines as intrinsic and exogenous regulators of pathogenesis in experimental autoimmune encephalomyelitis. *Res Immunol* 1998; 149(9):771–781.

162. Merrill JE, Ignarro LJ, Sherman MP, Melinek J, Lane TE. Microglial cell cytotoxicity of oligodendrocytes is mediated through nitric oxide. *J Immunol* 1993; 151(4):2132–2141.

163. Cross AH, Misko TP, Lin RF, et al. Aminoguanidine, an inhibitor of inducible nitric oxide synthase, ameliorates experimental autoimmune encephalomyelitis in SJL mice. *J Clin Invest* 1994; 93(6):2684–2690.

164. Racke MK, Cannella B, Albert P, et al. Evidence of endogenous regulatory function of transforming growth factor-beta 1 in experimental allergic encephalomyelitis. *Int Immunol* 1992; 4(5):615–620.

165. Weiner HL, Friedman A, Miller A, et al. Oral tolerance: Immunologic mechanisms and treatment of animal and human organ-specific autoimmune diseases by oral administration of autoantigens. *Annu Rev Immunol* 1994; 12:809–837.

166. Khoury SJ, Hancock WW, Weiner HL. Oral tolerance to myelin basic protein and natural recovery from experimental autoimmune encephalomyelitis are associated with downregulation of inflammatory cytokines and differential upregulation of transforming growth factor beta, interleukin 4, and prostaglandin E expression in the brain. *J Exp Med* 1992; 176(5):1355–1364.

167. Karpus WJ, Gould KE, Swanborg RH. CD4⁺ suppressor cells of autoimmune encephalomyelitis respond to T-cell receptor–associated determinants on effector cells by interleukin-4 secretion. *Eur J Immunol* 1992; 22(7):1757–1763.

168. van der Veen RC, Stohlman SA. Encephalitogenic Th1 cells are inhibited by Th2 cells with related peptide specificity: Relative roles of interleukin (IL)-4 and IL-10. *J Neuroimmunol* 1993; 48(2):213–220.

169. Inobe JI, Chen Y, Weiner HL. In vivo administration of IL-4 induces TGF-beta–producing cells and protects animals from experimental autoimmune encephalomyelitis. *Ann NY Acad Sci* 1996; 778:390–392.

170. Shaw MK, Lorens JB, Dhawan A, et al. Local delivery of interleukin 4 by retrovirus-transduced T lymphocytes ameliorates experimental autoimmune encephalomyelitis. *J Exp Med* 1997; 185(9):1711–1714.

171. Khoruts A, Miller SD, Jenkins MK. Neuroantigen-specific Th2 cells are inefficient suppressors of experimental autoimmune encephalomyelitis induced by effector Th1 cells. *J Immunol* 1995; 155(10):5011–5017.

172. Falcone M, Bloom BR. A T helper cell 2 (Th2) immune response against non-self antigens modifies the cytokine profile of autoimmune T-cells and protects against experimental allergic encephalomyelitis. *J Exp Med* 1997; 185(5):901–907.

173. Karpus WJ, Kennedy KJ, Smith WS, Miller SD. Inhibition of relapsing experimental autoimmune encephalomyelitis in SJL mice by feeding the immunodominant PLP139-151 peptide. *J Neurosci Res* 1996; 45(4):410–423.

174. Racke MK, Burnett D, Pak SH, et at. Retinoid treatment of experimental allergic encephalomyelitis. IL-4 production correlates with improved disease course. *J Immunol* 1995; 154(1):450–458.

175. Liblau R, Steinman L, Brocke S. Experimental autoimmune encephalomyelitis in IL-4–deficient mice. *Int Immunol* 1997; 9(5):799–803.

176. Falcone M, Rajan AJ, Bloom BR, Brosnan CF. A critical role for IL-4 in regulating disease severity in experimental allergic encephalomyelitis as demonstrated in IL-4–deficient C57BL/6 mice and BALB/c mice. *J Immunol* 1998; 160(10):4822–4830.

177. Cannella B, Raine CS. The adhesion molecule and cytokine profile of multiple sclerosis lesions [see comments]. *Ann Neurol* 1995; 37(4):424–435.

178. Fiorentino DF, Zlotnik A, Mosmann TR, Howard M, O'Garra A. IL-10 inhibits cytokine production by activated macrophages. *J Immunol* 1991; 147(11):3815–3822.

179. Oswald IP, Gazzinelli RT, Sher A, James SL. IL-10 synergizes with IL-4 and transforming growth factor-beta to inhibit macrophage cytotoxic activity. *J Immunol* 1992; 148(11):3578–3582.

180. Frei K, Lins H, Schwerdel C, Fontana A. Antigen presentation in the central nervous system. the inhibitory effect of IL-10 on MHC class II expression and production of cytokines depends on the inducing signals and the type of cell analyzed. *J Immunol* 1994; 152(6):2720–2728.

181. Gerosa F, Paganin C, Peritt D, et al. Interleukin-12 primes human CD4 and CD8 T-cell clones for high production of both interferon-gamma and interleukin-10. *J Exp Med* 1996; 183(6):2559–2569.

182. Cannella B, Gao YL, Brosnan C, Raine CS. IL-10 fails to abrogate experimental autoimmune encephalomyelitis. *J Neurosci Res* 1996; 45(6):735–746.

183. Bettelli E, Das MP, Howard ED, et al. IL-10 is critical in the regulation of autoimmune encephalomyelitis as demonstrated by studies of IL-10- and IL-4–deficient and transgenic mice. *J Immunol* 1998; 161(7):3299–3306.

184. Mathisen PM, Yu M, Johnson JM, Drazba JA, Tuohy VK. Treatment of experimental autoimmune encephalomyelitis with genetically modified memory T-cells. *J Exp Med* 1997; 186(1):159–164.

185. Cua DJ, Groux H, Hinton DR, Stohlman SA, Coffman RL. Transgenic interleukin 10 prevents induction of experimental autoimmune encephalomyelitis. *J Exp Med* 1999; 189(6):1005–1510.

186. Racke MK, Dhib-Jalbut S, Cannella B, et al. Prevention and treatment of chronic relapsing experimental allergic encephalomyelitis by transforming growth factor-beta 1. *J Immunol* 1991; 146(9):3012–3017.

187. Johns LD, Flanders KC, Ranges GE, Sriram S. Successful treatment of experimental allergic encephalomyelitis with transforming growth factor-beta 1. *J Immunol* 1991; 147(6):1792–1796.

188. Johns LD, Sriram S. Experimental allergic encephalomyelitis: Neutralizing antibody to TGF beta 1 enhances the clinical severity of the disease. *J Neuroimmunol* 1993 ;47(1):1–7.

189. Weinberg AD, Whitham R, Swain SL, et al. Transforming growth factor-beta enhances the *in vivo* effector function and memory phenotype of antigen-specific T helper cells in experimental autoimmune encephalomyelitis. *J Immunol* 1992; 148(7):2109–2117.

190. Kuruvilla AP, Shah R, Hochwald GM, et al. Protective effect of transforming growth factor beta 1 on experimental autoimmune diseases in mice. *Proc Natl Acad Sci USA* 1991; 88(7):2918–2921.

191. Brandes ME, Allen JB, Ogawa Y, Wahl SM. Transforming growth factor beta 1 suppresses acute and chronic arthritis in experimental animals. *J Clin Invest* 1991; 87(3):1108–1113.

192. Wyss-Coray T, Borrow P, Brooker MJ, Mucke L. Astroglial overproduction of TGF-beta 1 enhances inflammatory central nervous system disease in transgenic mice. *J Neuroimmunol* 1997; 77(1):45–50.

193. Otten U, Ehrhard P, Peck R. Nerve growth factor induces growth and differentiation of human B lymphocytes. *Proc Natl Acad Sci USA* 1989; 86(24):10059–10063.

194. Ehrhard PB, Erb P, Graumann U, Otten U. Expression of nerve growth factor and nerve growth factor receptor tyrosine kinase Trk in activated CD4-positive T-cell clones. *Proc Natl Acad Sci USA* 1993; 90(23):10984–10988.

195. Lambiase A, Bracci-Laudiero L, et al. Human CD4$^+$ T-cell clones produce and release nerve growth factor and express high-affinity nerve growth factor receptors. *J Allergy Clin Immunol* 1997; 100(3):408–414.

196. Ehrhard PB, Erb P, Graumann U, Schmutz B, Otten U. Expression of functional Trk tyrosine kinase receptors after T-cell activation. *J Immunol* 1994; 152(6):2705–2709.

197. Santambrogio L, Benedetti M, Chao MV, et al. Nerve growth factor production by lymphocytes. *J Immunol* 1994; 153(10):4488–4495.

198. Torcia M, Bracci-Laudiero L, Lucibello M, et al. Nerve growth factor is an autocrine survival factor for memory B lymphocytes. *Cell* 1996; 85(3):345–356.

199. Braun A, Appel E, Baruch R, et al. Role of nerve growth factor in a mouse model of allergic airway inflammation and asthma. *Eur J Immunol* 1998; 28(10):3240–3251.

200. Micera A, De Simone R, Aloe L. Elevated levels of nerve growth factor in the thalamus and spinal cord of rats affected by experimental allergic encephalomyelitis. *Arch Ital Biol* 1995; 133(2):131–142.

201. Micera A, Properzi F, Triaca V, Aloe L. Nerve growth factor antibody exacerbates neuropathological signs of experimental allergic encephalomyelitis in adult Lewis rats. *J Neuroimmunol* 2000; 104(2):116–123.

202. Roth GA, Jorgensen VH, Bornstein MB. Effect of insulin, proinsulin and pancreatic extract on myelination and remyelination in organotypic nerve tissue in culture. *J Neurol Sci* 1985; 71(2-3):339–350.

203. McMorris FA, Smith TM, DeSalvo S, Furlanetto RW. Insulin-like growth factor I/somatomedin C: A potent inducer of oligodendrocyte development. *Proc Natl Acad Sci USA* 1986; 83(3):822–826.

204. Mozell RL, McMorris FA. Insulin-like growth factor I stimulates oligodendrocyte development and myelination in rat brain aggregate cultures. *J Neurosci Res* 1991; 30(2):382–390.

205. McMorris FA, Mozell, RL, Carson MJ, et al. Regulation of oligodendrocyte development and central nervous system myelination by insulin-like growth factors. *Ann NY Acad Sci* 1993; 692:321–334.

206. Roth GA, Spada V, Hamill K, Bornstein MB. Insulin-like growth factor I increases myelination and inhibits demyelination in cultured organotypic nerve tissue. *Brain Res Dev Brain Res* 1995; 88(1):102–108.

207. Liu X, Yao DL, Webster H. Insulin-like growth factor I treatment reduces clinical deficits and lesion severity in acute demyelinating experimental autoimmune encephalomyelitis. *Mult Scler* 1995; 1(1):2–9.

208. Yao DL, Liu X, Hudson LD, Webster HD. Insulin-like growth factor I treatment reduces demyelination and up-regulates gene expression of myelin-related proteins in experimental autoimmune encephalomyelitis. *Proc Natl Acad Sci USA* 1995; 92(13):6190–6194.

209. Liu X, Linnington C, Webster HD, et al. Insulin-like growth factor-I treatment reduces immune cell responses in acute nondemyelinative experimental autoimmune encephalomyelitis. *J Neurosci Res* 1997; 47(5):531–538.

210. Lovett-Racke AE, Bittner P, Cross AH, Carlino JA, Racke MK. Regulation of experimental autoimmune encephalomyelitis with insulin-like growth factor (IGF-1) and IGF-1/IGF-binding protein-3 complex (IGF-1/IGFBP3). *J Clin Invest* 1998; 101(8):1797–1804.

211. Cannella B, Hoban CJ, Gao YL, et al. The neuregulin, glial growth factor 2, diminishes autoimmune demyelination and enhances remyelination in a chronic relapsing model for multiple sclerosis. *Proc Natl Acad Sci USA* 1998; 95(17):10100–10105.

212. Marchionni MA, Cannella B, Hoban C, et al. Neuregulin in neuron/glial interactions in the central nervous system. GGF2 diminishes autoimmune demyelination, promotes oligodendrocyte progenitor expansion, and enhances remyelination. *Adv Exp Med Biol* 1999; 468:283–295.

213. Mathisen PM, Yu M, Yin L, et al. Th2 T-cells expressing transgene PDGF-A serve as vectors for gene therapy in autoimmune demyelinating disease. *J Autoimmun* 1999; 13(1):31–38.

214. Cua DJ, Hinton DR, Stohlman SA. Self-antigen–induced Th2 responses in experimental allergic encephalomyelitis (EAE)–resistant mice. Th2-mediated suppression of autoimmune disease. *J Immunol* 1995; 155(8):4052–4059.

215. Lafaille JJ, Keere FV, Hsu AL, et al. Myelin basic protein–specific T helper 2 (Th2) cells cause experimental autoimmune encephalomyelitis in immunodeficient hosts rather than protect them from the disease. *J Exp Med* 1997; 186(2):307–312.

216. Chen Y, Kuchroo VK, Inobe J, Hafler DA, Weiner HL. Regulatory T-cell clones induced by oral tolerance: suppression of autoimmune encephalomyelitis. *Science* 1994; 265(5176):1237–1240.

217. Khoury SJ, Akalin E, Chandraker A, et al. CD28-B7 costimulatory blockade by CTLA4Ig prevents actively induced experimental autoimmune encephalomyelitis and inhibits Th1 but spares Th2 cytokines in the central nervous system. *J Immunol* 1995; 155(10):4521–4524.

218. Karpus WJ, Ransohoff RM. Chemokine regulation of experimental autoimmune encephalomyelitis: Temporal and spatial expression patterns govern disease pathogenesis. *J Immunol* 1998; 161(6):2667–2671.

219. Glabinski AR, Tani M, Strieter RM, Tuohy VK, Ransohoff RM. Synchronous synthesis of alpha- and beta-chemokines by cells of diverse lineage in the central nervous system of mice with relapses of chronic experimental autoimmune encephalomyelitis. *Am J Pathol* 1997; 150(2):617–630.

220. Glabinski AR, Tani M, Tuohy VK, Tuthill RJ, Ransohoff RM. Central nervous system chemokine mRNA accumulation follows initial leukocyte entry at the onset of acute murine experimental autoimmune encephalomyelitis. *Brain Behav Immun* 1995; 9(4):315–330.

221. Glabinski AR, Tuohy VK, Ransohoff RM. Expression of chemokines RANTES, MIP-1alpha and GRO-Alpha correlates with inflammation in acute experimental autoimmune encephalomyelitis. *Neuroimmunomodulation* 1998; 5(3–4):166–171.

222. Ransohoff RM, Glabinski A, Tani M. Chemokines in immune-mediated inflammation of the central nervous system. *Cytokine Growth Factor Rev* 1996; 7(1):35–46.

223. Ransohoff RM, Hamilton TA, Tani M, et al. Astrocyte expression of MRNA encoding cytokines IP-10 and JE/MCP-1 in experimental autoimmune encephalomyelitis. *FASEB J* 1993; 7(6):592–600.

224. Godiska R, Chantry D, Dietsch GN, Gray PW. Chemokine expression in murine experimental allergic encephalomyelitis. *J Neuroimmunol* 1995; 58(2):167–176.

225. Matejuk A, Vandenbark AA, Burrows GG, Bebo BF Jr, Offner H. Reduced chemokine and chemokine receptor expression in spinal cords of TCR BV8S2 transgenic mice protected against experimental autoimmune encephalomyelitis with BV8S2 protein. *J Immunol* 2000; 164(7):3924–3931.

226. Karpus WJ, Lukacs NW, McRae BL, et al. An important role for the chemokine macrophage inflammatory protein-1 alpha in the pathogenesis of the T-cell–mediated autoimmune disease, experimental autoimmune encephalomyelitis. *J Immunol* 1995; 155(10):5003–5010.

227. Kennedy KJ, Strieter RM, Kunkel SL, Lukacs NW, Karpus WJ. Acute and relapsing experimental autoimmune encephalomyelitis are regulated by differential expression of the CC chemokines macrophage inflammatory protein-1alpha and monocyte chemotactic protein-1. *J Neuroimmunol* 1998; 92(1-2):98–108.

228. Lukacs NW, Strieter RM, Elner V, et al. Production of chemokines, interleukin-8 and monocyte chemoattractant protein-1, during monocyte: endothelial cell interactions. *Blood* 1995; 86(7):2767–2773.

229. Goebeler M, Yoshimura T, Toksoy A, et al. The chemokine repertoire of human dermal microvascular endothelial cells and its regulation by inflammatory cytokines. *J Invest Dermatol* 1997; 108(4):445–451.

230. Zach O, Bauer HC, Richter K, et al. Expression of a chemotactic cytokine (MCP-1) in cerebral capillary endothelial cells *in vitro*. *Endothelium* 1997; 5(3):143–153.

231. Glabinski AR, Balasingam V, Tani M, et al. Chemokine monocyte chemoattractant protein-1 is expressed by astrocytes after mechanical injury to the brain. *J Immunol* 1996; 156(11):4363–4368.

232. Sun D, Hu X, Liu X, Whitaker JN, Walker WS. Expression of chemokine genes in rat glial cells: the effect of myelin basic protein–reactive encephalitogenic T-cells. *J Neurosci Res* 1997; 48(3):192–200.

233. Bacon KB, Premack BA, Gardner P, Schall TJ. Activation of dual T-cell signaling pathways by the chemokine RANTES. *Science* 1995; 269(5231):1727–1730.

234. Turner L, Ward SG, Westwick J. RANTES-activated human T lymphocytes. A role for phosphoinositide 3- kinase. *J Immunol* 1995; 155(5):2437–2444.

235. Taub DD, Ortaldo JR, Turcovski-Corrales SM, et al. Beta chemokines costimulate lymphocyte cytolysis, proliferation, and lymphokine production. *J Leukoc Biol* 1996; 59(1):81–89.

236. Taub DD, Turcovski-Corrales SM, Key ML, Longo DL, Murphy WJ. Chemokines and T lymphocyte activation: I. Beta chemokines costimulate human T lymphocyte activation *in vitro*. *J Immunol* 1996; 156(6):2095–2103.

237. Turner L, Ward SG, Sansom D, Westwick JA Role for RANTES in T lymphocyte proliferation. *Biochem Soc Trans* 1996; 24(1):93S.

238. Gilat D, Hershkoviz R, Mekori YA, Vlodavsky I, Lider O. Regulation of adhesion of CD4+ T lymphocytes to intact or heparinase-treated subendothelial extracellular matrix by diffusible or anchored RANTES and MIP-1 beta. *J Immunol* 1994; 153(11): 4899–4906.

239. Bacon KB, Szabo MC, Yssel H, Bolen JB, Schall TJ. RANTES induces tyrosine kinase activity of stably complexed P125FAK and ZAP-70 in human T-cells. *J Exp Med* 1996; 184(3):873–882.

240. Kawabe Y, Ochi A. Programmed cell death and extrathymic reduction of Vbeta8+ CD4+ T-cells in mice tolerant to staphylococcus aureus enterotoxin B [see comments]. *Nature* 1991; 349(6306):245–248.

241. Lenardo MJ. Interleukin-2 programs mouse alpha beta T lymphocytes for apoptosis. *Nature* 1991; 353(6347):858–861.

242. Russell JH, White CL, Loh DY, Meleedy-Rey P. Receptor-stimulated death pathway is opened by antigen in mature T-cells. *Proc Natl Acad Sci USA* 1991; 88(6):2151–2155.

243. Boehme SA, Lenardo MJ. Ligand-induced apoptosis of mature T lymphocytes (propriocidal regulation) occurs at distinct stages of the cell cycle. *Leukemia* 1993; 7 (suppl 2):S45–S49.

244. Boehme SA, Lenardo MJ. Propriocidal apoptosis of mature T lymphocytes occurs at S phase of the cell cycle. *Eur J Immunol* 1993; 23(7):1552–1560.

245. Webb S, Morris C, Sprent J. Extrathymic tolerance of mature T-cells: clonal elimination as a consequence of immunity. *Cell* 1990; 63(6):1249–1256.

246. Nagata M, Santamaria P, Kawamura T, Utsugi T, Yoon JW. Evidence for the role of CD8+ cytotoxic T-cells in the destruction of pancreatic beta-cells in nonobese diabetic mice. *J Immunol* 1994; 152(4):2042–2050.

247. Suda T, Tanaka M, Miwa K, Nagata S. Apoptosis of mouse naive T-cells induced by recombinant soluble Fas ligand and activation-induced resistance to Fas ligand. *J Immunol* 1996; 157(9): 3918–3924.

248. Raine CS, Traugott U, Stone SH. suppression of chronic allergic encephalomyelitis: relevance to multiple sclerosis. *Science* 1978; 201(4354):445–448.

249. Kennedy MK, Tan LJ, Dal Canto MC, et al. Inhibition of murine relapsing experimental autoimmune encephalomyelitis by immune tolerance to proteolipid protein and its encephalitogenic peptides. *J Immunol* 1990; 144(3):909–915.

250. Su XM, Sriram S. Treatment of chronic relapsing experimental allergic encephalomyelitis with the intravenous administration of splenocytes coupled to encephalitogenic peptide 91-103 of myelin basic protein. *J Neuroimmunol* 1991; 34(2-3):181–190.

251. Gaur A, Wiers B, Liu A, Rothbard J, Fathman CG. Amelioration of autoimmune encephalomyelitis by myelin basic protein synthetic peptide–induced anergy. *Science* 1992; 258(5087):1491–1494.

252. Genain CP, Abel K, Belmar N, et al. Late complications of immune deviation therapy in a nonhuman primate [see comments]. *Science* 1996; 274(5295):2054–2057.

253. Bitar DM, Whitacre CC. Suppression of experimental autoimmune encephalomyelitis by the oral administration of myelin basic protein. *Cell Immunol* 1988; 112(2):364–370.

254. Higgins PJ, Weiner HL. Suppression of experimental autoimmune encephalomyelitis by oral administration of myelin basic protein and its fragments. *J Immunol* 1988; 140(2):440–445.

255. Whitacre CC, Gienapp IE, Meyer A, Cox KL, Javed N. Oral tolerance in experimental autoimmune encephalomyelitis. *Ann NY Acad Sci* 1996; 778:217–227.

256. Whitacre CC, Gienapp IE, Orosz CG, Bitar DM. Oral tolerance in experimental autoimmune encephalomyelitis. III. Evidence for clonal anergy. *J Immunol* 1991; 147(7):2155–2163.

257. Friedman A, Weiner HL. Induction of anergy or active suppression following oral tolerance is determined by antigen dosage. *Proc Natl Acad Sci USA* 199491(14):6688–6692.

258. Lider O, Santos LM, Lee CS, Higgins PJ, Weiner HL. Suppression of experimental autoimmune encephalomyelitis by oral administration of myelin basic protein. II. Suppression of disease and *in vitro* immune responses is mediated by antigen-specific CD8+ T lymphocytes. *J Immunol* 1989; 142(3):748–752.

259. Miller A, Lider O, Weiner HL. Antigen-driven bystander suppression after oral administration of antigens. *J Exp Med* 1991; 174(4):791–798.

260. Miller A, Lider O, Roberts AB, Sporn MB, Weiner HL. Suppressor T-cells generated by oral tolerization to myelin basic protein suppress both *in vitro* and *in vivo* immune responses by the release of transforming growth factor beta after antigen-specific triggering. *Proc Natl Acad Sci USA* 199289(1):421–425.

261. Chen Y, Inobe J, Marks R, et al. Peripheral deletion of antigen-reactive T-cells in oral tolerance [published erratum appears in *Nature* 1995; 377(6546):257]. *Nature* 1995; 376(6536): 177–180.

262. Al Sabbagh A, Miller A, Santos LM, Weiner HL. Antigen-driven tissue-specific suppression following oral tolerance: orally administered myelin basic protein suppresses proteolipid protein-induced experimental autoimmune encephalomyelitis in the SJL mouse. *Eur J Immunol* 1994; 24(9):2104–2109.

263. Grima B, Zelenika D, Javoy-Agid F, Pessac B. Identification of new human myelin basic protein transcripts in the immune and central nervous systems. *Neurobiol Dis* 1994; 1(1-2):61–66.

264. Pribyl TM, Campagnoni CW, Kampf K, et al. Expression of the myelin proteolipid protein gene in the human fetal thymus. *J Neuroimmunol* 1996; 67(2):125–130.

265. MacKenzie-Graham AJ, Pribyl TM, Kim S, et al. Myelin protein expression is increased in lymph nodes of mice with relapsing experimental autoimmune encephalomyelitis. *J Immunol* 1997; 159(9):4602–4610.

266. Schmied M, Breitschopf H, Gold R, et al. Apoptosis of T lymphocytes in experimental autoimmune encephalomyelitis. evidence for programmed cell death as a mechanism to control inflammation in the brain. *Am J Pathol* 1993; 143(2):446–452.

267. Zeine R, Owens T. Loss rather than downregulation of CD4+ T-cells as a mechanism for remission from experimental allergic encephalomyelitis. *J Neuroimmunol* 1993; 44(2):193–198.

268. Tabi Z, McCombe PA, Pender MP. Apoptotic elimination of V beta 8.2+ cells from the central nervous system during recovery from experimental autoimmune encephalomyelitis induced by the passive transfer of V beta 8.2+ encephalitogenic T-cells. *Eur J Immunol* 1994; 24(11):2609–2617.

269. Tabi Z, McCombe PA, Pender MP. Antigen-specific down-regulation of myelin basic protein-reactive T-cells during spontaneous recovery from experimental autoimmune encephalomyelitis: further evidence of apoptotic deletion of autoreactive T-cells in the central nervous system. *Int Immunol* 1995; 7(6):967–973.

270. Sabelko-Downes KA, Cross AH, Russell JH. Dual role for Fas ligand in the initiation of and recovery from experimental allergic encephalomyelitis. *J Exp Med* 1999; 189(8):1195–1205.

271. Dittel BN, Merchant RM, Janeway CA Jr. Evidence for Fas-dependent and Fas-independent mechanisms in the pathogenesis of experimental autoimmune encephalomyelitis. *J Immunol* 1999; 162(11):6392–6400.

272. McCarron RM, Fallis RJ, McFarlin DE. Alterations in T-cell antigen specificity and class ii restriction during the course of chronic relapsing experimental allergic encephalomyelitis. *J Neuroimmunol* 1990; 29(1-3):73–79.

273. Perry LL, Barzaga-Gilbert E, Trotter JL. T-cell sensitization to proteolipid protein in myelin basic protein–induced relapsing experimental allergic encephalomyelitis. J Neuroimmunol 1991; 33(1):7–15.

274. Miller SD, Vanderlugt CL, Begolka WS, et al. Epitope spreading leads to myelin-specific autoimmune responses in SJL mice chronically infected with Theiler's virus. J Neurovirol 1997; 3(suppl 1):S62–S65.

275. Katz-Levy Y, Neville KL, Girvin AM, et al. Endogenous presentation of self myelin epitopes by CNS-resident APCs in Theiler's virus-infected mice [see comments]. J Clin Invest 1999; 104(5):599–610.

276. Vanderlugt CL, Neville KL, Nikcevich KM, et al. Pathologic role and temporal appearance of newly emerging autoepitopes in relapsing experimental autoimmune encephalomyelitis. J Immunol 2000; 164(2):670–678.

277. Vanderlugt CL, Karandikar NJ, Lenschow DJ, et al. Treatment with intact anti-B7-1 mAb during disease remission enhances epitope spreading and exacerbates relapses in R-EAE. J Neuroimmunol 1997; 79(2):113–118.

278. Rodriguez M, Oleszak E, Leibowitz J. Theiler's murine encephalomyelitis: a model of demyelination and persistence of virus. Crit Rev Immunol 1987; 7(4):325–365.

279. Melvold RW, Jokinen DM, Knobler RL, Lipton HL. Variations in genetic control of susceptibility to Theiler's murine encephalomyelitis virus (TMEV)-induced demyelinating disease. I. Differences between susceptible SJL/J and resistant BALB/c strains map near the T-cell beta-chain constant gene on chromosome 6. J Immunol 1987; 138(5):1429–1433.

280. Kappel CA, Melvold RW, Kim BS. Influence of sex on susceptibility in the Theiler's murine encephalomyelitis virus model for multiple sclerosis. J Neuroimmunol 1990; 29(1-3):15–19.

281. Brahic M, Bureau JF. Genetics of susceptibility to Theiler's virus infection. Bioessays 1998; 20(8):627–633.

282. Miller SD, Gerety SJ, Kennedy MK, et al. Class II–restricted T-cell responses in Theiler's murine encephalomyelitis virus (TMEV)–induced demyelinating disease. III. failure of neuroantigen-specific immune tolerance to affect the clinical course of demyelination. J Neuroimmunol 1990; 26(1):9–23.

283. Lipton HL, Dal Canto MC. Chronic neurologic disease in Theiler's virus infection of SJL/J mice. J Neurol Sci 1976; 30(1):201–207.

284. Dal Canto MC, Lipton HL. Schwann cell remyelination and recurrent demyelination in the central nervous system of mice infected with attenuated Theiler's virus. Am J Pathol 1980; 98(1):101–122.

285. Karpus WJ, Pope JG, Peterson JD, Dal Canto MC, Miller SD. Inhibition of Theiler's virus–mediated demyelination by peripheral immune tolerance induction [published erratum in J Immunol 1996; 156(8):after 3088]. J Immunol 1995; 155(2):947–957.

286. Peterson JD, Waltenbaugh C, Miller SD. IgG subclass responses to Theiler's murine encephalomyelitis virus infection and immunization suggest a dominant role for Th1 cells in susceptible mouse strains. Immunology 1992; 75(4):652–658.

287. Peterson JD, Karpus WJ, Clatch RJ, Miller SD. Split tolerance of Th1 and Th2 cells in tolerance to Theiler's murine encephalomyelitis virus. Eur J Immunol 1993; 23(1):46–55.

288. Gerety SJ, Karpus WJ, Cubbon AR, et al. Class II–restricted T-cell responses in Theiler's murine encephalomyelitis virus–induced demyelinating disease. V. Mapping of a dominant immunopathologic VP2 T-cell epitope in susceptible SJL/J mice. J Immunol 1994; 152(2):908–918.

289. Gerety SJ, Rundell MK, Dal Canto MC, Miller SD. Class II–restricted T-cell responses in Theiler's murine encephalomyelitis virus–induced demyelinating disease. VI. Potentiation of demyelination with and characterization of an immunopathologic CD4+ T-cell line specific for an immunodominant VP2 epitope. J Immunol 1994; 152(2):919–929.

290. Ebers GC, Bulman DE, Sadovnick AD, et al. Population-based study of multiple sclerosis in twins. N Engl J Med 1986; 315(26):1638–1642.

291. Sibley WA, Bamford CR, Clark K. Clinical viral infections and multiple sclerosis. Lancet 1985; 1(8441):1313–1315.

292. Oldstone MB. Molecular mimicry as a mechanism for the cause and a probe uncovering etiologic agent(s) of autoimmune disease. Curr Topics Microbiol Immunol 1989; 145:127–135.

293. Kurtzke JF. Epidemiologic evidence for multiple sclerosis as an infection [published erratum in Clin Microbiol Rev 1994; 7(1):141]. Clin Microbiol Rev 1993; 6(4):382–427.

294. Panitch HS. Influence of infection on exacerbations of multiple sclerosis. Ann Neurol 1994; 36(suppl):S25–S28.

295. Gamble DR. The epidemiology of insulin dependent diabetes with particular reference to the relationship of virus infection to its etiology. Epidemiol Rev 1980; 2:49–70.

296. Yoon JW, Notkins AL. Virus-induced diabetes in mice. Metabolism 1983; 32(suppl 1):37–40.

297. Hafler DA. The Distinction blurs between an autoimmune versus microbial hypothesis in multiple sclerosis [comment]. J Clin Invest 1999; 104(5):527–529.

298. Taurog JD, Richardson JA, Croft JT, et al. The germfree state prevents development of gut and joint inflammatory disease in HLA-B27 transgenic rats. J Exp Med 1994; 180(6):2359–2364.

299. Fujinami RS, Oldstone MB. Amino acid homology between the encephalitogenic site of myelin basic protein and virus: Mechanism for autoimmunity. Science 1985; 230(4729):1043–1045.

300. van Eden W, Holoshitz J, Nevo Z, et al. Arthritis induced by a T-lymphocyte clone that responds to mycobacterium tuberculosis and to cartilage proteoglycans. Proc Natl Acad Sci USA 1985; 82(15):5117–5120.

301. Hemmer B, Vergelli M, Tranquill L, et al. Human T-cell response to myelin basic protein peptide (83-99): Extensive heterogeneity in antigen recognition, function, and phenotype. Neurology 1997; 49(4):1116–1126.

302. Grogan JL, Kramer A, Nogai A, et al. Cross-reactivity of myelin basic protein–specific T-cells with multiple microbial peptides: Experimental autoimmune encephalomyelitis induction in TCR transgenic mice. J Immunol 1999; 163(7):3764–3770.

303. Garza KM, Tung KS. Frequency of molecular mimicry among T-cell peptides as the basis for autoimmune disease and autoantibody induction. J Immunol 1995; 155(11):5444–5448.

304. Alldinger S, Fonfara S, Kremmer E, Baumgartner W. Up-regulation of the hyaluronate receptor CD44 in canine distemper demyelinated plaques. Acta Neuropathol (Berl) 2000; 99(2):138–146.

305. Talbot PJ, Paquette JS, Ciurli C, Antel JP, Ouellet F. Myelin basic protein and human coronavirus 229E cross-reactive T-cells in multiple sclerosis. Ann Neurol 1996; 39(2):233–240.

306. Gautam AM, Liblau R, Chelvanayagam G, Steinman L, Boston T. A viral peptide with limited homology to a self peptide can induce clinical signs of experimental autoimmune encephalomyelitis. J Immunol 1998; 161(1):60–64.

307. Mokhtarian F, Zhang Z, Shi Y, Gonzales E, Sobel RA. Molecular mimicry between a viral peptide and a myelin oligodendrocyte glycoprotein peptide induces autoimmune demyelinating disease in mice. J Neuroimmunol 1999; 95(1-2):43–54.

308. Ruiz PJ, Garren H, Hirschberg DL, et al. Microbial epitopes act as altered peptide ligands to prevent experimental autoimmune encephalomyelitis. J Exp Med 1999; 189(8):1275–1284.

309. Oldstone MB. Virus–induced autoimmunity: molecular mimicry as a route to autoimmune disease. J Autoimmun 1989; 2 (suppl):187–194.

310. Oldstone MB. Molecular mimicry and immune-mediated diseases. FASEB J 1998; 12(13):1255–1265.

311. Oldstone MB. Molecular mimicry and autoimmune disease [published erratum in Cell 1987; 51(5):878]. Cell 1987; 50(6):819–820.

312. Ufret-Vincenty RL, Quigley L, Tresser N, et al. In vivo survival of viral antigen-specific T-cells that induce experimental autoimmune encephalomyelitis. J Exp Med 1998; 188(9):1725–1738.

313. Arredondo LR, Deng C, Ratts RB, et al. Role of nerve growth factor in experimental autoimmune encephalomyelitis. Eur J Immunol 2001; 31:625–633.

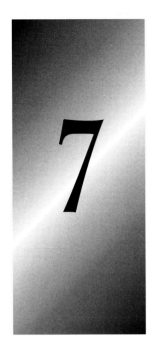

# 7

# Tissue Culture Studies of Demyelination and Remyelination

*Fredrick J. Seil, M.D.*

Tissue culture studies of serum antimyelin factors were initiated with Bornstein's and Appel's description almost four decades ago of demyelination of rat organotypic cerebellar cultures by sera from rabbits with experimental allergic encephalomyelitis (EAE) induced by inoculation with whole central nervous system (CNS) tissue combined with complete Freund adjuvant (CFA) (1). After application of sera to myelinated cultures, neuroglia became swollen and myelin sheaths increased in brightness. Some myelin sheaths then developed fusiform swellings and eventually fragmented, whereas others were described as "melting" away and fading into the glial background. Axons were unaffected and remyelinated after replacement of the demyelinating sera with normal medium. Demyelination was complement dependent, because heating sera to 56°C eliminated the demyelinating activity, which was restored by addition of fresh guinea pig serum. Myelinated cultures of rat spinal ganglia were unaffected because the demyelination was specific for CNS myelin.

In a subsequent study, Bornstein reported similar demyelinating activity in 68 percent of sera from human subjects with active multiple sclerosis (MS), whereas most normal human sera did not demyelinate CNS cultures (2). Remyelination also occurred as a consequence of reapplication of normal nutrient medium. The results of these tissue culture studies of serum demyelinating factors sug-

gested a role for humoral factors, possibly antibodies, in the pathogenesis of experimental and human demyelinating disease. Subsequent studies were aimed at the further characterization and identification of specific factors in sera from animals with EAE and human subjects with MS that induced demyelination. Discussion of the electrophysiologic effects of serum factors in tissue culture studies of demyelinating disease was included in previous reviews (3,4) and is not addressed further in this chapter.

## EAE AND SERUM DEMYELINATING FACTORS

### Characterization of Antimyelin Factors

Demyelinating activity in sera from rabbits with EAE induced by inoculation with whole CNS tissue (anti-CNS sera) was found in the immunoglobulin G2 (IgG2) fraction and was abolished by absorption with homologous or heterologous brain but not with other tissues such as lung, liver, kidney, or red blood cells (5). With immunofluorescent techniques, globulins in demyelinating anti-CNS sera were localized on myelin sheaths of cerebellar cultures, a localization subsequently supported with immunoperoxidase methods (6). The finding of demyelinating activity in the IgG2 fraction of anti-CNS sera was confirmed by Lebar et al. who did not find similar activity in serum IgG1 or IgM fractions

(7). Demyelinating activity was reduced by the removal of most of the IgG from anti-CNS sera, and the isolated IgG fraction was capable of demyelinating CNS cultures (8). These studies supported the antibody nature of the demyelinating factor. The complement dependence of the serum demyelinating activity was confirmed in a study by Liu et al. who also demonstrated a requirement for the terminal complement proteins (9). These results were interpreted as implying that activation of the membrane attack complex of complement, C5b-9, may be the factor responsible for myelin damage.

Whereas remyelination occurred after removal of demyelinating anti-CNS sera from CNS cultures, Bornstein and Raine found that remyelination was prevented by continued exposure to low concentrations of anti-CNS serum, concentrations that were insufficient to produce the initial demyelination (10). They also noted that, when anti-CNS sera were applied to mouse spinal cord and dorsal root ganglia cultures before myelination, glial differentiation and central myelin formation were inhibited. The inhibition of myelination was complement dependent and reversible and was specific for CNS myelin. Myelination inhibition also occurred with low concentrations of serum and thus was considered to be a more sensitive assay of serum antimyelin activity than demyelination.

Examination of CNS cultures by electron microscopy after application of anti-CNS sera in the presence of complement found two patterns of demyelination (11). One consisted of intramyelinic swellings with splitting of major and minor dense lines, and the second was characterized by a "smudging" of the myelin sheaths, with altered periodicity and the development of fingerprintlike configurations. These patterns of demyelination corresponded to patterns previously observed by light microscopy (1). Myelin debris was found initially extracellularly but then found in macrophages and astrocytes. Many oligodendrocytes showed degenerative changes, and dense oligodendrocytes disappeared. If cultures were exposed to decomplemented anti-CNS sera, demyelination did not occur, but there was a doubling of the space between the major dense lines, and the minor dense lines contained four rather than two electron-dense leaflets (12). The doubling of the myelin period corresponded to the increased brightness of the myelin sheaths noted by light microscopy (1). This complement-independent step was considered the first stage of the demyelinating reaction consequent to exposure to anti-CNS serum (12).

No differentiated glia were observed in cultures exposed to anti-CNS sera before myelination (10). Dense oligodendrocytes, myelin, and typical astroglia did not appear until several days after removal of the anti-CNS sera. Application of decomplemented antisera to CNS cultures before myelination did not inhibit

oligodendrocyte differentiation, but these cells produced a profusion of cytoplasmic processes that formed myelin with doubled periodicity and which frequently failed to ensheath axons (13,14).

## Specificity of Antimyelin Factors

The described tissue culture studies supporting a possible role for antimyelin antibodies in the pathogenesis of EAE were done with sera from animals with EAE induced by sensitization with whole CNS or CNS white matter. Because EAE also could be induced by inoculation of myelin components, it was of interest to assess the demyelinating and myelination inhibiting capacity of sera from animals sensitized with specific myelin fractions.

The first such attempt was made by Lumsden, who applied sera from animals inoculated with a diffusible encephalitogenic peptide to myelinated organotypic CNS cultures (15). The sera failed to demyelinate the cultures, which Lumsden attributed to a lack of "antigenicity" of his peptide. Subsequently, my colleagues and I exposed myelinated mouse cerebellar cultures to sera from guinea pigs with EAE induced by sensitization with myelin basic protein (MBP) combined with CFA (16). MBP was the first established encephalitogenic myelin protein (17,18). We also inoculated some guinea pigs initially with MBP in combination with incomplete Freund adjuvant (without *Mycobacterium tuberculosis*), followed by a challenge dose of MBP with CFA, which resulted in the production of high titers of antibody to MBP. As a positive control, we also exposed cultures to sera from guinea pigs with EAE induced by inoculation with whole CNS plus CFA. Neither the sera from the animals with EAE induced by MBP nor the sera from the hyperimmunized animals demyelinated cerebellar cultures. Cultures were demyelinated by sera from guinea pigs with EAE induced by sensitization with whole CNS, but none of these sera had detectable levels of antibody to MBP.

We subsequently assessed myelination inhibiting activity of sera from animals sensitized or hyperimmunized with MBP in a series of studies. In the first of these studies, most sera from guinea pigs inoculated with bovine MBP and containing high titers of anti-MBP antibody did not inhibit myelination in mouse cerebellar cultures, whereas most sera from guinea pigs inoculated with equivalent amounts of whole CNS and containing low titers of antibody to MBP did inhibit myelination (19). Sera from subhuman primates with EAE induced by sensitization with MBP also failed to inhibit myelination in cerebellar cultures, whereas anti-CNS sera from subhuman primates were positive for myelination inhibition (20). Similar results were obtained with sera from Lewis rats sensitized with guinea pig MBP or guinea pig whole CNS, with sera from the former being negative and sera from the latter being positive for inhibition of myelination in CNS cultures (21). In the final study of this series, myelination inhibiting capabilities of sera from rabbits sensitized with bovine whole CNS tissue and sensitized or hyperimmunized with MBP from five different species (bovine, guinea pig, rabbit, monkey, and human) were compared (22). All the rabbits inoculated with whole CNS tissue plus CFA developed EAE, and all their sera inhibited myelination in mouse cerebellar cultures without detectable titers of precipitating antibody to MBP. The rabbits sensitized or hyperimmunized with MBP developed all possible combinations of EAE and precipitating antibody. Serum from one of these animals inhibited myelination, and this animal had neither EAE nor detectable anti-MBP antibody, whereas sera from the remaining eight animals, including those with EAE and high titers of antibody to MBP, were negative for myelination inhibition. Thus, there was a complete dissociation of myelination inhibiting activity, induction of EAE, and formation of anti-MBP antibody.

Tissue culture demyelinating activity was found by Dubois-Dalcq et al. in sera from rabbits inoculated with CFA and cerebroside, a nonencephalitogenic glycolipid component of myelin (23). Demyelination was not restricted to CNS myelin in spinal cord and dorsal root ganglion cultures because some peripherally myelinated fibers also were affected. The demyelinating activity of sera from cerebroside-sensitized rabbits was confirmed by Fry et al., who also showed that these sera inhibited myelination in CNS cultures (24). These investigators found anticerebroside antibodies in rabbit anti-CNS sera and in anticerebroside sera, and they abolished the demyelinating and myelination inhibiting activities of both sera by absorption with cerebroside. Sera from Lewis rats sensitized with cerebroside did not inhibit myelination of cerebellar cultures (21), and demyelinating activity was not obtained with sera from cerebroside-inoculated guinea pigs (7) because antimyelin effects appeared to be restricted to rabbit antisera. Hruby et al. demonstrated myelination inhibition in CNS cultures by sera from rabbits sensitized with synthetic galactocerebrosides (GC), thus ruling out any possible contamination with other myelin components (25). Myelination inhibition was not obtained with rabbit antisera directed against glucocerebrosides, thereby establishing that the antimyelin activity was specific to anti-GC sera.

The peripheral demyelinating property of rabbit anti-GC sera was confirmed by Saida et al. (26). In a later study, Ranscht et al. described inhibition of myelination of cultured dorsal root ganglion neurons by Schwann cells with a mouse-derived monoclonal antibody to GC (27). The action of anti-GC antibodies against peripheral myelin stands apart from the repeatedly described (1,10, 28–30) specificity of anti-CNS sera for central myelin.

As an encephalitogenic myelin protein, MBP, did not induce antimyelin antibodies and as antisera to GC,

a nonencephalitogenic myelin glycolipid, demyelinated and inhibited myelination of CNS cultures, the antigenic properties of other myelin components were investigated. Proteolipid protein (PLP), the major CNS myelin protein, induced a chronic form of EAE (31,32), but sera from animals sensitized with PLP neither demyelinated nor inhibited myelination when applied to CNS cultures (29,33). Myelin-associated glycoprotein (MAG), a minor component of CNS myelin, did not induce EAE, but its localization at the myelin membrane surface (34,35) made it a candidate for induction of antimyelin antibodies. Rabbit antisera to MAG did not demyelinate or inhibit myelination of CNS cultures (30). Mouse monoclonal antibodies to MAG interfered with neuron–oligodendrocyte adhesion in dissociated cell cultures (36). By immunoabsorption and fractionation experiments and complement fixation studies, Lebar et al. characterized tissue culture demyelinating factors in sera from whole CNS-sensitized or CNS myelin-sensitized guinea pigs as antibodies to an antigen designated "M2" (7,37). M2, which was different from MBP and GC and not present in peripheral myelin, was later identified as a glycoprotein component of oligodendrocyte membrane (38).

Immunization of rabbits with gangliosides, glycolipid components of neuronal and myelin membranes, induced a demyelinating disease (39–41). Roth et al. claimed that antisera to GM1, a major ganglioside, caused demyelination of spinal cord tissue cultures (42). The reported myelin reduction was only 20 to 25 percent, and was not supported in a follow-up study from the same laboratory (43). Another group of investigators found no demyelinating or myelination inhibiting activity in spinal cord and dorsal root ganglia cultures exposed to four high titer rabbit anti-GM1 sera (44).

## Antibodies to CMIP and MOG

Extraction of CNS myelin with chlorform-methanol selectively removes PLP, almost all of the MBP, and most lipids (45). The remaining chloroform-methanol insoluble protein (CMIP) fraction contains a large number of low- and high-molecular-weight proteins, among them Wolfgram protein (acidic PLP), MAG, and other glycoproteins, including M2 and the myelin oligodendrocyte glycoprotein (MOG) (46–48). MOG is a minor myelin protein localized at the external surfaces of myelin sheaths and oligodendrocyte membranes (49). Rabbits inoculated with the CMIP fraction and CFA did not develop clinical EAE, but histopathologic examination showed occasional focal mononuclear inflammatory infiltrates in perivascular spaces or sometimes spread into the surrounding parenchyma (50). Antibodies were elicited to a large number of proteins, but anti-GC antibodies were not evident by enzyme-linked immunosorbent assay or immunoblot assays (H.C. Agrawal, unpublished observations). Anti-CMIP sera inhibited myelination of cerebellar cultures and demyelinated centrally myelinated fibers in spinal cord and dorsal root ganglia cultures but spared peripherally myelinated fibers (50). The specific action against CNS myelin was similar to that reported for anti-CNS sera. It was subsequently shown that the demyelination and myelin inhibition are rapidly reversed with removal of anti-CMIP sera from the cultures (F.J. Seil and H.C. Agrawal, unpublished observations). In an initial attempt to identify the CMIP component that elicited antimyelin antibodies, the most likely suspect, Wolfgram protein, was ruled out (F.J. Seil, D.N. Bourdette, and H.C. Agrawal, unpublished observations).

Ultrastructural studies of anti-CMIP serum-induced demyelination and myelination inhibition (R.M. Herndon, F.J. Seil, and H.C. Agrawal, unpublished observations) revealed some differences from the changes described with anti-CNS sera (10,11). Whereas oligodendrocytes were extensively destroyed by anti-CNS sera, many survived in cultures demyelinated by anti-CMIP sera. When anti-CNS sera were applied to cultures before myelination, oligodendrocyte differentiation was profoundly inhibited and few oligodendrocytes could be identified. Light, intermediate, and dark oligodendroglia were evident in cultures in which myelination was inhibited by anti-CMIP sera. Many of the oligodendrocytes were vacuolated to some degree, with the most severe vacuolar changes appearing in the dark (most differentiated) oligodendroglia. However, oligodendrocytes were clearly differentiated and present in substantial numbers. Anti-CMIP sera appeared to interfere with glial–axonal interactions to inhibit myelin formation rather than with oligodendrocyte maturation.

Immunization of rodents with MOG induced acute and chronic EAE (51–53). Recently, it was shown that, by changing immunization protocols and using different inbred rat strains, a variety of chronic disease courses could be produced (54). Before the encephalitogenicity of MOG had been defined, a correlation was found between in vivo demyelinating activity in guinea pigs with chronic EAE and titers of antibody to MOG (55). Moreover, demyelination was greatly augmented in acute EAE in rats by intravenous injection of a monoclonal anti-MOG antibody (56). Application of this monoclonal anti-MOG antibody to myelinated reaggregating brain cell cultures induced reversible complement-dependent demyelination (57). Myelination inhibition was not assayed, the antibody was not tested against peripherally myelinated fibers, and no ultrastructural examination of patterns of demyelination in tissue culture has been reported. Because MOG is present in the CMIP fraction of myelin, the behavior of anti-MOG sera likely would be similar in all of these respects to those described for anti-CMIP sera. It is also probable that MOG and M2 are the same glycoproteins.

**TABLE 7.1**
*EAE and Antibody Induction by CNS Antigens*

| | | ANTIBODIES | | |
| | | DEMYELINATING | | MYELINATION INHIBITING |
| ANTIGEN | EAE | CNS | PNS | CNS |
| --- | --- | --- | --- | --- |
| Whole CNS | + | + | − | + |
| MBP | + | − | − | − |
| GC | − | + | + | + |
| PLP | + | − | − | − |
| MAG | − | − | − | − |
| CMIP | ±* | + | − | + |
| M2 | ND | + | ND† | ND |
| MOG | + | + | ND | ND |
| GM1 | ±‡ | − | − | − |

CMIP; chloroform-methanol insoluble protein fraction of myelin; CNS; central nervous system; EAE; experimental allergic encephalomyelitis; GC; galactocerebroside; GM1; GM1 ganglioside; M2; a CNS myelin glycoprotein identified as an antigen that induced demyelinating antibodies found in anti-CNS and anti-CNS myelin sera; MAG; myelin-associated glycoprotein; MBP; myelin basic protein; MOG; myelin oligodendrocyte glycoprotein; ND; not determined; PLP; myelin proteolipid protein; PNS; peripheral nervous system.

*No clinical EAE but occasional perivascular inflammatory infiltrates histologically.

†Sera containing anti-M2 antibodies did not bind to PNS myelin.

‡Several reports of induction of an experimental demyelinating disease in rabbits.

Table 7.1 presents a summary of CNS and myelin antigens and their ability to induce EAE and/or antimyelin factors active in tissue cultures.

## MS AND SERUM DEMYELINATING FACTORS

After Bornstein's initial study (2), Bornstein and Hummelgard reported on serum demyelinating activity in an expanded series of human subjects with MS (58). Demyelinating activity was found in 64 percent of sera from patients with definitely active disease, 41 percent of sera from patients in whom disease activity was not clearly evident at the time of serum sampling, 11 percent of sera from patients without disease activity, and 7 percent of sera from normal subjects. When the overall course of the disease was considered, they found that 71 percent of sera from patients with active exacerbating and remitting MS demyelinated CNS tissue cultures compared with 48 percent of sera from patients with a chronic–progressive course. In other reported series, Ulrich and Lardi found serum demyelinating activity in 36 percent of MS subjects with active disease and in 6 percent without disease activity (59), and Seil et al. reported that 40 percent of sera from patients with active disease demyelinated spinal cord cultures compared with 5 percent of sera from patients during stationary periods (60). Bradbury et al. found demyelinating activity in 74 percent of sera from subjects with MS, in 68 percent of sera from patients with a wide range of diseases other than MS, and in 22 percent of sera from normal human subjects (61). The occurrence of demyelinating activity in a significant number of sera from patients with other neurologic diseases, especially amyotrophic lateral sclerosis (ALS), had been reported by others (2,59,62).

Sera from subjects with MS specifically demyelinated CNS cultures and did not affect peripherally myelinated fibers (28). Curiously, demyelinating MS sera did not inhibit myelination in spinal cord and cerebellar cultures (59,60). The ultrastructural characteristics of demyelination induced by MS sera were similar to those described for anti-CNS sera, except that demyelination proceeded more slowly and was less extensive (63). The most frequently observed change was an alteration of the myelin periodicity, with breakdown into smudged or fingerprintlike areas. Astrocytic processes surrounded and phagocytosed the degenerating myelin. A portion of the population of oligodendrocytes degenerated acutely or subacutely and were phagocytosed by astrocytes. A late change noted in some of the sheaths was a doubling of the myelin period.

Demyelinating activity of MS sera was removed by absorption with brain tissue (2) and a nonmyelin CNS tissue pellet that included oligodendrocytes but not with purified myelin (64). No immunostained myelin was found when demyelinating MS sera were applied to CNS cultures and fixed and treated with peroxidase-conjugated anti-human globulin, suggesting that the demyelinating activity of MS sera was not associated with a myelin-binding immunoglobulin (6). Depletion of MS sera of all γ-globulin did not decrease their tissue culture demyelinating capability, and isolated Ig fractions from most MS sera did not demyelinate CNS cultures (65,66). These findings further support the notion that demyelinating activity in most MS sera is associated with some serum factor other than γ-globulin.

Of interest is a report of the detection of anti-MOG antibodies in the sera of 8 of 16 MS patients and the identification of anti-MOG antibody-producing B lymphocytes in their cerebrospinal fluid (67). This was not specific for MS, however, because patients with other neurologic diseases also had elevated plasma and cerebrospinal fluid levels of antibody to MOG (68). Recently, anti-MOG antibodies were detected by a sensitive immunocytochemical technique as bound to dis-

integrating myelin sheaths in acute lesions from 3 patients with MS (69). The vesicular demyelination and the anti-MOG antibody binding were identical to those seen in marmosets with EAE induced by inoculation with MOG and CFA (69,70). Thus, MOG could be a target for antibody-mediated demyelination in at least some cases of MS (71).

## POSSIBLE SIGNIFICANCE OF ANTIMYELIN FACTORS

Raine and coworkers compared histopathologic changes in EAE induced in guinea pigs by inoculation of CFA and whole white matter or MBP, MBP plus GC, or MBP plus total myelin lipids (72). Clinically, EAE induced by whole white matter and MBP were similar, but whole white matter provoked inflammatory and demyelinating lesions, whereas only inflammatory lesions were observed in MBP-induced EAE. GC or total myelin lipids, when given separately, induced neither EAE nor histopathologic changes. When GC or total myelin lipids were injected in combination with MBP, EAE with inflammatory and demyelinating lesions was induced. The lipid haptens appeared to have an augmenting effect on MBP, and the investigators speculated that MBP triggers the T-cell component of the immune response in EAE and that B-cell–secreted factors induced by GC or other lipid haptens are necessary for demyelination to occur.

In a similar vein, Bourdette et al. subjected guinea pigs to a suboptimal transfer (insufficient to transfer EAE) of lymphocytes sensitized to MBP, followed by immunization with CFA and MBP, chicken brain alone, or MBP plus chicken brain or myelin (73). Chicken MBP is not encephalitogenic in guinea pigs (74), so that the chicken brain functioned as a source of all of the non-MBP components of whole CNS, including lipids and glycoproteins. Myelination inhibiting activity of sera collected from the guinea pigs was correlated with the degree of histologically graded demyelination of spinal cord and brain sections. Moderate to severe demyelination and myelination inhibiting antibodies were found only in animals receiving both MBP and chicken brain or myelin, and not with MBP or chicken brain alone. These results were consistent with the notion that antibodies directed against non-MBP (nonencephalitogenic) components of CNS augment the extent of demyelination in EAE.

Antibody to MOG can augment demyelination when injected intravenously during induction of EAE by transfer of MBP-sensitized T-cells (56). The concept of a combined action of cellular and humoral mechanisms to produce inflammatory demyelinating lesions in EAE was further supported by the finding that MOG, which induced EAE with inflammatory and demyelinating components, elicited a T-cell–mediated immune reaction and a B-cell–secreted demyelinating antibody response (51–53). The combined action of cellular and antibody mechanisms does not appear to be an invariable requirement for demyelination in EAE, however, because extensive demyelination can occur in some species or strains and in some circumstances without augmentation by antibodies. For instance, in chronic EAE induced in SJL/J mice by passive transfer with MBP sensitized T-cells, considerable demyelination can occur, even with the initial episode, in the absence of antibodies that bind to myelin (75).

MS has come to be regarded as an autoimmune inflammatory demyelinating disease with heterogeneous pathology and pathogenesis (71,76,77). Recent reports of binding of anti-MOG antibodies to myelin undergoing vesicular disintegration in acute lesions from three cases of MS suggested one mechanism for demyelination in MS (69,70). MOG is a logical target for demyelination, and antibody-augmented or antibody-induced demyelination is consistent with the concept of combined T-cell and B-cell mechanisms in the pathogenesis of the animal model of MS, i.e., EAE. However, serum demyelinating factors in most cases of MS do not appear to be antibodies (6,65,66), which has lent support to the notion that B-cell–dependent demyelination may be restricted to a small subgroup of MS patients (78–80). Moreover, serum demyelinating factors correlated with disease activity in some cases of MS (2,58–61) but are not specific for MS, because demyelinating activity was reported in sera from a significant proportion of patients with other neurologic diseases (2,59,61,62). Three patients represent a very small sampling of the total spectrum of MS, so much additional work is needed as a follow-up to the promising start of Genain et al. (69) in defining the extent of an antibody role for demyelination in MS (also see comments by Karni et al. 68 and Wekerle 81). Perhaps a reexamination of the relationship of tissue culture demyelinating factors in MS to Ig should be included.

## Acknowledgments

Studies from the author's laboratory were supported by the Medical Research Service of the Department of Veterans Affairs.

## References

1. Bornstein MB, Appel SH. The application of tissue culture to the study of experimental "allergic" encephalomyelitis. *J Neuropathol Exp Neurol* 1961; 20:141–157.
2. Bornstein MB. A tissue culture approach to the demyelinative disorders. *NCI Monogr* 1963; 11:197–214.
3. Seil FJ. Tissue culture studies of demyelinating diseases: a critical review. *Ann Neurol* 1977; 2:345–355.
4. Seil FJ. Tissue culture studies of neuroelectric blocking factors. In: Waxman SG, Ritchie JM (eds.), *Demyelinating Disease: Basic And Clinical Electrophysiology*. New York: Raven Press; 1981; 281–288.
5. Appel SH, Bornstein MB. The application of tissue culture to the study of experimental allergic encephalomyelitis. II. Serum factors responsible for demyelination. *J Exp Med* 1964; 119:303–312.
6. Johnson AB, Bornstein MB. Myelin-binding antibodies in vitro. Immunoperoxidase studies with experimental allergic encephalomyelitis, anti-galactocerebroside and multiple sclerosis sera. *Brain Res* 1978; 159:173–182.
7. Lebar R, Boutry J-M, Vincent C, Robineaux R, Voisin A. Studies on autoimmune encephalomyelitis in the guinea pig. II. An in vitro investigation on the nature, properties, and specificity of the serum-demyelinating factor. *J Immunol* 1976; 116:1439–1446.
8. Grundke-Iqbal I, Raine CS, Johnson AB, Brosnan CF, Bornstein MB. Experimental allergic encephalomyelitis. Characterization of serum factors causing demyelination and swelling of myelin. *J Neurol Sci* 1981; 50:63–79.
9. Liu WT, Vanguri P, Shin ML. Studies on demyelination in vitro: the requirement of membrane attack components of the complement system. *J Immunol* 1983; 131:778–782.
10. Bornstein MB, Raine CS. Experimental allergic encephalomyelitis: antiserum inhibition of myelination in vitro. *Lab Invest* 1970; 23:536–542.
11. Raine CS, Bornstein MB. Experimental allergic encephalomyelitis: an ultrastructural study of experimental demyelination in vitro. *J Neuropathol Exp Neurol* 1970; 29:177–191.
12. Bornstein MB, Raine CS. The initial lesion in serum-induced demyelination in vitro. *Lab Invest* 1976; 35:391–401.
13. Diaz M, Bornstein MB, Raine CS. Disorganization of myelinogenesis in tissue culture by anti-CNS serum. *Brain Res* 1978; 154:231–239.
14. Raine CS, Diaz M, Pakingan M, Bornstein MB. Antiserum-induced dissociation of myelinogenesis in vitro. An ultrastructural study. *Lab Invest* 1978; 38:397–403.
15. Lumsden CE. Immunopathological events in multiple sclerosis. *Int Congr Ser Excerpta Med* 1966; 100:231–239.
16. Seil FJ, Falk GA, Kies MW, Alvord EC Jr. The in vitro demyelinating activity of sera from guinea pigs sensitized with whole CNS and with purified encephalitogen. *Exp Neurol* 1968; 22:545–55.
17. Kies MW, Alvord EC Jr. Encephalitogenic activity in guinea pigs of water-soluble protein fractions of nervous tissue. In: Kies MW, Alvord EC Jr. (eds.), *"Allergic" Encephalomyelitis*. Springfield: Thomas; 1959; 293–299.
18. Kies MW, Thompson EB, Alvord EC Jr. The relationship of myelin proteins to experimental allergic encephalomyelitis. *Ann NY Acad Sci* 1965; 122:146–160.
19. Kies MW, Driscoll BF, Seil FJ, Alvord EC Jr. Myelination inhibition factor: dissociation from induction of experimental allergic encephalomyelitis. *Science* 1973; 179:689–690.
20. Seil FJ, Rauch HC, Einstein ER, Hamilton AE. Myelination inhibition factor: its absence in sera from subhuman primates sensitized with myelin basic protein. *J Immunol* 1973;111:96–100.
21. Seil FJ, Smith ME, Leiman AL, Kelly JM. Myelination inhibiting and neuroelectric blocking factors in experimental allergic encephalomyelitis. *Science* 1975;187:951-953.
22. Seil FJ, Kies MW, Bacon, ML. Neural antigens and induction of myelination inhibition factor. *J Immunol* 1975; 114:630–634.
23. Dubois-Dalcq M, Niedieck B, Buyse M. Action of anti-cerebroside sera on myelinated tissue cultures. *Pathol Eur* 1970; 5:331–347.
24. Fry JM, Weissbarth S, Lehrer GM, Bornstein MB. Cerebroside antibody inhibits sulfatide synthesis and myelination and demyelinates in cord tissue cultures. *Science* 1974; 183:540–542.
25. Hruby S, Alvord EC Jr, Seil FJ. Synthetic galactocerebrosides evoke myelination-inhibiting antibodies. *Science* 1977; 195:173–175.
26. Saida T, Silberberg DH, Fry JM, Manning MC. Demyelinating antigalactocerebroside antibodies in EAN and EAE. *J Neuropathol Exp Neurol* 1977; 36:627.
27. Ranscht B, Wood PM, Bunge RB. Inhibition of in vitro peripheral myelin formation by monoclonal anti-galactocerebroside. *J Neurosci* 1987; 7:2936–2947.
28. Bornstein MB, Raine CS. Multiple sclerosis and experimental allergic encephalomyelitis: specific demyelination of CNS in culture. *Neuropathol Appl Neurobiol* 1977; 3:359–367.
29. Seil FJ, Agrawal HC. Myelin-proteolipid protein does not induce

demyelinating or myelination-inhibiting antibodies. *Brain Res* 1980; 194:273–277.

30. Seil FJ, Quarles RH, Johnson D, Brady RO. Immunization with purified myelin-associated glycoprotein does not evoke myelination-inhibiting or demyelinating antibodies. *Brain Res* 1981; 209:470–475.

31. Williams RM, Lees MB, Cambi F, Macklin WB. Chronic experimental allergic encephalomyelitis induced in rabbits with bovine white matter proteolipid apoprotein. *J Neuropathol Exp Neurol* 1982; 41:508–521.

32. Cambi F, Lees MB, Williams RM, Macklin WB. Chronic experimental allergic encephalomyelitis produced by bovine proteolipid apoprotein: immunological studies in rabbits. *Ann Neurol* 1983; 13:303–308.

33. Mithen F, Bunge R, Agrawal H. Proteolipid protein antiserum does not affect CNS myelin in rat spinal cord culture. *Brain Res* 1980; 197:477–483.

34. Quarles RH, Everly JL, Brady RO. Demonstration of a glycoprotein which is associated with a purified myelin fraction from rat brain. *Biochem Biophys Res Commun* 1972; 47:491–497.

35. Poduslo JF, Quarles RH, Brady RO. External labeling of galactose in surface membrane glycoproteins of the intact myelin sheath. *J Biol Chem* 1976; 251:153–158.

36. Poltorak M, Sadoul R, Keilhauer G, et al. Myelin-associated glycoprotein, a member of the L2/HNK-1 family of neural cell adhesion molecules, is involved in neuron-oligodendrocyte and oligodendrocyte-oligodendrocyte interaction. *J Cell Biol* 1987; 105:1893–1899.

37. Lebar R, Vincent C, Fischer-le Boubennec E. Studies on autoimmune encephalomyelitis in the guinea pig. III. A comparative study of two autoantigens of central nervous system myelin. *J Neurochem* 1979; 33:1451–1460.

38. Lebar R, Lubetzki C, Vincent C, Lombrail P, Boutry J-M. The M2 autoantigen of central nervous system myelin, a glycoprotein present in oligodendrocyte membrane. *Clin Exp Immunol* 1986; 66:423–443.

39. Nagai Y, Momoi T, Saito M, Mitsuzawa E, Ohtani S. Ganglioside syndrome, a new autoimmune neurologic disorder, experimentally induced with brain gangliosides. *Neurosci Lett* 1976; 2:107–111.

40. Cohen O, Schwartz M, Cohen IR, Sela B-A, Eshhar N. Multiple sclerosis-like disease in rabbits by immunization with brain gangliosides. *Isr J Med Sci* 1981; 17:711–714.

41. Konat G, Offner H, Lev-Ram V, et al. Abnormalities in brain myelin of rabbits with experimental autoimmune multiple sclerosis-like disease induced by immunization to gangliosides. *Acta Neurol Scand* 1982; 66:568–574.

42. Roth GA, Roytta M, Yu RK, Raine CS, Bornstein MB. Antisera to different glycolipids induce myelin alterations in mouse spinal cord tissue cultures. *Brain Res* 1985; 339:9–18.

43. Saito M, Macala LJ, Roth GA, Bornstein MB, Yu RK. Effect of antiglycolipid antisera on the lipid composition of cultured mouse spinal cord. *Exp Neurol* 1986; 92:752–756.

44. Bourdette DN, Zalc B, Baumann N, Seil FJ. Antisera to the ganglioside GM1 do not have anti-myelin or anti-axon activities in vitro. *Brain Res* 1989; 478:175–180.

45. Gonzales-Sastre F. The protein composition of isolated myelin. *J Neurochem* 1970; 17:1049–1056.

46. Wolfgram F, Kotorii K. The composition of the myelin proteins of the central nervous system. *J Neurochem* 1968; 15:1281–1290.

47. Quarles RH, Pasnak CF. A rapid procedure for selectively isolating the major glycoprotein from purified rat brain myelin. *Biochem J* 1977; 163:635–637.

48. Reig JA, Rames JM, Cozar M, et al. Purification and chemical characterization of a W2 protein from rat brain myelin. *J Neurochem* 1982; 39:507–511.

49. Brunner C, Lassmann H, Waehneldt TV, Matthieu J-M, Linington C. Differential ultrastructural localization of myelin basic protein, myelin/oligodendrocyte glycoprotein, and 2', 3'-cyclic nucleotide 3'-phosphodiesterase in the CNS of adult rats. *J Neurochem* 1989; 52:296–304.

50. Seil FJ, Garwood MM, Clark HB, Agrawal HC. Demyelinating and myelination-inhibiting factors induced by chloroform-methanol insoluble proteins of myelin. *Brain Res* 1983; 288:384–388.

51. Armor S, Groome N, Linington C, et al. Identification of epitopes of myelin oligodendrocyte glycoprotein for the induction of experimental allergic encephalomyelitis in SJL and Biozzi AB/H mice. *J Immunol* 1994; 153:4349–4356.

52. Adelmann M, Wood J, Benzel I, et al. The N-terminal domain of the myelin oligodendrocyte glycoprotein (MOG) induces acute demyelinating experimental autoimmune encephalomyelitis in the Lewis rat. *J Neuroimmunol* 1995; 63:17–27.

53. Johns TG, Kerlero de Rosbo N, Menon KK, et al. Myelin oligodendrocyte glycoprotein induces a demyelinating encephalomyelitis resembling multiple sclerosis. *J Immunol* 1995; 154:5536–5541.

54. Storch MK, Stefferl A, Brehm U, et al. Autoimmunity to myelin oligodendrocyte glycoprotein in rats mimics the spectrum of multiple sclerosis pathology. *Brain Pathol* 1998; 8:681–694.

55. Linington C, Lassmann H. Antibody responses in chronic relapsing experimental allergic encephalomyelitis: Correlation of serum demyelinating activity with antibody titre to the myelin/oligodendrocyte glycoprotein (MOG). *J Neuroimmunol* 1987; 17:61–69.

56. Linington C, Bradl M, Lassmann H, Brunner C, Vass K. Augmentation of demyelination in rat acute encephalomyelitis by circulating mouse monoclonal antibodies directed against a myelin/oligodendrocyte glycoprotein. *Am J Pathol* 1988; 130:443–454.

57. Kerlero de Rosbo N, Honneger P, Lassmann H, Mattieu J-M. Demyelination induced in aggregating brain cell cultures by a monoclonal antibody against myelin/oligodendrocyte glycoprotein. *J Neurochem* 1990; 55:583–587.

58. Bornstein MB, Hummelgard A. Multiple sclerosis: serum induced demyelination in tissue culture. In: Shiraki H, Yonezawa T, Kuroiwa Y (eds.), *The Aetiology and Pathogenesis of the Demyelinating Diseases.* Tokyo: Japan Science Press; 1976; 341–350.

59. Ulrich J, Lardi H. Multiple sclerosis: demyelination and myelination inhibition of organotypic tissue cultures of spinal cord by sera of patients with multiple sclerosis and other neurological diseases. *J Neurol* 1978; 218:7–16.

60. Seil FJ, Westall FC, Romine JS, Salk J. Serum demyelinating factors in multiple sclerosis. *Ann Neurol* 1983; 13:664–667.

61. Bradbury K, Aparicio SR, Sumner DW, et al. Comparison of in vitro demyelination and cytotoxicity of humoral factors in multiple sclerosis and other neurological diseases. *J Neurol Sci* 1985; 70:167–181.

62. Hughes D, Field EJ. Myelinotoxicity of serum and spinal fluid in multiple sclerosis: a critical assessment. *Clin Exp Immunol* 1967; 2:295–309.

63. Raine CS, Hummelgard A, Swanson E, Bornstein MB. Multiple sclerosis: serum-induced demyelination in vitro: a light and electron microscopic study. *J Neurol Sci* 1973; 20:127–148.

64. Wolfgram F, Duquette P. Demyelinating antibodies in multiple sclerosis. *Neurology* 1976; 26(6, pt 2):68–69.

65. Grundke Iqbal I, Bornstein MB. Multiple sclerosis: immunochemical studies on the demyelinating serum factor. *Brain Res* 1979; 160:489–503.

66. Grundke-Iqbal I, Bornstein MB. Multiple sclerosis: serum gamma globulin and demyelination in organ culture. *Neurology* 1980; 30:749–754.

67. Sun J, Olsson T, Xiao B-G, et al. T- and B-cell responses to myelin-oligodendrocyte glycoprotein in multiple sclerosis. *J Immunol* 1991; 146:1490–1495.

68. Karni A, Bakimer-Kleiner R, Abramsky O, Ben-Nun A. Elevated levels of antibody to myelin oligodendrocyte glycoprotein is not specific for patients with multiple sclerosis. *Arch Neurol* 1999; 56:311–315.

69. Genain CP, Cannella B, Hauser SL, Raine CS. Identification of autoantibodies associated with myelin damage in multiple sclerosis. *Nat Med* 1999; 5:170–175.

70. Raine CS, Cannella B, Hauser SL, Genain CP. Demyelination in primate autoimmune encephalomyelitis and acute multiple sclerosis: a case for antigen-specific antibody mediation. *Ann Neurol* 1999; 46:144–160.

71. Storch M, Lassmann H. Pathology and pathogenesis of demyelinating diseases. *Curr Opin Neurol* 1997; 10:186–192.

72. Raine CS, Traugott U, Farooq M, Bornstein MB, Norton WT. Augmentation of immune-mediated demyelination by lipid haptens. *Lab Invest* 1981; 45:174–182.

73. Bourdette DN, Driscoll BF, Seil FJ, Kies MW, Alvord EC Jr. Severity of demyelination in vivo correlates with serum myelination inhibition activity in guinea pigs having a new form of experimental allergic encephalomyelitis. *Neurochem Pathol* 1986; 4:1–9.

74. Martenson RE, Deibler GE, Kies MW, Levine S, Alvord EC Jr. Myelin basic proteins of mammalian and submammalian vertebrates: Encephalitogenic activities in guinea pigs and rats. *J Immunol* 1972; 109:262–270.

75. Whitham RH, Nilaver G, Bourdette DN, Seil FJ. Serum anti-myelin antibodies in chronic relapsing experimental allergic encephalomyelitis. *J Neuroimmunol* 1988; 18:155–170.

76. Lucchinetti CF, Brück W, Rodriguez M, Lassmann H. Distinct patterns of multiple sclerosis pathology indicates heterogeneity in pathogenesis. *Brain Pathol* 1996; 6:259–274.

77. Luchinetti C, Brück W, Parisi J, et al. Heterogeneity of multiple sclerosis lesions: implications for the pathogenesis of demyelination. *Ann Neurol* 2000; 47:707–717.

78. Storch MK, Piddlesden S, Haltia M, et al. Multiple sclerosis: in situ evidence for antibody- and complement-mediated demyelination. *Ann Neurol* 1998; 43:465–471.

79. Archelos JJ, Storch MK, Hartnung H-P. The role of B cells and autoantibodies in multiple sclerosis. *Ann Neurol* 2000; 47:694–706.

80. Seil FJ. Demyelinating antibodies in multiple sclerosis [letter]. *Ann Neurol* 2000; 48:948.

81. Wekerle H. Remembering MOG: autoantibody mediated demyelination in multiple sclerosis? *Nat Med* 1999; 5:153–154.

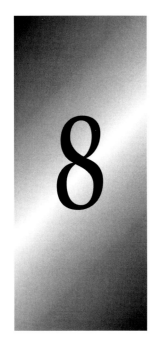

# 8 Multiple Sclerosis: The Role of Pathogens in Demyelination

*John W. Rose, M.D.*
*John E. Greenlee, M.D.*

Multiple sclerosis (MS) is an inflammatory disease and, from the time the disease was described by Charcot, clinicians have questioned whether the disease might be caused by an infectious agent. The record of clinical investigations in MS has been punctuated by numerous attempts to detect a causative agent by using currently available technology. Thus, over the years, multiple organisms, ranging from bacteria and spirochetes to viruses, have been proposed as possible etiologic agents (Table 8.1). However, no reported isolation of an infectious agent from MS tissue has received consistent independent confirmation (1–4).

Within the past several decades, three lines of evidence have been invoked to support the hypothesis that an infectious agent causes MS. The first of these, as discussed in Chapter 7, is that a number of viral agents can cause demyelinating disorders in experimental animals. The second line of evidence comes from epidemiologic studies suggesting that MS arises after time-limited exposure to an environmental factor, presumably a pathogen. The third line of evidence, derived from human disease, is that a number of infectious agents may be associated with peripheral (PNS) or central (CNS) nervous system demyelinating disease.

In this chapter, we review the pathogens that are known to cause demyelination, the mechanisms by which viruses or other pathogens may produce demyelination, the evidence supporting a role for pathogens in MS, and the candidate pathogens suspected of having a role in MS. We conclude by discussing the criteria to establish an etiologic role for a pathogen in MS and future directions for research in this important field.

## INFECTIOUS AGENTS OF HUMANS KNOWN TO CAUSE PNS OR CNS DEMYELINATION

Viruses and pathogens known to cause demyelination in the CNS are shown in Table 8.2 with the specific conditions produced by the infection. Several of these organisms may be associated with demyelination in the PNS or CNS. A number of organisms including viruses such as human immunodeficiency virus (HIV), Epstein-Barr virus (EBV), and cytomegalovirus (CMV), mycoplasma, and the bacteria *Campylobacter jejuni* are associated with acute inflammatory demyelinating polyneuropathy (AIDP). In this condition, the infection is antecedent to the onset of neurologic symptoms, and neuropathy is the result of an immunologic response with cross-reactivity to peripheral myelin.

CNS demyelination may be produced directly by viral infections with papovavirus (JC virus) or the chronic measles virus infection, subacute sclerosing panen-

**TABLE 8.1**
*Viruses and Pathogens Isolated from Patients with Multiple Sclerosis\**

| YEAR | VIRUS | TISSUE |
|---|---|---|
| 1946 | Rabies | Brain |
| 1964 | Herpes simplex, type 2 | Brain |
| 1964 | Scrapie | Brain |
| 1972 | Measles virus | Brain |
| 1978 | Simian virus 5 | Brain |
| 1979 | Chimpanzee cytomegalo-virus | Brain |
| 1980 | Coronavirus | Brain |
| 1982 | Subacute myelo-opticoneuropathy–like virus | Brain |
| 1982 | Tick-borne encephalitis Flavivirus | Brain |
| 1986 | HTLV-I | CSF mono-nuclear cells |
| 1989 | LM7 (retrovirus) | CSF/blood |
| 1989 | Herpes simplex, type 1 | CSF |
| 1992 | Epstein-barr virus | CSF/blood |
| 1994 | Human herpes virus-6 | Blood |
| 2000 | *Chlamydia pneumoniae* | CSF |

\*Adapted from *Viral Infections of the Nervous System*, 2nd ed. New York: LIppincott-Raven; 1998; 248–257.
CSF, cerebrospinal fluid; HTLV-I, human T-lymphotropic virus -I.

cephalitis (SSPE). A postinfectious encephalomyelitis may occur after exposure to pathogens including mycoplasma, measles virus, human herpes virus 6 (HHV-6), EBV, and CMV. Thus, there is overlap between the pathogens associated with postinfectious peripheral and central demyelination (Table 8.2). In addition, a single organism such as measles virus may cause CNS demyelination by direct infection, as in SSPE, or as a result of an immune response to a cleared infection cross-reacting with myelin, as in postinfectious encephalomyelitis (5).

## KNOWN MECHANISMS OF VIRUS-INDUCED CNS DEMYELINATION IN HUMANS

Two major mechanisms of virus-induced CNS demyelination are viral destruction of oligodendrocytes and postinfectious immune-mediated demyelination. A third and apparently rare, mechanism of CNS demyelination is immune complex–mediated vasculopathy. These mechanisms are considered below, followed by a discussion of the theoretical mechanisms of pathogen-induced demyelination.

## Viral Lysis of Oligodendrocytes

This is the only direct mechanism through which viruses may produce demyelination and is known to occur in two human conditions. In progressive multifocal leukoencephalopathy (PML), a disorder seen in approximately 4 percent of patients with HIV infection, progressive demyelination of brain results from lytic infection of oligodendrocytes by the polyomavirus, JC virus (6). In SSPE, a rare, late complication of systemic measles infection, infection of oligodendrocytes with secondary demyelination occurs as a minor component of a more widespread neurologic process involving astrocytes and neurons (7).

## Postinfectious Immune–mediated Demyelination

Episodes of acute demyelination, termed *neuroparalytic accidents*, were observed after immunization with early brain-derived rabies vaccines, and demyelination as an immune response to myelin basic protein (MBP) was first reported in 1935 by Rivers and Swenker (8). We now know that similar episodes of demyelination can follow a number of human infections, and immune mechanisms are believed to represent a final common pathway through which a variety of infectious agents can induce a fairly uniform syndrome of demyelinating disease (9). An essentially identical pattern of CNS white matter injury may be seen after infection with EBV, measles virus, CMV, *Mycoplasma pneumoniae*, and, very likely, a variety of other infectious agents. In these disorders, the autoimmune response to white matter may be induced in at least two ways. In EBV infection, nonproductive infection of B lymphocytes produces a wide variety of autoantibodies, the prototype of which is the heterophile antibody response. Demyelination in this setting may occur as part of a widespread perturbation of immune function. In infection by other agents, including measles virus, CMV, and M pneumoniae, autoimmune demyelination may result as a consequence of "molecular mimicry," a process in which host immune response to a foreign antigen cross-reacts with a self-antigen to produce autoimmune disease (10). As discussed in the preceding chapter, molecular mimicry with its attendant autoimmune response has been used to induce CNS demyelination in experimental animals (10). In humans, injury of peripheral nerves in AIDP after *C. jejuni* infection is thought to occur by this mechanism. Although molecular mimicry has not been proven to be of etiologic significance in human CNS demyelination, this mechanism has been suggested in syndromes of postinfectious polyneuropathy and encephalomyelitis seen in some patients after infection with measles virus, cytomegalovirus, or *M. pneumoniae*.

**TABLE 8.2**
*Viruses and Pathogens Causing Demyelination in Peripheral and Central Nervous Systems*

| PATHOGEN | SYNDROMES INVOLVING PERIPHERAL NERVE | SYNDROMES INVOLVING BRAIN AND SPINAL CORD |
|---|---|---|
| **Viruses** | | |
| HIV | AIDP/CIDP | Vacuolar myelopathy |
| HTLV-I | None known | Tropical spastic paraparesis |
| JC virus | None known | Progressive multifocal leukoencephalopathy |
| Human herpes virus 6 | None known | Encephalomyelitis: possibly acute and postinfectious |
| Measles virus | AIDP | Postinfectious encephalomyelitis, subacute sclerosing panencephalitis |
| Rubella virus | AIDP | Postinfectious encephalomyelitis, progressive rubella panencephalitis |
| Epstein-Barr virus | AIDP | Postinfectious encephalomyelitis |
| Cytomegalovirus | AIDP | Postinfectious encephalomyelitis |
| **Mycoplasma** | | |
| *Mycoplasma pneumoniae* | AIDP | Postinfectious encephalomyelitis, transverse myelitis |
| **Spirochetes** | | |
| Lyme disease | — | Encephalomyelitis |
| **Bacteria** | | |
| *Campylobacter jejeuni* | AIDP | None known |

AIDP, acute inflammatory demyelinating polyneuropathy; CIDP, chronic inflammatory demyelinating polyneuropathy; HIV, human immunodeficiency virus; HTLV-I, human T-lymphotropic virus-I.

## Immune Complex Vasculopathy

In rare cases, rubella virus infection is followed by a delayed, progressive condition accompanied by white matter injury. Evaluation of affected brains has not shown evidence of viral infection but rather of microvascular changes that appear to be due to immune complex deposition (11). This mechanism of demyelination has not been associated with other human infectious agents. Of note, progressive rubella panencephalitis also has been associated with significant parenchymal inflammation that may contribute to the demyelination (12).

## Overview of Potential Mechanisms of Virus-Induced CNS Demyelination

A substantial number of mechanisms has been suggested to cause or contribute to CNS demyelination (Table 8.3). Whether these mechanisms participate in the pathogenesis of MS remains speculative. These mechanisms are paired with examples from human disease, animal models, or in vitro experiments in Table 8.3. Mechanisms of demyelination not previously detailed in this section are discussed below.

Theoretically, oligodendrocytes also may undergo cell death due to the altered homeostasis produced by a nonlytic viral infection. This may occur in several of the experimental models of viral-induced demyelination.

Involvement of oligodendrocytes by latent viral infection could elicit an immune response directly targeting these cells. In addition, oligodendrocytes are relatively sensitive to toxic conditions produced during inflammation. Nonspecific immune responses triggered by viral infections in other cells also might result in demyelination as a consequence of collateral apoptotic or necrotic death of oligodendrocytes. In addition, the immune response to a particular pathogen may stimulate the production of proinflammatory cytokines, interferons, and reactive small molecules such as peroxynitrite, thereby augmenting demyelination (13).

Proteins from a pathogen also might serve as superantigens capable of stimulating T-cells bearing specific T-cell receptors. This can result in nonspecific stimulation of autoreactive cell populations (14). Viruses and other pathogens may infect or damage CNS endothelial cells, resulting in a breakdown of the blood–brain barrier (BBB). Disruption of the BBB may cause antigens to be exposed, which would otherwise remain sequestered, thereby facilitating injury to myelin and potentiating antigenic spread (15). In addition, pathogens might produce proteins that alter the immune response or toxins contributing to demyelination (14,16). Some viruses have cytokines encoded in their nucleic acid, which may alter the immune response and favor viral persistence (14). Viral infection in the CNS may stimulate host cells to produce a protein that is not ordinarily exposed to the immune system (15,17).

**TABLE 8.3**
*Potential Mechanisms of Virus-Induced Demyelination of the Central Nervous System*

| MECHANISM | DISEASE/EXAMPLE |
|---|---|
| Lytic infection of oligodendrocytes | Human: SSPE (measles virus) and PML (JC virus) |
| Persistent infection of oligodendrocytes with resultant abnormal homeostasis and cell death | Animal: Theiler murine encephalomyelitis virus |
| Molecular mimicry: immunologic cross-reactivity between viral antigens and oligodendrocyte or myelin proteins | Human: EBV/HSV-1 epitopes cross-react with transaldolase in CNS* |
| | Animal: Viral antigen-induced experimental allergic encephalomyelitis |
| Demyelination induced by virus-encoded toxins | Human: Theoretical for retroviral infection |
| Oligodendrocyte death due to inflammatory environment elicited by nonlethal oligodendrocyte infection | Human: HHV-6 in PML |
| | Animal: JHMV |
| Bystander death of oligodendrocytes in an inflammatory environment elicited by infection of other cell types | Animal: JHMV |
| Virus acts as a "superantigen," inducing a nonspecific T-cell response that reacts with components of myelin | Theoretical |
| Autoimmune response to a nontolerized protein produced by virus-infected cells | Human (theoretical): EBV and a-b crystallin |
| Disruption of the blood–brain barrier with unmasking of normally sequestered brain antigens | Human: Postinfectious encephalomyelitis and SSPE |
| Coexistence of viral infections produces or accentuates demyelination | Human (theoretical): Papovavirus and HHV-6 in PML |

*From *J Immunol* 1999; 163:4027–4032.
CNS, central nervous system; EBV, Epstein-Barr virus; HHV-6, human herpes virus-6; HSV-I, herpes simplex virus-I; PML, progressive multifocal leukoencephalopathy; SSPE, subacute sclerosing panencephalitis.

Recent work has suggested that simultaneous infection with 2 viruses may be a significant factor in disease pathogenesis of PML and possibly MS (18). In addition, a growing body of evidence, including recent studies of axonal injury in MS brains, suggests that MS may not be a solely demyelinating condition, and several of these processes may be involved in disease pathogenesis affecting myelin and axons.

### Route of Infection

For CNS demyelination, the route of viral infection may be by one of four different pathways: (1) ascent along nerves into the CNS (herpes simplex virus [HSV] and varicella zoster virus [VZV]), (2) expression in the CNS of an endogenous virus encoded in the genome (retrovirus or MS-associated retrovirus [MSRV]; see next section), (3) penetration into the CNS by infected macrophages (HIV and HHV-6), or (4) hematogenous spread to the CNS (infected B cells in EBV). If a virus or other pathogen initiates MS then understanding the route of viral penetration into the CNS would be therapeutically important.

## DO PATHOGENS CAUSE OR CONTRIBUTE TO MS?

Evidence for an infectious cause of MS includes data from epidemiologic and clinical investigations.

### Epidemiologic Evidence

The most suggestive evidence associating MS with exposure to an infectious agent comes from an important body of epidemiologic studies. The basis for these studies is the observation that MS has a higher incidence in temperate climates and that the prevalence of MS diminishes as one moves south toward the equator. There is also some evidence that the incidence of the disorder may be higher in temperate regions at as one moves farther from the equator in the southern hemisphere. Migration studies have indicated that individuals emigrating to Israel and South Africa after adolescence have an incidence of MS similar to that seen in their countries of origin. In contrast, individuals moving before adolescence have an incidence similar to that seen in the country to which they immigrate (19,20). These data suggest that MS may be associated with childhood exposure to some unknown agent or agents. Although investigators suggested that the increase in familial MS might be explainable by shared environment, a 1995 study by the Canadian collaborative group failed to find evidence that duration of common habitation could explain the existence of MS in families (21). Two apparent epidemics of MS have been reported. The first of these occurred in the Faroe Islands. By report, MS was not known to the inhabitants of these islands before World War II. Between 1943 and 1949, however, 16 cases were reported, with another 16 cases reported between 1950 and 1973. Although disease prevalence in 1977 was 34 per 100,000 populations, no cases were reported between 1973 and 1981. These findings suggest a point-source epidemic, with exposure of a naive population during a period when the islands were occupied by foreign troops, followed by a period of latency before the appearance of demyelinating disease (22). Somewhat similar data exist for Iceland, where increases in disease prevalence occurred in 1922 and 1945, the latter rise occurring after occupation by American and British armed forces (23).

## Mediators of Inflammation in Clinical Materials

These clinical studies showed that interferon-α and interferon-α–inducible protein, MxA, are increased in MS patients, possibly consistent with an infectious process (24). In addition, there is expression of class I of the major histocompatibility complex (MHC) antigen on oligodendrocytes during infection, which could promote CD8$^+$ T-cell–mediated cytotoxicity (25).

## Attempts to Detect Infectious Agents by Serological Methods

These investigations date to studies in 1962 by Adams and Ishigawa, who found an antibody to the measles virus the cerebrospinal fluid (CSF) of patients with MS (26). Over the years, however, efforts to detect antiviral antibodies in serum and CSF of MS patients have been largely inconclusive, and no consistent or clear pattern of viral infection has emerged from this line of investigation. Titers for candidate viruses including measles, EBV, and human T-lymphotropic virus-I (HTLV-I) were not substantially elevated in MS patients compared with control subjects (27,28). The possibility also exists, as discussed below, that elevated titers of antiviral antibody do not reflect causation but rather nonspecific perturbation of the patient's immune response.

## PATHOGENS OF CURRENT INTEREST IN MS

### Human Herpes Virus-6

HHV-6 is lymphotropic and neurotropic (29) and has been shown in vitro to infect oligodendrocytes and microglia in culture and peripheral blood mononuclear cells (PBMCs) in vivo (30,31). The virus may be latent in monocytes and bone marrow progenitor cells, and latency may be associated with integration of the full-length viral genome into the short arm of chromosome 17 (Chr 17p13.3) (32–34). The virus genome has been shown to integrate into the human genome on chromosome 17, thus allowing the virus to persist despite intact host immune response (32). The virus is the etiologic agent of the childhood condition exanthem subitum. In addition, the virus has been associated with febrile convulsions and rare cases of encephalitis, in particular in the setting of impaired host immunity such as HIV infection or organ transplantation (32). The virulence of HHV-6 may increase significantly in the presence of coinfecting viruses such as CMV or HIV (35–38). Studies of HHV-6 in MS have included immunologic, immunohistochemical, and molecular investigations.

### Immunological Evidence of HHV-6 in MS

Elevated titers to HHV-6 have been detected in the serum and CSF of some MS patients (39–42). HHV-6 DNA has been found in the serum of patients (42). Cellular immunity to the virus also may be found in these individuals (42). Elevated levels of the virus receptor, soluble CD46, have been found in MS patients (43,44). According to a recent investigation, HHV-6 DNA can be isolated from PBMCs of some MS patients but not of controls (45). A study of CSF antibody titers favored HHV-6B over HHV-6A in MS (46). Elevated titers of immunoglobulin G (IgG) and IgM antibodies to HHV-6 in MS compared with healthy controls were found in the studies by Albashi et al. (39,47). However, they also reported similar findings in patients with the much more nebulous entity, chronic fatigue syndrome (47). In addition, those investigators cultured HHV-6B from MS and HHV-6A from chronic fatigue syndrome PBMCs, respectively (47). This raises the questions about the virus: Does it cause several human diseases or is it nonspecifically activated in patients with other illnesses and/or immunosuppressive therapies?

### Immunohistochemical and Molecular Biological Evidence

In 1993, Sola et al. used polymerase chain reaction (PCR) to find HHV-6 DNA in PBMCs from an MS patient (48). Numerous studies subsequently evaluated serum and CSF antibody titers for HHV-6 and PCR of PBMCs and CSF, with highly variable results (39,46,49–60). Challoner et al. used molecular virologic techniques to show viral nucleic acid of HHV-6B in the brains of MS and control subjects (61). These data indicate that the virus may be resident in the human CNS. PCR for HHV-6 structural protein 101 was positive in 36 percent of MS brain sections and 13 percent of control brains (29). In situ PCR associated the virus with oligodendrocytes and, to a lesser extent, neurons (18,61). In MS brains, immunohisto-chemical techniques showed a preponderance of virus-specific staining around demyelinating lesions, with localization to oligodendrocytes, and with much less staining in normal-appearing white matter (61). PCR studies of MS brain tissue found a greater association of HHV-6 with active than with inactive plaques (62). Interestingly, HSV and VZV also were detected (62). HHV-6 was found around areas of demyelination in MS and PML (63). HHV-6 was identified as a pathogen in fulminant demyelinating disease and encephalitis in MS patients (64-66). Therefore, HHV-6 may be etiologic in MS or, like other viruses, may contribute indirectly to the clinical course of MS patients.

### Summary of HHV-6 in MS

Although these studies suggest an association between HHV-6 and demyelinating illness in some patients, overall the evidence at present is inconsistent (52–60). Specifically, other laboratories have not found serologic evidence supporting a role for HHV-6 in MS (52,60). In other studies, PCR for multiple regions of the HHV-6 genome has not demonstrated a significant difference between the CSF of control subjects and the CSF of subjects with relapsing–remitting MS or chronic progressive MS (52). It is unlikely that HHV-6 is a primary pathogen in the majority of patients. However, it is possible that, in some of the cases of MS, HHV-6 is the primary pathogen, whereas in others it may facilitate disease progression. Overall, HHV-6 remains a viable candidate pathogen that might contribute to the pathogenesis of MS in at least some cases. It is a common virus with the potential for significant effects in the CNS. The finding of this virus in association with the demyelinating lesions of MS and PML is intriguing, although the significance of this observation in terms of clinical disease is unknown (18). The virus may be responsible for inducing MS alone or in concert with other viruses. Nonspecific reactivation is an alternative explanation for expression of HHV-6 in demyelinating lesions. Further investigations should show whether the virus is truly a pathogen in MS or a latent virus incidentally found in the brain. At present, there are no data supporting the use of antiviral therapy directed at HHV-6 in MS patients outside of clinical trials.

## EBV and Other Herpes Viruses

### EBV in MS

EBV is a ubiquitous virus that infects 90 percent of the population. EBV has been postulated repeatedly as a causative agent of MS. Many studies have found significant elevations of EBV-specific antibodies in MS patients, which may antedate the clinical expression of MS (67). The data supporting EBV as a precursor to MS includes the results of epidemiologic studies of common viruses in large populations (68). Late infection, after age 15 years, with EBV, measles, or mumps was associated with increased risk of MS (69). Investigation of a Danish cluster of MS patients showed that all affected individuals were exposed to a subtype of EBV not found in healthy controls (70). Additional serologic investigations have been interpreted as being consistent with a role for EBV in MS. A case control study of Norwegian MS patients versus age-, sex-, and geographically matched controls showed that IgG antibodies to EBV capsid antigen, nuclear antigen, and early antigen were significantly elevated in patients with MS (68). Elevated titers to EBV were found in the sera of 18 women who subsequently developed MS (67). In addition, higher titers to EBV were found in 126 MS patients compared with control individuals (67). Titers to HSV, herpes zoster (HZ), and CMV were not elevated in the MS patients. Antigen specific immunoblotting technique showed the presence of EBV-specific immunoglobulins in the CSF of 5 of 15 MS patients and 0 of 12 controls (71). Viral nucleic acid can be detected in PBMCs from MS patients, and EBV transformed cell lines can occur spontaneously in cells from CSF of MS patients. To date there has been no demonstration of EBV in the CNS of MS patients (72,73).

### Other Herpes Viruses

Other herpes viruses have been considered as potentially causative for MS (4). Herpes virus, EBV, CMV, and specific CD8+ T-cells have been isolated from tissues and blood of patients with autoimmune diseases including MS (74). HSV-1, HSV-2 and VZV also have been considered as agents capable of initiating MS (75). Magnetic resonance imaging (MRI) in Japanese MS patients visualized brainstem lesions suggestive of ascent of virus along the tracts of the trigeminal nerve, as can occur with HSV and VZV infections (76). Investigations of HHV-7 and HHV-8 found no evidence for their involvement in MS (56).

A study using PCR to examine herpes viruses in postmortem brain found that HSV, HHV-6, and VZV are detected with greater frequency in MS patients than in controls. However, those results were not statistically significant and EBV was detected with greater frequency in controls (62).

One placebo-controlled study of the antiviral drug valcyclovir found no beneficial effect for it in MS (77).

A subgroup analysis of a small number of patients with high MRI activity suggested reduced subsequent MRI activity in the valcyclovir-treated patients compared with placebo-treated patients (77). Further study of this observation may be warranted (78). If a herpes virus is identified as the cause of MS, the choice of antiviral therapy is not as simple as might be expected. Effective therapy could require specificity for virus type and strain.

## Endogenous Retrovirus

Considerable interest exists in a retroviral etiology for MS (79,80). Because HTLV-I, another retrovirus, causes an inflammatory demyelinating myelopathy known as tropical spastic paraparesis or HTLV-I associated myelopathy, a retrovirus is a candidate pathogen in MS. Additional evidence that retrovirus can cause CNS demyelination comes from a neurologic disease of sheep, visna, which is caused by a lentivirus (81–83).

Human endogenous retrovirus (HERV-W) is a family of endogenous retroviruses whose members may have the capacity to alter gene function and thereby influence disease course (84). MSRV can be isolated as retrovirus-like particles from patients. The HERV-W sequences are located on at least 11 human chromosomes (85–88). One sequence is on chromosome 14 in the region of the T-cell receptor a-gene (86).

MSRV may have a role in the pathogenesis of MS (86–88). MSRV peptides have been detected in CSF (88). Virus-specific RNA was found in the sera of MS patients (89). A recent investigation found extracellular RNA in peripheral blood encoding the MSRV-pol gene in 25 of 25 MS patients and 3 of 25 control individuals (90). MSRV expression in inflammatory brain diseases might be increased by the presence of activated macrophages (91). A specific haplotype of the putative autoantigen appears to confer risk for the development of MS regardless of HLA-DR type (92,93). A CD4$^+$ T-cell–mediated immune response to HERV peptides was found in acute but not in stable MS (94). In addition, endogenous retrovirus may contribute to the death of oligodendrocytes (95) by producing gliotoxins or by other mechanisms (16).

Circumspection is advisable before assigning a role for MSRV in the pathogenesis of MS. For example, other investigators examined the possibility of a retroviral etiology and found no evidence for reverse transcriptase in the CNS of MS patients (96). In addition, much effort was expended trying to confirm initially exciting results implicating HTLV-1, with the ultimate consensus that this retrovirus is not involved in MS (97,98).

## Coronavirus

Coronaviruses were recovered from MS brains by intracerebral injection of mice without antibody to known pathogens. This agent has not received consistent independent confirmation through isolation in other laboratories. The likelihood is high that these viruses were contaminants (99). Of interest are subsequent studies showing that coronaviruses may infect and cause demyelination in the primate brain (100–102). One report found coronavirus RNA and antigen in the MS brain, but another study did not (103). Further, no significant difference between MS patients and control was found with regard to the presence of coronavirus RNA (104).

## Other Viruses

A number of other infectious agents ranging from rabies virus to primate viruses and tick-borne encephalitis virus have been reported in different contexts (4,105) (Table 8.1). These are largely sporadic reports, without substantial confirmatory findings in other laboratories. For example, JC virus DNA was detected in the CSF of MS patients in one study, but that finding was not confirmed in another investigation (106,107).

## Nonviral Agents

The interesting studies associating *Chlamydia pneumoniae*, an obligate intracellular pathogen, with MS are discussed in Chapter 9. There is considerable controversy among investigators studying this organism and its relation to MS. Of particular importance is the finding that the nucleic acid of this organism can be detected in MS CSF, and under specific conditions the organism also can be cultured from the CSF (108). Contradictory results have been reported by different groups of investigators, and it is clear that establishing standards for the detection of the nucleic acid and culture of the organism is essential (109,110). Establishing these findings as specific for MS and determining whether they occur at the onset of the disease or in the early stages of the disease are major goals of ongoing research. The demonstration of adsorption of CSF oligoclonal bands from MS patients by the *C. pneumoniae*–specific antigens, including the elementary body, is an important observation (111) (Figure 8.1). The magnitude of the adsorption seems to be very significant in many patients (discussed in Chapter 9). The adsorption of pathogen-specific antibodies from the CSF of patients with chronic CNS infections has been observed in several other diseases and, hence, may be a major confirmatory observation in the MS patients. Other investigators have found some adsorption of MS CSF immunoglobulins with *C. pneumoniae* antigen but questioned whether the quantity and affinity of the antibodies are of the magnitude seen in other CNS infectious disorders (112). It would be of particular interest to determine whether there is significant intrathecal synthesis of immunoglobulins specific for *C. pneumoniae*. Current clinical trials are using antibiotic therapy directed against this

**FIGURE 8.1**

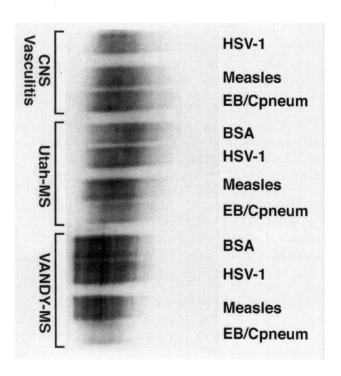

Isoelectric focusing gel of CSF immunoglobulins from three patients adsorbed against pathogen-specific antigens. The first patient is a control with CNS vasculitis, and CSF immunoglobulins are not adsorbed by HSV-1, measles virus, or EB/Cpneum. The second patient has MS (Utah-MS) with partial adsorption of CSF immunoglobulins by EB/Cpneum but not by BSA, measles virus, or HSV-1. Another patient with MS (Vandy MS) shows dramatic adsorption of immunoglobulins by EB/Cpneum and no adsorption with BSA or the viral antigens.

From Sriram and Rose, unpublished data. BSA, bovine serum albumin; CNS, central nervous system; CSF, cerebrospinal fluid; EB/Cpneum, elementary bodies from *Chlamydia pneumoniae*; HSV-I, herpes simplex virus-I; MS, multiple sclerosis.

agent. These trials, if successful, would provide strong supportive evidence of a role for this human pathogen.

## CONCLUSION

Over the past three decades, many infectious agents have been proposed as pathogens producing MS. However, essentially all of the attempts to associate specific pathogens with MS have been marred by inconsistency in the data from laboratory to laboratory and by the absence of a systematic approach to the problem. Transmission of demyelinating disease to an animal will be difficult and might require a transgenic animal expressing human receptors for a pathogen. It is probable that we will never be able to fulfill Koch's postulates regarding MS (113,114). Nonetheless, it will be of critical importance to consider criteria that might be used to establish the role

## TABLE 8.4
*Criteria for Establishing the Role of a Virus or Pathogen in Multiple Sclerosis*

| CRITERIA | PATHOGEN | | | |
|---|---|---|---|---|
| | HHV-6 | EBV | MSRV | CP |
| Reproducible detection by multiple laboratories | ? | ? | ? | ? |
| Pathogen-specific humoral immune responses | + | + | ND | + |
| Pathogen-specific immune response | + | + | + | ND |
| Detection of viral nucleic acid in the CSF | + | + | + | + |
| Detection of viral nucleic acid in MS lesions | + | ND | ND | ND |
| Pathogen cultured from the CSF | ND | + | ND | + |
| Pathogen cultured from the brain | ND | ND | ND | ND |
| Pathogen isolated from demyelinating but not from control regions | ND | ND | ND | ND |
| Transmission of disease to experimental animals* | ND | ND | ND | ND |
| Effective and specific antimicrobial treatment | ND | ND | ND | ND |

* Successful transmission to an animal model depends heavily on species specificity of the pathogens.
CP, *Chlamydia pneumoniae*; CSF, cerebrospinal fluid; EBV, Epstein-Barr virus; HHV-6, human herpes virus-6; MSRV, MS-associated retrovirus; MS, multiple sclerosis; ND, not determined; +, positive findings.

of a given virus or pathogen in disease pathogenesis. Potential criteria and their applications to current candidate agents are listed in Table 8.4. Assessing the candidate pathogens in the context of these criteria will help to define their validity in MS. For example, simply detecting an elevation of immunoglobulins to a pathogen in sera will not suffice. Nonspecific elevations might occur as a result of altered immune responses in MS patients or as the result of nonpathogenic viral reactivation. As the field evolves, the application of these criteria will help to separate pathogenesis from epiphenomenon.

Our current knowledge indicates that MS is a multifactorial condition, with environmental, genetic, and immunologic components. The disorder is heterogeneous in its clinical course, pathology, and response to treatment. Thus, when diagnosing a patient as having MS, we may be dealing with any of several discrete disease entities. Many other possible factors also come into play. For example, the interaction of two different viruses or pathogens might be required to produce disease in some patients. In this setting, an ordinarily latent virus could become pathogenic in environments altered by a second infection. This sort of interaction could be extremely difficult to detect. Further, MS could be caused by one or more undescribed viruses not amenable to current methods of isolation.

To establish the role of a pathogen, it will be necessary to investigate larger populations of patients and normal and other disease patient controls to determine the specificity of immunologic and molecular biologic evidence of infection. The MS patient should be investigated before receiving immunomodulatory or immunosuppressive treatments. In addition, patients treated with these therapies will need special controls if they are included in studies attempting to find pathogens. The use of standardized techniques for measurement of antibody titers and performance of PCR will ensure reproducibility of the findings in other laboratories. For detection of viral DNA in CSF, all cells should be eliminated to prevent contamination from peripheral cells infected with the virus. At present, no virus or combination of viruses has been definitively associated with MS, and much work needs to be done before such an association can be proven.

## Acknowledgment

The writing of this chapter was supported by the resources of the Neurovirology Research Laboratory at the VASLCHCS.

## References

1. Johnson RT. Possible viral cause of multiple sclerosis. In: *Viral Infections of the Nervous System* 2nd ed., New York: Lippincott-Raven; 1998; 248–257.

2. Greenlee J, Rose J. Controversies in neurological infectious diseases. *Sem Neurology* 2001; 20:375–386.

3. Azoulay-Cayla A. Is multiple sclerosis a disease of viral origin? *Pathol Biol (Paris)* 2000; 48:4–14.

4. Vastag B. Not so fast: research on infectious links to MS questioned. *JAMA* 2001; 285:279–281.

5. Johnson RT, Griffin D, Hirsch R, et al. Measles encephalomyelitis: clinical and immunological studies. *N Engl J Med* 1984; 310:137–141.

6. Greenlee JE. Progressive multifocal leukoencephalopathy. In: Aminoff MJ, Goetz CG (ed.), *Handbook of Clinical Neurology*. Elsevier Science BV; 1998: 399–430.

7. Allen I, McQuaid S, McMahon J, Kirk J, McConnell R. The significance of measles virus antigen and genome distribution in the CNS in SSPE for mechanisms of viral spread and demyelination. *J Neuropathol Exp Neurol* 1996; 55:471–480.

8. Rivers TM, Swenker FF. Encephalomyelitis accompanied by myelin destruction experimentally produced in monkeys. *J Exp Med* 1935; 61:689–702.

9. Stohlman SA, Hinton DR. Viral induced demyelination. *Brain Pathol* 2001; 11: 92-106

10. Fujinami R, Oldstone M. Amino acid homology between the encephalitogenic site of myelin basic protein and virus: mechanism for autoimmunity. *Science* 1985; 230:1043–1045.

11. Wolinsy JS. Progressive rubella panencephalitis. In: McKendall RR (ed.), *Viral Diseases. Handbook of Clinical Neurology*, New Series, Vinken PJ, Bruyn GW, Klawans HL (series eds.). Chapter 25, 1988; 56: 401–416.

12. Townsend JJ, Stroop WG, Baringer JR, et al. The neuropathology of progressive rubella panencephalitis after childhood rubella. *Neurology* 1982; 32:185–190.

13. Rose J, Hill K, Wada Y, et al. Nitric oxide synthase inhibitor, aminoguanidine, reduces inflammation and demyelination produced by Theiler's virus infection. *J Neuroimmunol* 1998; 81:82–89.

14. Rose J. Pathogenesis of viral immune-mediated syndromes. In: Mckendall R, Stroop W (eds.), *Handbook of Neurovirology*. Dekker; 1994; 95–102.

15. Miller S, Vadwelugt C, Begolka W, et al. Persistent infection with Theiler's virus leads to CNS autoimmunity via epitope spreading. *Nat Med* 1997; 3:1133–1136.

16. Perron H. MSRV retrovirus and gliotoxin protein: Potential biological markers in multiple sclerosis? *Ann Biol Clin (Paris)* 1998; 56:427–438.

17. van Sechel AC, Bajramovic JJ, van Stipdonk MJ, et al. EBV-induced expression and HLA-DR-restricted presentation by human B cells of alpha B-crystallin, a candidate autoantigen in multiple sclerosis. *J Immunol* 1999; 162:129–135.

18. Blumberg BM, Mock DJ, Powers JM, et al. The HHV6 paradox: ubiquitous commensal or insidious pathogen? A two-step in situ PCR approach. *J Clin Virol* 2000; 16:159–178.

19. Alter M, Liebowitz U, Speer J. Risk of multiple sclerosis related to age of immigration to Israel. *Arch Neurol* 1966; 15:234–237.

20. Dean G. The annual incidence, prevalence and mortality in white South African-born and white immigrants to South Africa. *BMJ* 1967; 2:724–730.

21. Kurtzke JF. Epidemiologic evidence for multiple sclerosis as an infection. *Clin Microbiol Rev* 1993; 6:382–427.

22. Kurtzke JF, Gudmundsson K, Bergmann S. Multiple sclerosis in Iceland. I. Evidence of a postwar epidemic. *Neurology* 1982; 32:143–150.

23. Chieux V, Chehadeh W, Hautecoeur P, et al. Increased levels of antiviral MxA protein in peripheral blood of patients with a chronic disease of unknown etiology. *J Med Virol* 2001; 65(2):301–308.

25. Redwine J, Buchmeier M, Evans C. In vivo expression of major histocompatiblity complex molecules on oligodendrocytes and neurons during viral infection. *Am J Pathol* 2001; 159:1219–1224.

26. Adams J, Imagawa D. Measles antibodies in multiple sclerosis. *Proc Soc Exp Biol Med* 1962; 111:562–566.

27. Bergkvist M, Sandberg-Wollheim M. Serological differences in monozygotic twin pairs discordant for multiple sclerosis. *Acta Neurol Scand* 2001; 104:262–265.

28. Alperovitch A, Berr C, Cambom-Thomsen A, et al. Viral antibody titers, immunogenetic markers, and their interrelations in multiple sclerosis patients and controls. *Hum Immunol* 1991; 31:94–99.

29. Friedman JE, Lyons MJ, Cu G, et al. The association of the human herpes virus-6 and MS. *Mult Scler* 1999; 5:355–362.

30. Albright AV, Lavi E, Black JB, et al. The effect of human herpes virus-6 (HHV-6) on cultured human neural cells: oligodendrocytes and microglia. *J Neurovirol* 1998; 4:86–94.

31. Soldan SS, Leist TP, Juhng KN, McFarland HF, Jacobson S. Increased lymphoproliferative response to human herpesvirus type 6A variant in multiple sclerosis patients. *Ann Neurol* 2000; 47:306–313.

32. Toreli G, Barozzi P, Marasca R, et al. Targeted integration of human herpes virus-6 in the p arm of chromosome 17 of peripheral blood lymphocytes. *J Med Virol* 1995; 46:178–188.

33. Luppi M, Barozzi P, Morris CM, Merelli E, Torelli G. Integration of human herpes virus-6 genome in human chromosomes. *Lancet* 1998; 352:1707–1708.

34. Morris C, Luppi M, McDonald M, Barozzi P, Torelli G. Fine mapping of an apparently targeted latent human herpes virus type 6 integration site in chromosome band 17p13.3. *J Med Virol* 1999; 58:69–75.

35. Yoshikawa T, Asano Y. Central nervous system complications in human herpes virus-6 infection. *Brain Dev* 2000; 22:307–314.

36. Clark DA. Human herpes virus-6. *Rev Med Virol* 2000; 10:155–173.

37. Dockrell DH, Smith TF, Paya CV. Human herpesvirus 6. *Mayo Clin Proc* 1999; 74:163–170.

38. Kimberlin DW, Whitley RJ. Human herpesvirus-6: neurologic implications of a newly-described viral pathogen. *J Neurovirol* 1998; 4:474–485.

39. Ablashi DV, Lapps W, Kaplan M, et al. Human Herpes virus-6 (HHV-6) infection in multiple sclerosis: a preliminary report. *Mult Scler* 1998; 4:490–496.

40. Nielsen L, Larsen AM, Munk M, Vestergaard BF. Human herpes virus-6 immunoglobulin G antibodies in patients with multiple sclerosis. *Acta Neurol Scand* 1997; (suppl)169:76–78.

41. Soldan SS, Berti R, Salem N, et al. Association of human herpes virus-6 (HHV-6) with multiple sclerosis: Increased IgM response to HHV-6 early antigen and detection of serum HHV-6 DNA. *Nat Med* 1997; 3:1394–1399.

42. Berti R, Soldan SS, Akhyani N, McFarland HF, Jacobson S. Extended observations on the association of HHV-6 and multiple sclerosis. *J Neurovirol* 2000; (suppl 2):S85–S87.

43. Santoro F, Kennedy PE, Locatelli G, et al. CD46 is a cellular receptor for human herpes virus-6. *Cell* 1999; 99:817–827.

44. Soldan SS, Fogdell-Hahn A, Brennan MB, et al. Elevated serum and cerebrospinal fluid levels of soluble human herpes virus type 6 cellular receptor, membrane cofactor protein, in patients with multiple sclerosis. *Ann Neurol* 2001; 50:486–493.

45. Kim JS, Lee KS, Park JH, Kim MY, Shin WS. Detection of human herpes virus 6-variant A in peripheral blood mononuclear cells from multiple sclerosis patients. *Eur Neurol* 2000; 43:170–173.

46. Ongradi J, Rajda C, Maordi C, et al. A pilot study on the antibodies to HHV-6 variants and HHV-7 in CSF of MS patients. *J Neurovirol* 1999; 5:529–532.

47. Ablashi DV, Eastman HB, Owen CB, et al. Frequent HHV-6 reactivation in multiple sclerosis (MS) and chronic fatigue syndrome (CFS) patients. *J Clin Virol* 2000; 16:179–191.

48. Sola P, Merelli E, Marasca R, et al. Human herpes virus-6 and multiple sclerosis: Survey of anti-HHV-6 antibodies by immunoflourescence and viral sequences by polymerase chain reaction. *J Neurol Neurosurg Psychiatry* 1993; 56:917–919.

49. Nielsen L, Larsen A, Vestergaard B. Human herpes virus-6 immunoglobulin G antibodies in patients with multiple sclerosis. *Acta Neurol Scand* 1997; 169:S76–S78.

50. Wilborn F, Schmidt C, Brinkman V, et al. A potential role for human herpes virus-6 in nervous system disease. *J Neuroimmunol* 1994; 49:213–221.

51. Goldberg S, Albright A, Lisak R, et al. Polymerase chain reaction analysis of human herpes virus-6 sequences in the sera and cerebrospinal fluid of patients with multiple sclerosis. *J Neurovirol* 1995; 6:545–549.

52. Enbom M, Wang FZ, Fredrikson S, et al. Similar humoral and cellular immunological reactivities to human herpes virus-6 in patients with multiple sclerosis and controls. *Clin Diagn Lab Immunol* 1999; 6:545–549.

53. Mirandola P, Stefan A, Brambilla E, Campadelli-Fiume G, Grimaldi LM. Absence of human herpes virus-6 and 7 from spinal fluid and serum of multiple sclerosis patients. *Neurology* 1999; 53:1367–1368.

54. Mayne M, Krishnan J, Metz L, et al. Infrequent detection of human herpes virus-6 DNA in peripheral blood mononuclear cells from multiple sclerosis patients. *Ann Neurol* 1998; 44:391–394.

55. Merille E, Bedin R, Sola P, et al. Human herpes virus-6 and human herpes virus-8 DNA sequences in brains of multiple sclerosis patients, normal adults and children. *J Neurol* 1997; 244:450–454.

56. Martin C, Embom M, Soderstrom M, et al. Absence of seven human herpes viruses, including HHV-6, by polymerase chain reaction in CSF and blood from patients with multiple sclerosis and optic neuritis. *Acta Neurol Scand* 1997; 95:280–283.

57. Rotola A, Caselli E, Cassai E, et al. Novel human herpes viruses and multiple sclerosis. *J Neurovirol* 2000; (suppl 2):S88–S91.

58. Rotola A, Cassai E, Tola MR, Granieri E, Di Luca D. Human herpes virus-6 is latent in peripheral blood of patients with relapsing-remitting multiple sclerosis. *J Neurol Neurosurg Psychiatry* 1999; 67:529–531.

59. Hay KA, Tenser RB. Leukotropic herpesviruses in multiple sclerosis. *Mult Scler* 2000; 6:66–68.

60. Taus C, Pucci E, Cartechini E, et al. Absence of HHV-6 and HHV-7 in cerebrospinal fluid in relapsing-remitting multiple sclerosis. *Acta Neurol Scan* 2000; 101:224–228.

61. Challoner P, Smith K, Parker J, et al. Plaque-associated expression of human herpes virus-6 in multiple sclerosis. *Proc Natl Acad Sci USA* 1995; 92:7440–7444.

62. Sanders V, Felisan S, Waddell A, et al. Detection of herpesviridae in postmortem multiple sclerosis brain tissue and controls by polymerase chain reaction. *J Neurovirol* 1996; 2:249–258.

63. Mock D, Powers C, Goodman A, et al. Association of human herpes virus-6 with the demyelinative lesions of progressive multifocal leukoencephalopathy. *J Neurovirol* 1999; 5:363–373.

64. Merelli E, Sola P, Barozzi P, Torelli G. An encephalitic episode in a multiple sclerosis patient with human herpes virus-6 latent infection. *J Neurol Sci* 1996; 137:42–46.

65. Carrigan D, Harrington D, Knox K. Subacute leukoencephalitis caused by CNS infection with human herpes virus-6 manifesting as acute multiple sclerosis. *Neurology* 1996; 47:145–148.

66. Novoa L, Nagra A, Nakawatse T, et al. Fulminant demyelinating encephalomyelitis associated with productive HHV-6 infection. *J Med Virol* 1997; 52:301–308.

67. Ascherio A, Munger K, Lennette E, et al. Epstein-Barr virus antibodies and risk of multiple sclerosis a prospective study. *JAMA* 2001; 268:3083–3088.

68. Myhr KM, Riise T, Barrett-Connor E, et al. Altered antibody pattern to Epstein-Barr virus but not to other herpes viruses in multiple sclerosis: A population based case-control study from western Norway. *J Neurol Neurosurg Psychiatry* 1998; 64:539–542.

69. Hernan MA, Zhang SM, Lipworth L, Olek MJ, Ascherio A. Multiple sclerosis and age at infection with common viruses. *Epidemiology* 2001; 12:301–306.

70. Munch M, Hvas J, Christensen T, Moller-Larsen A, Haahr S. A single subtype of Epstein-Barr virus in members of multiple sclerosis clusters. *Acta Neurol Scand* 1998; 98:395–399.

71. Rand KH, Houck H, Denslow ND, Heilman KM. Epstein-Barr virus nuclear antigen-1 (EBNA-1) associated oligoclonal bands in patients with multiple sclerosis. *J Neurol Sci* 2000; 173:32–39.

72. Haahr S, Munch M. The association between multiple sclerosis and infection with Epstein-Barr virus and retrovirus. *J Neurovirol* 2000; (suppl 2):S76–S79.

73. Morre SA, van Beek J, De Groot CJ, et al. Is Epstein-Barr virus present in the CNS of patients with MS? *Neurology* 2001; 56:692.

74. Scotet E, Peyrat M, Saulquin X, et al. Frequent enrichment for CD8 T cells reactive against common herpes viruses in chronic inflammatory lesions: towards a reassessment of the physiopathological significance of T-cell clonal expansions found in

autoimmune inflammatory processes. *Eur J Immunol* 1999; 29:973–985.

75. Nakashima I, Fujihara K, Kimpara T, et al. Linear pontine trigeminal root lesions in multiple sclerosis: clinical and magnetic resonance imaging studies in 5 cases. *Arch Neurol* 2001; 58:101–104.

76. Bergstrom T. Herpes viruses—a rationale for antiviral treatment in multiple sclerosis. *Antiviral Res* 1999; 41:1–19.

77. Bech E, Lycke J,Gadenberg P, et al. A randomized, double blind, placebo controlled MRI study of anti-herpes virus therapy in MS. *Neurology* 2002; 58:31–36.

78. Goodman A, Miller D. Infections and MS: clinical trials move to center stage. *Neurology* 2002; 58:7–8.

79. Rasmussen HB, Lucotte G, Clausen J. Endogenous retroviruses and multiple sclerosis. J Neurovirol 2000; (suppl 2):S80–S84.

80. Fujinami RS, Libbey JE. Endogenous retroviruses: are they the cause of multiple sclerosis? *J Neurovirol* 2000; (suppl 2):S80–S84.

81. Sigurdsson B, Palsson P. Visna of sheep. A slow demyelinating infection. *Brit J Exp Pathol* 1958; 39:519–528.

82. Zink M, Narayan O, Kennedy P, Clements J. Pathogenesis of VISNA/MAEDI and caprine arthritis-encephalitis: New leads on the mechanism of restricted virus replication and persistent inflammation. *Vet Immunol Immunopathol* 1987; 15:167–180.

83. Clements J, Gdovin S, Montelaro R, Narayan O. Antigenic variation in lentiviral diseases. *Ann Rev of Immunol.* 1988; 6:139–159.

84. Blond JL, Beseme F, Duret L, et al. Molecular characterization and placental expression of HERV-W, a new human endogenous retrovirus family. *J Virol* 1999; 73:1175–1185.

85. Kim HS, Lee WH. Human endogenous retrovirus HERV-W family: Chromosomal localization, identification, and phylogeny. *AIDS Res Hum Retroviruses* 2001; 17:643–648.

86. Alliel PM, Perin JP, Pierig R, Rieger F. An endogenous retrovirus with nucleic acid sequences similar to those of the multiple sclerosis associated retrovirus at the human T-cell receptor alpha, delta gene locus. *Cell Mol Biol (Noisy-le-grand)* 1998; 44:927–931.

87. Perron H, Perin JP, Rieger F, Aslliel PM. Particle-associated retroviral RNA and tandem RGH/HERV-W copies on human chromosome 7q: Possible components of a 'chain-reaction' triggered by infectious agents in multiple sclerosis? *J Neurovirol* 2000; (suppl 2):S67–S75.

88. Alliel PM, Perin JP, Peirig R, et al. Endogenous retroviruses and multiple sclerosis. II. HERV-7q. *C R Acad Sci III* 1998; 321:857–863.

89. Garson JA, Tuke PW, Giraud P, et al. Detection of virion-associated MSRV-RNA in serum of patients with multiple sclerosis. *Lancet* 1998; 351:33.

90. Serra C, Sotgiu S, Mameli G, et al. Multiple sclerosis and multiple sclerosis-associated retrovirus in Sardinia. *Neurol Sci* 2001; 22:171–173.

91. Johnston JB, Silva C, Holden J, et al. Monocyte activation and differentiation augment human endogenous retrovirus expression: implications for inflammatory brain diseases. *Ann Neurol* 2001; 50:429–430.

92. Rassmussen HB, Clausen J. A novel haplotype of the endogenous retrovirus, HRES-1, in patients with multiple sclerosis and healthy individuals. *Autoimmunity* 1999; 29:141–145.

93. Rasmussen HB, Kelly MA, Francis DA, Clausen J. Association between the endogenous retrovirus HRES-1 and multiple sclerosis in the United Kingdom—evidence of genetically different disease subsets? *Dis Markers* 2000; 16:101–104.

94. Clerici M, Fusi ML, Caputo D, et al. Immune responses to antigens of human endogenous retroviruses in patients with acute or stable multiple sclerosis. *J Neuroimmunol* 1999; 99:173–182.

95. Rieger F, Pierig R, Cifuentes-Diaz C, et al. New perspectives in multiple sclerosis: retroviral involvement and glial cell death. *Pathol Biol (Paris)* 2000; 48:15–24.

96. Deb-Rinker P, Klempan TA, O'Reilly RL, Torrey EF, Singh SM. Molecular characterization of a MSRV-like sequence identified by RDA from monozygotic twin pairs discordant for schizophrenia. *Genomics* 1999; 6:133–144.

97. Hackett J, Swanson P, Leahy D, et al. search for retrovirus in patients with multiple sclerosis. *Ann Neurol* 1996; 40:805–809.

98. Hauser S, Aubert C, Burks J, et al. Analysis of human T-lymphotropic virus sequences in multiple sclerosis tissue. *Nature* 1986; 322:176–177.

99. Weiss S. Coronaviruses SD and SK share extensive nucleotide homology with murine coronaviruses. *Virology* 1983; 126:669–677.

100. Murray R, Cai G-Y, Hoel K, et al. Coronavirus infects and causes demyelination in primate central nervous system. *Virology* 188: 274-284, 1992

101. Murray R, Cai G-Y, Cabriac G. Autoimmune demyelination in primates following coronavirus infection [abstract]. *Neurology* 1992; (suppl 3):326.

102. Murray R, Brown B, Brian D, Cabriac G. Detection of coronavirus RNA and antigen in multiple sclerosis brain. *Ann Neurol* 1992; 3:525–533.

103. Sorensen O, Collins A, Flintoff W, Ebers G, Dales S. Probing for the human coronavirus OC43 in multiple sclerosis. *Neurology* 1986; 36:1604–1606.

104. Dessau R, Lisby G, Freidriksen J. Coronaviruses in spinal fluid of patients with monosymptomatic optic neuritis. *Acta Neurol Scand* 1999; 100:88–91.

105. Johnson R. The virology of demyelinating diseases. *Ann Neurol* 1994; 36:S54–S60.

106. Ferrante P, Omodero-Zorini E, Caldarelli-Stefano R, et al. Detection of JC virus DNA in cerebrospinal fluid from multiple sclerosis patients. *Mult Scler* 1998; 4:49–54.

107. Bogdanovic G, Priftakis P, Hammarin A, et al. Detection of JC virus in cerebrospinal fluid (CSF) samples from patients with progressive multifocal leukoencephalopathy but not in CSF samples from patients with herpes simplex encephalitis, enterovirus meningitis or multiple sclerosis. *J Clin Microbiol* 1998; 36:1137–1138.

108. Sriram S, Stratton C, Yao S, et al. Chlamydia pneumoniae infection of the central nervous system in multiple sclerosis. *Ann Neurol* 1999; 46:6–14.

109. Trieb J, Haas A, Stille W, et al. Multiple sclerosis and *Chlamydia pneumoniae*. *Ann Neurol* 2000; 47:408.

110. Gieffers J, Pohl D, Trieb J, et al. Presence of *Chlamydia pneumoniae* DNA in the cerebrospinal fluid is a common phenomenon in a variety of neurological diseases and not restricted to multiple sclerosis. *Ann Neurol* 2001; 49:585–589.

111. Yao S, Stratton C, Mitchell W, Sriram S. CSF oligoclonal bancs in MS include antibodies against *Chlamydophila* antigens. *Neurology* 2001; 56:1168–1176.

112. Derfuss T, Gurkov R, Then Bergh F, et al. Intrathecal antibody production against *Chlamydia pneumoniae* in multiple sclerosis is part of a polyspecific immune response. *Brain* 2001; 124:1325–1335.

113. Rivers T. Viruses and Koch's postulates. *J Bacteriol* 1937; 33:1–12.

114. Johnson R, Gibbs C. Koch's postulates and slow infections of the nervous system. *Arch Neurol* 1974; 30:36–38.

115. Esposito M, Venkatesh V, Otvos L, Weng Z, Vajda S, Banki K, Perl A. Human transaldolase and cross-reactive viral epitopes identified by autoantibodies of multiple scleosis patients. *J Immunol* 1999; 163:4027–4032.

# 9 Viral Demyelinating Diseases in Experimental Animals

*Jane E. Libbey, M.S.*
*Robert S. Fujinami, Ph.D.*

Multiple sclerosis (MS) is the most common demyelinating disease in humans. It is considered to be an autoimmune disease of the central nervous system (CNS) characterized by inflammatory demyelinating lesions that coalesce into large plaque regions within white matter. Contrary to the autoimmune nature of MS, epidemiologic studies have pointed to a viral or microbial infection as the etiology (1). Risk of MS increases as the distance from the equator increases. Migration studies of individuals moving between high-risk and low-risk areas have found that individuals carry the risk of the area from which they migrated if the individual moves after age 15 years. However, they acquire the risk of the new area to which they migrated if the individual moves before age 15 years (2) (Figure 9.1). Such epidemiologic studies have suggested that exposure to an agent or repeated infections before puberty contributes to MS in high-risk areas or protects against MS in low-risk areas. Also in support of a role for an infectious agent in MS, epidemiologic studies of isolated populations with no reported cases of MS found an initial wave of MS followed by secondary cases arising in small epidemics after contact with Europeans or North Americans (3). There has also been a correlation between viral infections and the exacerbation of MS (4–7). Lastly, in contrast to many other autoimmune diseases, such as diabetes, arthritis,

and thyroiditis, MS occurs only in humans, with no naturally occurring animal counterpart. This suggests a pathogen with a limited host range as the cause of MS.

Over the past 100 years, viruses have been suggested to be the cause of MS, yet no single virus has been identified as the causative agent. Table 9.1 lists viral or prion agents including rabies virus, several members of the herpesvirus family, several members of the paramyxovirus family, and retroviral agents recently from MS tissue (8–12).

Viral infections can cause demyelinating disease (8). Current animal models for viral-induced demyelinating disease are listed in Table 9.2. Infection can result in focal areas to large plaques of demyelination. Due to the similarities between these viral-induced demyelinating diseases and MS, many of these animal infections have been used as models to study MS. Some of the similarities between MS and these experimental animal models follow: (1) genetic susceptibility plays a role in the development of MS and virus-induced demyelination; (2) MS can be of the relapsing–remitting type or the progressive type, and animal models are now available that display a relapsing–remitting or a progressive course of disease; and (3) similarities in neuropathology.

The primary target in MS is thought to be the oligodendrocyte, which forms myelin in the CNS. White matter inflammatory demyelinating lesions with glial scarring

**TABLE 9.1**
*Viruses Recovered from Patients
with Multiple Sclerosis\**

| Agent | Year |
|---|---|
| Rabies virus | 1946 |
| Herpes simplex virus, type 2 | 1964 |
| Scrapie agent | 1965 |
| MS-associated agent | 1972 |
| Parainfluenza virus, type 1 | 1972 |
| Measles virus | 1972 |
| Simian virus-5 | 1978 |
| Chimpanzee cytomegalovirus | 1979 |
| Coronavirus | 1980 |
| SMON-like virus | 1982 |
| Tick-borne encephalitis flavivirus | 1982 |
| Human T-cell lymphotrophic virus, type 1 | 1986 |
| LM7 (retrovirus) | 1989 |
| Herpes simplex virus, type 1 | 1989 |
| Human herpesvirus-6 | 1994 |

\*Adapted from *Viral Infections of the Nervous System*. New York: Lippincott-Raven; 1998.
MS, multiple sclerosis; SMON, subacute myelo-opticoneuropathy.

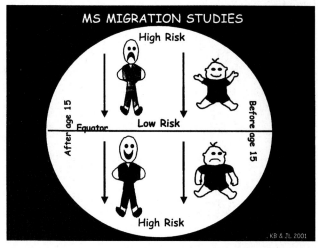

**FIGURE 9.1**

MS migration studies. Migration after age 15 years results in retaining the risk of the region from which has moved. Migration before age 15 years results in acquiring the risk of the region to which has moved. MS, multiple sclerosis.

characterize the neuropathology of MS (13). The lesions are multifocal in time and space, appearing in the optic nerve, brainstem, spinal cord, and periventricular white matter. These lesions could be the result of an immune response recognizing viral determinants in infected oligodendrocytes and killing these infected cells or by lymphocytes producing oligodendrocyte toxic factors such as tumor necrosis factor (TNF) or lymphotoxin that lead to oligodendrocyte death. Multiple pathologic mechanisms may lead to myelin destruction, resulting in the characteristic white matter plaques.

## BACKGROUND

### Theiler's Murine Encephalomyelitis Virus (TMEV)

TMEV was isolated from the CNS of mice with spontaneous flaccid paralysis of the hind limbs (14,15). This virus was found to be a naturally occurring enteric pathogen of mice (16). Demyelination during TMEV infection was first reported by Daniels et al. (17). Little notice was paid to this animal model for demyelination until Lipton described a biphasic disease leading to demyelination (18). TMEV has been divided into two subgroups based on neurovirulence. The Theiler's Original (TO) subgroup, which includes the DA, TO, WW and BeAn strains, among others, causes an acute

encephalomyelitis followed by CNS demyelination and viral persistence. The GDVII subgroup, which includes the GDVII and FA strains, causes an acute fatal polioencephalomyelitis (19). Infection of mice with strains from the TO subgroup is a favored animal model for MS (20).

TMEV belongs to the family *Picornaviridae*, genus *Cardiovirus*. TMEV is a nonenveloped, positive sense, single-stranded RNA virus with a genome of approximately 8100 nucleotides (Figure 9.2). A small virally encoded protein, VPg, is covalently bound to the viral RNA at the 5' end, and the 3' end of the genome is polyadenylated. The viral RNA is first translated into a single large precursor polyprotein that is posttranslationally cleaved by a virally encoded protease into various structural capsid proteins, VP1–4, and at least six nonstructural proteins. A virally encoded polymerase allows for the replication of negative sense RNA from the viral genome and subsequent replication of additional positive sense RNA, which in turn is incorporated into viral capsids leading to infectious virus progeny (21). Viruses of both subgroups, although different in biological activity, are 90 percent identical at the nucleotide level and 95 percent identical at the amino acid level (22). The receptors used by TMEV to enter cells are not known, although P0 may be a receptor used outside the CNS (23).

The ability of TMEV to cause disease in mice and the characteristics of the disease depend on the strain (24), sex (25), and age (26,27) of the mouse and on the dose and strain of the virus. C57BL/6 and BALB/c mice are resistant to infection with TMEV, whereas SJL/J mice

**TABLE 9.2**
*Animal Models of Demyelinating Diseases\**

| Virus Family | Virus | Host Animal |
|---|---|---|
| Papovavirus | SV40 | Monkeys |
| Coronavirus | MHV | Mice |
| | | Rats |
| Picornavirus | TMEV | Mice |
| | Encephalomyocarditis virus | Mice |
| Rhabdovirus | Chandipura virus | Mice |
| | Vesicular stomatitis virus | Mice |
| Togavirus | Semliki Forest virus | Mice |
| | Venezuelan equine encephalitis virus | Mice |
| | Ross River virus | Mice |
| Paramyxovirus | Canine distemper virus | Dogs |
| Lentivirus | Visna virus | Sheep |
| | Caprine arthritis–encephalitis virus | Goats |

\*Adapted from *Viral Infections of the Nervous System.* New York: Lippincott-Raven; 1998.
MHV, mouse hepatitis virus; SV40, simian virus-40; TMEV, Theiler's murine encephalomyelitis virus.

are susceptible (24). Resistance maps genetically to the H-2D region (28,29), to the constant-region β-chain gene locus of the T-cell receptor (30), and a locus on chromosome 3 (31).

The demyelination induced by infection of a susceptible strain of mouse with the DA strain of TMEV is characterized by destruction of the myelin sheaths with relative sparing of the axons (32), although axonal loss has been associated with progressive disease (33). Virus persists and can be localized to neurons (34), oligodendrocytes (35), astrocytes (36), and microglia/macrophages (37). The clinical symptoms of weakness of the extremities, spasticity, incontinence, and eventual paralysis are very similar to what is seen in MS (18).

### Mouse Hepatitis Virus (MHV)

MHV was isolated from the CNS of mice with spontaneous paralysis of the hind limbs (38). This virus was found to cause demyelination during infection (38,39).

A systematic study of the ability of MHV to produce demyelination was performed by Weiner (40). MHV was found to be a naturally occurring respiratory or enteric pathogen of mice (41). Infection of mice with neuroadapted strains of MHV is a favored animal model for MS.

MHV belongs to the family *Coronaviridae*, genus *Coronavirus*. MHV is an enveloped, positive sense, single-stranded RNA virus with a genome of approximately 31000 nucleotides (Figure 9.3). The 5' end is capped and the 3' end is polyadenylated. The viral RNA is first translated into a virally encoded polymerase. The virally encoded polymerase allows for the replication of negative sense RNA from the viral genome and subsequent replication of additional positive sense RNA, which in turn is incorporated into infectious virus progeny. The negative sense RNA acts as a template for the synthesis of a 3' coterminal nested set of subgenomic mRNAs by means of a process of discontinuous transcription. Each of these mRNAs has a leader sequence that corresponds to the viral 5' terminus. These subgenomic mRNAs encode the struc-

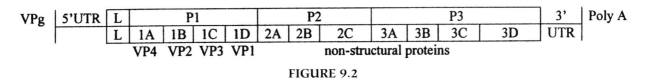

**FIGURE 9.2**

TMEV genome. Structure of the TMEV RNA and cleavages to the polyprotein producing the viral proteins. Adapted from *Fields Virology.* New York: Lippincott-Raven; 1996:609–654. L, leader sequence; P1–3, proteins 1 to 3; Poly A, polyadenylated tail; TMEV, Theiler's murine encephalomyelitis virus; UTR, untranslater region; VP1–4, capsid proteins 1 to 4; VPg, virally encoded protein.

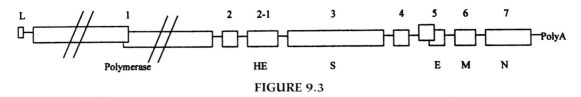

**FIGURE 9.3**

MHV genome. Structure of the MHV RNA and open reading frames encoding the viral proteins. Adapted from *Fields Virology*. New York: Lippincott-Raven; 1996:1075–1093. 1–7, open reading frames 1 to 7; E, virally encoded small membrane protein; HE, hemagglutinin-esterase protein; L, leader sequence; M, virally encoded membrane or matrix protein; MHV, mouse hepatitis virus; N, nucleocapsid protein; Poly A, polyadenylated tail; S, spike protein.

tural and nonstructural viral proteins. The viral genomic RNA is associated with the nucleocapsid protein within the virion. The nucleocapsid is surrounded by a host cell–derived envelope that contains three virally encoded proteins: spike protein (S), membrane or matrix protein, and the small membrane protein. Some MHV strains also encode the hemagglutinin-esterase protein, which is also embedded in the envelope. Nonstructural proteins, including the polymerase and two proteases, are encoded by the remainder of the MHV genome (42). The receptor used by MHV to enter cells is a cell surface molecules of the biliary glycoprotein and carcinoembryonic family (43).

The ability of MHV to cause disease in mice and the characteristics of the disease depend on the strain and age of the mouse (44) and the dose, route of inoculation, and strain of the virus. BALB/c and C57BL/6 mice develop fatal encephalitis with infection with the JHM strain of MHV. Rare survivors develop a chronic demyelinating disease (45). In contrast, SJL/J mice are resistant to the development of encephalitis and demyelinating disease due to a polymorphism in the receptor (43). Many neuroattenuated strains of MHV do not cause a fatal encephalitis but do cause chronic demyelination (45).

Chronic demyelination induced by infection of a susceptible strain of mouse with MHV is characterized by destruction of the myelin sheaths with sparing of the axons (46). Virus can be localized to neurons, oligodendrocytes, astrocytes, and microglia and macrophages (46). The clinical symptoms are incoordination and the development of hind limb paralysis and, in some animals, tetraplegia (41,45).

## IMMUNE RESPONSE AND IMMUNOPATHOLOGY

A key element in the development of demyelination appears to be viral persistence. The level of virus or viral products is proportional to the amount of demyelination and clinical disease. Demyelination could occur by means of four different mechanisms (Table 9.3) or a combination of any of the four (47).

The immune response to viral infection of the CNS may contribute to the pathogenesis of demyelination in TMEV and MHV infections. One means to study the role of the host immune system in viral-induced demyelination is to infect immunodeficient mice. Nude mice, partially immunodeficient, and severe combined immunodeficient (SCID) mice, profoundly immunosuppressed, have been used for this purpose. Another means to study the role of the host immune system in viral-induced demyelination is to infect immune knockout mice. When considering the immune system, one also must consider the major histocompatibility complex (MHC) class I and II molecules and the role, if any, they play in viral-induced demyelination.

### TMEV—Nude and SCID Mice

The role of the immune system in demyelination has been studied for TMEV infection. Intracranial inoculation of immunocompetent susceptible mice with the DA strain of TMEV resulted in demyelination apparent at 1 month postinfection. Intracranial inoculation of nude mice with DA virus resulted in demyelination apparent as soon as 7 days postinfection (48–50). In addition, intraocular and intravenous inoculations of nude mice with the DA strain resulted in demyelination 3 weeks postinfection (51). The data suggest that the immunocompetent mice are protected against demyelination during the acute phase of infection by the immune system and that the route of

---

**TABLE 9.3**
*Mechanisms of Demyelination*

1. Direct viral lysis of infected oligodendrocytes (cells myelinate axons in the central nervous system)
2. Direct immune response against infected oligodendrocytes
3. Autoimmune response against uninfected oligodendrocytes triggered by infection
4. Indirect nonspecific bystander immune response in vicinity of infection

inoculation in the immunodeficient mice affects the time required for the development of lesions but not the distribution of the lesions.

Intracranial infection of SCID mice resulted in death 17 days postinoculation, without clearance of the virus and without demyelination (52). Adoptive transfer of splenocytes from immunocompetent resistant mice to SCID mice produced results based on the number of splenocytes transferred. If too few cells were transferred, the mice died from the lethal challenge without demyelination. If 1.8 to 7.5 × 10$^6$ cells were transferred, persistence of the virus within the white matter of the spinal cord and demyelination resulted. If too many cells were transferred, the virus was cleared without demyelination. Demyelination appeared to depend on a critical balance between persistent viral infection and lymphocytes. Adoptive transfer of splenocytes from SCID mice to SCID mice resulted in the death of the mice from the lethal challenge. This finding indicated that T- and B-cells are required for protection and that macrophages and natural killer cells, normally present in SCID spleens, are not. If the splenocytes from the immunocompetent resistant mice, at concentrations that protect against demyelination, were depleted of CD4$^+$ or CD8$^+$ T-cells, demyelination occurred subsequent to their transfer into SCID mice. The lesions were more severe if the splenocytes were depleted of CD4$^+$ T-cells, suggesting that CD8$^+$ T-cells may be particularly effective in promoting demyelination. Depletion of CD4$^+$ and CD8$^+$ T-cells resulted in death from the lethal challenge, thus confirming the protection by T-cells.

The roles of MHC class I and II molecules have been studied for TMEV infection. The role of MHC class I molecules remains controversial due to conflicting reports. MHC class I expression persisted in the CNS of susceptible mice throughout the chronic demyelinating disease but returned to normal undetectable levels by 28 days postinfection in resistant mice (53). This upregulation of class I was mediated by interferon-α/β and not by the direct effect of TMEV infection (54). SCID mice expressed class I in the CNS after infection, so functional T- or B-cells are not required for this upregulation (54). Class I–restricted CD8$^+$ cytotoxic T lymphocytes were TMEV specific at 7 days postinfection in resistant but not in susceptible strains of mice (55). The susceptible mice have cells that are cytotoxic; they are just not virus specific (55). Thus, the TMEV-specific cytotoxic T-cells may play a role in the clearance of the virus, and the non–virus-specific cytotoxic T-cells may play a role in demyelination. In contrast, demyelination can occur in MHC class I knockout resistant mice that lack functional CD8$^+$ T-cells (56). Demyelination was observed in resistant CD8 knockout mice, and demyelination similar to that in controls was observed in susceptible CD8 knockout mice (57,58). However, demyelination was partly

suppressed in susceptible mice treated with anti-CD8 antibodies (59).

As with MHC class I molecules, there are conflicting reports for MHC class II molecules. MHC class II molecules are induced on astrocytes during TMEV infection (60). In contrast, demyelination can occur in MHC class II knockout resistant mice that lack functional CD4$^+$ T-cells (61). Demyelination was observed in resistant CD4 knockout mice, and severe demyelination as compared with control mice was observed in susceptible CD4 knockout mice (57,58). However, demyelination was partly suppressed in mice treated with anti-MHC class II antibodies (62,63).

Taken together, these data suggest that CD8$^+$ (class I restricted) and CD4$^+$ (class II restricted) T-cells contribute to virus-induced demyelination but that neither is individually absolutely necessary for demyelination to occur. Demyelination may be promoted by either T-cell population, independently, in the presence of virus, or some other factors may mediate demyelination.

## MHV—Nude and SCID Mice

The role of the immune system in demyelination has been studied for MHV infection (64). Intracranial infection of immunocompetent susceptible mice with a neuroattenuated MHV strain resulted in clearance of virus and demyelination. Intracranial inoculation of nude mice with a wild-type MHV strain resulted in incomplete clearance of virus and demyelination. However, intracranial infection of SCID mice resulted in death 12 days postinfection without clearance of the virus and without demyelination. Further, clearance of virus and demyelination resulted from the adoptive transfer of splenocytes from immunocompetent susceptible mice to SCID mice. An immunologic basis for viral-induced demyelination is supported by these studies, and the immune system components required for demyelination may be separate from those required for viral clearance. Conventional T-cells do not appear to be required for demyelination, as shown by the presence of demyelinating disease in nude mice; therefore, γ-δ T-cells, natural killer cells, and cytokines may participate in the demyelination process (64). However, conventional CD4$^+$ and CD8$^+$ T-cells have been shown, through the use of an adoptive transfer model, to be independently capable of producing MHV-induced demyelination, although neither subset is required for demyelination (65).

The roles of MHC class I and II molecules have been studied for MHV infection. Similar to the role of MHC class I in TMEV infection, the role of MHC class I remains controversial in MHV infections due to conflicting reports. Class I expression on astrocytes increased when primary cells were infected, decreased when cells were persistently infected, and showed no expression when cells were taken from chronically infected mice experiencing demyelinating disease (66–68). Demyelination occurred in mice that lacked functional CD8$^+$ T-cells or the stable expression of MHC class I (64,69), which is in agreement with the adoptive transfer model showing no requirement for CD8$^+$ T-cells in demyelination (65).

As with MHC class I, the expression of MHC class II increased with infection of astrocytes with MHV; however, demyelination can occur in MHC class II-deficient mice (64,70), which is in agreement with the adoptive transfer model showing no requirement for CD4$^+$ T-cells in demyelination (65). Thus, the resulting MHV-induced demyelination may be controlled by genes other than MHC classes I and II.

## CD4 versus CD8—Protection and Clearance

The host immune system plays an important role in protection against and clearance of the infecting virus. In TMEV infection, cellular immune responses play a role in viral clearance. Lindsley and Rodriguez suggested that CD8$^+$ T-cells play a critical role in clearance of the virus in resistant mice (71). They found that CD8$^+$ T-cells accumulate in the CNS of resistant mice, at approximately 7 days postinfection, and that very few CD8$^+$ T-cells accumulate in susceptible mice before 14 days postinfection. The inability of the susceptible mice to clear the virus may result in viral persistence and demyelination. Mice depleted of T-cells by the administration of anti-CD3, anti-CD4, or anti-CD8 monoclonal antibodies at the time of infection were unable to clear the virus and succumbed to the viral infection (59,72–74). CD4 or CD8 knockout mice in a resistant or susceptible background were unable to clear the virus, and a persistent infection and demyelination resulted (57,58). Also, adoptively transferred CD8$^+$ T-cells from resistant mice conferred resistance to susceptible strains of mice (75).

In MHV infection, whole-body irradiation of susceptible mice prevented viral clearance and confirmed the role of the host immune system in the reduction of viral replication; there was a reduction in viral titer in nonirradiated mice after 7 days postinfection, although the response was too late to prevent death (76). Virus-specific CD4$^+$ or CD8$^+$ T-cells do not effectively clear the virus while protecting the mice against a lethal challenge; however, virus-specific CD4$^+$ and CD8$^+$ T-cells together did protect mice and clear the virus (47). Mice deficient in CD4$^+$ or CD8$^+$ T-cells were unable to clear virus and succumbed to the lethal challenge (76,77). Clearance of virus appeared to be mediated by CD8$^+$ T-cells in a CD4$^+$ T-cell–dependent fashion (76). Thus, protection against a lethal challenge with MHV and clearance of virus seem to be independent.

## Antibodies—Protection and Clearance

Humoral immunity plays a role in protection against and clearance of the infecting virus. Antiviral antibodies might control virus infection by binding to the virus and thus directly inactivating the virus or activating the classic complement pathway. Another mechanism for antibody control of infection is antibody-dependent cell-mediated cytotoxicity. However, antibodies also may be involved in generating the demyelination seen with virus infection.

TMEV-infected susceptible mice show increased immunoglobulin (Ig) in the cerebrospinal fluid, which was directed against virus (78). Knockout mice deficient in antibody production succumbed to the lethal challenge with TMEV infection (79). Depletion of Ig by anti-IgM antibodies or expression of the *xid* gene mutation increased demyelination in susceptible mice (80). Complement depletion of susceptible mice also increased demyelination (78). These results support a role for antibody and complement in clearance of virus in TMEV infection.

Yamada et al. generated a neutralizing monoclonal antibody to TMEV that showed specificity for oligodendrocytes and myelin structures (81). This antibody displayed an in vivo demyelinating effect. Also, the sera of mice chronically infected with TMEV had antibody with the same specificity as the monoclonal antibody. Thus, antibody to virus can augment demyelination in vivo, and antibody produced in mice may actively take part in the process of TMEV-induced demyelination.

In MHV infection, antiviral antibodies to the three viral structural proteins do not effectively clear the virus, resulting in a persistent CNS infection while protecting the mice from a lethal challenge (47). Immunization with a recombinant *Vaccinia* virus producing the S protein of MHV induced neutralizing antibodies specific for S protein (82). Subsequent challenge with MHV at 7 days postimmunization, at a time before the appearance of the S-specific antibodies, cleared the virus, with no demyelination. However, challenge with MHV at 21 days postimmunization, at a time when the production of S-specific antibodies has peaked, cleared the virus but left extensive demyelination. Thus, antibodies specific for virus appear to protect against lethal challenge and contribute to demyelination. These results are supported by work with recombinant tobacco mosaic virus producing epitopes of the S protein of MHV, which induced neutralizing antibodies that protected mice against a lethal challenge with MHV (83). Also, antiviral antibodies controlled the recurrence of infectious MHV during persistent CNS infection as seen by the reemergence of virus within the CNS of B-cell–deficient mice (46,84).

**TABLE 9.4**
*Comparison of TMEV and MHV*

| TMEV | MHV |
|---|---|
| **Similarities** ||
| Natural host: mouse ||
| Demyelination ||
| Clinical symptoms of paralysis ||
| Destruction of the myelin sheaths with sparing of the axons ||
| Animal model for MS ||
| Positive sense, single-stranded RNA ||
| Infects neurons, oligodendrocytes, astrocytes, and microglia/macrophages ||
| CD8$^+$ (MHC class I) and CD4$^+$ (MHC class II) T cells contribute to virus-induced demyelination ||
| **Differences** ||
| Genome of approximately 8100 nucleotides | Genome of approximately 31000 nucleotides |
| Nonenveloped virus | Enveloped virus |
| Biphasic disease | Monophasic disease |
| Infectious persistence | Noninfectious persistence |
| C57BL/6 and BALB/c mice are resistant | SJL/J mice are resistant |
| SJL/J mice are susceptible | BALB/c and C57BL/6 mice are susceptible |
| CD8$^+$ T-cells play a critical role in clearance of the virus | Clearance of virus is mediated by CD8$^+$ T-cells in a CD4$^+$ T-cell–dependent fashion |
| Antibody and complement play a role in clearance of virus | Antiviral antibodies control the recurrence of infectious MHV during persistent CNS infection |

CNS, central nervous system; MHC, major histocompatibility complex; MHV, mouse hepatitis virus; TMEV, Theiler murine encephalomyelitis virus.

## CONCLUSION

Although not perfect, TMEV and MHV infections of the mouse are reasonable models for MS (Table 9.4). The TMEV and MHV models are good for the study of the pathogenic mechanisms of virus-induced demyelinating disease. The viral-induced demyelination observed in these infections resembles the demyelination seen in MS patients. The clinical symptoms observed in TMEV- and MHV-infected mice mirror some of the symptoms observed in MS patients. The host immune system contributes to the demyelination that results from TMEV and MHV infection in a manner similar to the demyelination seen in MS patients. In addition, virus infections may play a role in MS, as shown by the exacerbation of symptoms with viral infection and the epidemiologic data suggesting a viral cause of MS. Through the study of viral-induced demyelination by TMEV and MHV, insights might be gained into the mechanisms of demyelination in MS.

### Acknowledgments

We are grateful to Ms. Kathleen Borick for preparation of the manuscript. This research was supported by NIH grants AI42525 and NS34497.

## References

1. Kurtzke JF, Heltberg A. Multiple sclerosis in the Faroe Islands. An epitome. *J Clin Epidemiol* 2001; 54:1–22.
2. Kurtzke JF. Epidemiologic evidence for multiple sclerosis as an infection. *Clin Microbiol Rev* 1993; 6:382–427.
3. Kurtzke JF. The epidemiology of multiple sclerosis. In: Raine CS, McFarland HF, Tourtellotte WW (eds.), *Multiple Sclerosis: Clinical and Pathogenetic Basis.* London: Chapman & Hall, 1997; 91–140.
4. Sibley WA, Bamford CR, Clark K. Clinical viral infections and multiple sclerosis. *Lancet* 1985; 1:1313–1315.
5. Andersen O, Lygner P-E, Bergström T, Andersson M, Vahlne A. Viral infections trigger multiple sclerosis relapses: a prospective seroepidemiological study. *J Neurol* 1993; 240:417–422.
6. De Keyser J, Zwanikken C, Boon M. Effects of influenza vaccination and influenza illness on exacerbations in multiple sclerosis. *J Neurol Sci* 1998; 159:51–53.
7. Panitch HS. Influence of infection on exacerbations of multiple sclerosis. *Ann Neurol* 1994; 36(suppl):S25–S28.
8. Johnson RT. *Viral Infections of the Nervous System.* New York: Lippincott-Raven Publishers, 1998.
9. Munch M, Møller-Larsen A, Christensen T, et al. B-lymphoblastoid cell lines from multiple sclerosis patients and a healthy control producing a putative new human retrovirus and Epstein-Barr virus. *Mult Scler* 1995; 1:78–81.
10. Møller-Larsen A, Christensen T. Isolation of a retrovirus from multiple sclerosis patients in self-generated Iodixanol gradients. *J Virol Methods* 1998; 73:151–161.
11. Christensen T, Dissing SP, Riemann H, Hansen HJ, Møller-Larsen A. Expression of sequence variants of endogenous retrovirus RGH in particle form in multiple sclerosis. *Lancet* 1998; 352:1033.

12. Garson JA, Tuke PW, Giraud P, Paranhos BG, Perron H. Detection of virion-associated MSRV-RNA in serum of patients with multiple sclerosis. *Lancet* 1998; 351:33.

13. Lucchinetti CF, Bruck W, Rodriguez M, Lassmann H. Distinct patterns of multiple sclerosis pathology indicates heterogeneity on pathogenesis. *Brain Pathol* 1996; 6:259–274.

14. Theiler M. Spontaneous encephalomyelitis of mice: a new virus disease. *Science* 1934; 80:122.

15. Theiler M. Spontaneous encephalomyelitis of mice, a new virus disease. *J Exp Med* 1937; 65:705–719.

16. Theiler M, Gard S. Encephalomyelitis of mice. I. Characteristics and pathogenesis of the virus. *J Exp Med* 1940; 72:49–67.

17. Daniels JB, Pappenheimer AM, Richardson S. Observations on encephalomyelitis of mice (DA strain). *J Exp Med* 1952; 96:517–535.

18. Lipton HL. Theiler's virus infection in mice: an unusual biphasic disease process leading to demyelination. *Infect Immun* 1975; 11:1147–1155.

19. Tsunoda I, Fujinami RS. Theiler's murine encephalomyelitis virus. In: Ahmed R, Chen I, (eds.), *Persistent Viral Infections*. Chichester: John Wiley & Sons, 1999; 517–536.

20. Dal Canto MC, Lipton HL. Animal model: Theiler's virus infection in mice. *Am J Pathol* 1977; 88:497–500.

21. Rueckert RR. Picornaviridae: the viruses and their replication. In: Fields BN, Knipe DM, Howley PM, et al. (eds.), *Fields Virology*. New York: Lippincott-Raven, 1996; 609–654.

22. Pevear DC, Borkowski J, Calenoff M, et al. Insights into Theiler's virus neurovirulence based on a genomic comparison of the neurovirulent GDVII and less virulent BeAn strains. *Virology* 1988; 165:1–12.

23. Libbey JE, McCright IJ, Isunoda I, Wada Y, Fujinami RS. Peripheral nerve protein, P0, as a potential receptor for Theiler's murine encephalomyelitis virus. *J Neurovirol* 2001; 7:97–104.

24. Lipton HL, Dal Canto MC. Susceptibility of inbred mice to chronic central nervous system infection by Theiler's murine encephalomyelitis virus. *Infect Immun* 1979; 26:369–374.

25. Kappel CA, Melvold RW, Kim BS. Influence of sex on susceptibility in the Theiler's murine encephalomyelitis virus model for multiple sclerosis. *J Neuroimmunol* 1990; 29:15–19.

26. Steiner CM, Rozhon EJ, Lipton HL. Relationship between host age and persistence of Theiler's virus in the central nervous system of mice. *Infect Immun* 1984; 43:432–434.

27. Rodriguez M, Leibowitz JL, Powell HC, Lampert PW. Neonatal infection with the Daniels strain of Theiler's murine encephalomyelitis virus. *Lab Invest* 1983; 49:672–679.

28. Clatch RJ, Melvold RW, Miller SD, Lipton HL. Theiler's murine encephalomyelitis virus (TMEV)-induced demyelinating disease in mice is influenced by the H-2D region: correlation with TMEV-specific delayed-type hypersensitivity. *J Immunol* 1985; 135:1408–1414.

29. Rodriguez M, Leibowitz J, David CS. Susceptibility to Theiler's virus-induced demyelination. Mapping of the gene within the H-2D region. *J Exp Med* 1986; 163:620–631.

30. Melvold RW, Jokinen DM, Knobler RL, Lipton HL. Variations in genetic control of susceptibility to Theiler's murine encephalomyelitis virus (TMEV)-induced demyelinating disease. I. Differences between susceptible SJL/J and resistant BALB/c strains map near the T-cell beta-chain constant gene on chromosome 6. *J Immunol* 1987; 138:1429–1433.

31. Melvold RW, Jokinen DM, Miller SD, Dal Canto MC, Lipton HL. Identification of a locus on mouse chromosome 3 involved in differential susceptibility to Theiler's murine encephalomyelitis virus-induced demyelinating disease. *J Virol* 1990; 64:686–690.

32. Dal Canto MC, Lipton HL. Primary demyelination in Theiler's virus infection. An ultrastructural study. *Lab Invest* 1975; 33:626–637.

33. McGavern DB, Murray PD, Rodriguez M. Quantitation of spinal cord demyelination, remyelination, atrophy, and axonal loss in a model of progressive neurologic injury. *J Neurosci Res* 1999; 58:492–504.

34. Dal Canto MC, Lipton HL. Ultrastructural immunohistochemical localization of virus in acute and chronic demyelinating Theiler's virus infection. *Am J Pathol* 1982; 106:20–29.

35. Rodriguez M, Leibowitz JL, Lampert PW. Persistent infection of oligodendrocytes in Theiler's virus-induced encephalomyelitis. *Ann Neurol* 1983; 13:426–433.

36. Aubert C, Chamorro M, Brahic M. Identification of Theiler's virus infected cells in the central nervous system of the mouse during demyelinating disease. *Microb Pathog* 1987; 3:319–326.

37. Clatch RJ, Miller SD, Metzner R, Dal Canto MC, Lipton HL. Monocytes/macrophages isolated from the mouse central nervous system contain infectious Theiler's murine encephalomyelitis virus (TMEV). *Virology* 1990; 176:244–254.

38. Cheever FS, Daniels JB, Pappenheimer AM, Bailey OT. A murine virus (JHM) causing disseminated encephalomyelitis with extensive destruction of myelin. I. Isolation and biological properties of the virus. *J Exp Med* 1949; 90:181–194.

39. Bailey OT, Pappenheimer AM, Cheever FS, Daniels JB. A murine virus (JHM) causing disseminated encephalomyelitis with extensive destruction of myelin. II. Pathology. *J Exp Med* 1949; 90:195–212.

40. Weiner LP. Pathogenesis of demyelination induced by a mouse hepatitis. *Arch Neurol* 1973; 28:298–303.

41. Wege H, Siddell S, ter Meulen V. The biology and pathogenesis of coronaviruses. Curr Topics *Microbiol Immunol* 1982; 99:165–200.

42. Holmes KV, Lai MMC. Coronaviridae: The viruses and their replication. In: Fields BN, Knipe DM, Howley PM, et al. (eds.), *Fields Virology*. New York: Lippincott-Raven, 1996; 1075–1093.

43. Williams RK, Jiang GS, Snyder SW, Frana MF, Holmes KV. Purification of the 110-kilodalton glycoprotein receptor for mouse hepatitis virus (MHV)-A59 from mouse liver and identification of a nonfunctional, homologous protein in MHV-resistant SJL/J mice. *J Virol* 1990; 64:3817–3823.

44. Stohlman SA, Frelinger JA, Weiner LP. Resistance to fatal central nervous system disease by mouse hepatitis virus, strain JHM. II. Adherent cell-mediated protection. *J Immunol* 1980; 124:1733–1739.

45. Lane TE, Buchmeier MJ. Murine coronavirus infection: a paradigm for virus-induced demyelinating disease. *Trends Microbiol* 1997; 5:9–14.

46. Stohlman SA, Hinton DR. Viral induced demyelination. *Brain Pathol* 2001; 11:92–106.

47. Houtman JJ, Fleming JO. Pathogenesis of mouse hepatitis virus-induced demyelination. *J Neurovirol* 1996; 2:361–376.

48. Roos RP, Wollmann R. DA strain of Theiler's murine encephalomyelitis virus induces demyelination in nude mice. *Ann Neurol* 1984; 15:494–499.

49. Rosenthal A, Fujinami RS, Lampert PW. Mechanism of Theiler's virus-induced demyelination in nude mice. *Lab Invest* 1986; 54:515–522.

50. Fujinami RS, Rosenthal A, Lampert PW, Zurbriggen A, Yamada M. Survival of athymic (nu/nu) mice after Theiler's murine encephalomyelitis virus infection by passive administration of neutralizing monoclonal antibody. *J Virol* 1989; 63:2081–2087.

51. Love S. Distribution of Theiler's virus in the CNS of athymic nude mice: effect of varying the route of inoculation. *J Neurol Sci* 1987; 81:55–66.

52. Rodriguez M, Pavelko KD, Njenga MK, Logan WC, Wettstein PJ. The balance between persistent virus infection and immune cells determines demyelination. *J Immunol* 1996; 157:5699–5709.

53. Lindsley MD, Patick AK, Prayoonwiwat N, Rodriguez M. Coexpression of class I major histocmpatibility antigen and viral RNA in central nervous system of mice infected with Theiler's virus: a model for multiple sclerosis. *Mayo Clin Proc* 1992; 67:829–838.

54. Njenga MK, Pease LR, Wettstein P, Mak T, Rodriguez M. Interferon α/β mediates early virus-induced expression of H-2D and H-2K in the central nervous system. *Lab Invest* 1997; 77:71–84.

55. Lin X, Pease LR, Rodriguez M. Differential generation of class I H-2D- versus H-2K-restricted cytotoxicity against a demyelinating virus following central nervous system infection. *Eur J Immunol* 1997; 27:963–970.

56. Pullen LC, Miller SD, Dal Canto MC, Kim BS. Class I-deficient resistant mice intracerebrally inoculated with Theiler's virus show an increased T cell response to viral antigens and susceptibility to demyelination. *Eur J Immunol* 1993; 23:2287–2293.

57. Rodriguez M, Rivera-Quiñones C, Murray PD, et al. The role of CD4+ and CD8+ T-cells in demyelinating disease following Theiler's virus infection: a model for multiple sclerosis. *J Neurovirol* 1997; 3(suppl 1):S43–S45.

58. Murray PD, Pavelko KD, Leibowitz J, Lin X, Rodriguez M. CD4+ and CD8+ T-cells make discrete contributions to demyelination and neurologic disease in a viral model of multiple sclerosis. *J Virol* 1998; 72:7320–7329.

59. Rodriguez M, Sriram S. Successful therapy of Theiler's virus-induced demyelination (DA strain) with monoclonal anti-Lyt-2 antibody. *J Immunol* 1988; 140:2950–2955.

60. Borrow P, Nash AA. Susceptibility to Theiler's virus-induced demyelinating disease correlates with astrocyte class II induction and antigen presentation. *Immunology* 1992; 76:133–139.

61. Njenga MK, Pavelko KD, Baisch J, et al. Theiler's virus persistence and demyelination in major histocompatibility complex class II-deficient mice. *J Virol* 1996; 70:1729–1737.

62. Friedmann A, Frankel G, Lorch Y, Steinman L. Monoclonal anti-I-A antibody reverses chronic paralysis and demyelination in Theiler's virus–infected mice: critical importance of timing of treatment. *J Virol* 1987; 61:898–903.

63. Rodriguez M, Lafuse WP, Leibowitz J, David CS. Partial suppression of Theiler's virus-induced demyelination in vivo by administration of monoclonal antibodies to immune-response gene products (Ia antigens). *Neurology* 1986; 36:964–970.

64. Houtman JJ, Fleming JO. Dissociation of demyelination and viral clearance in congenitally immunodeficient mice infected with murine coronavirus JHM. *J Neurovirol* 1996; 2:101–110.

65. Wu GF, Dandekar AA, Pewe L, Perlman S. CD4 and CD8 T-cells have redundant but not identical roles in virus-induced demyelination. *J Immunol* 2000; 165:2278–2286.

66. Joseph J, Knobler RL, Lublin FD, Hart MN. Regulation of MHC class I and II antigens on cerebral endothelial cells and astrocytes following MHV-4 infection. *Adv Exp Med Biol* 1990; 276:579–591.

67. Gilmore W, Correale J, Weiner LP. Coronavirus induction of class I major histocompatibility complex expression in murine astrocytes is virus strain specific. *J Exp Med* 1994; 180:1013–1023.

68. Sun N, Grzybicki D, Castro RF, Murphy S, Perlman S. Activation of astrocytes in the spinal cord of mice chronically infected with a neurotropic coronavirus. *Virology* 1995; 213:482–493.

69. Gombold JL, Sutherland RM, Lavi E, Paterson Y, Weiss SR. Mouse hepatitis virus A59-induced demyelination can occur in the absence of CD8+ T-cells. *Microb Pathog* 1995; 18:211–221.

70. Massa PT, Brinkmann R, ter Meulen V. Inducibility of Ia antigen on astrocytes by murine coronavirus JHM is rat strain dependent. *J Exp Med* 1987; 166:259–264.

71. Lindsley MD, Rodriguez M. Characterization of the inflammatory response in the central nervous system of mice susceptible or resistant to demyelination by Theiler's virus. *J Immunol* 1989; 142:2677–2682.

72. Rodriguez M, Lindsley MD, Pierce ML. Role of T cells in resistance to Theiler's virus infection. *Microb Pathog* 1991; 11:269–281.

73. Welsh CJ, Tonks P, Nash AA, Blakemore WF. The effect of L3T4 T-cell depletion on the pathogenesis of Theiler's murine encephalomyelitis virus infection in CBA mice. *J Gen Virol* 1987; 68(pt 6):1659–1667.

74. Borrow P, Tonks P, Welsh CJ, Nash AA. The role of CD8+ T-cells in the acute and chronic phases of Theiler's murine encephalomyelitis virus-induced disease in mice. *J Gen Virol* 1992; 73(pt 7):1861–1865.

75. Nicholson SM, Dal Canto MC, Miller SD, Melvold RW. Adoptively transferred CD8+ T lymphocytes provide protection against TMEV-induced demyelinating disease in BALB/c mice. *J Immunol* 1996; 156:1276–1283.

76. Williamson JS, Stohlman SA. Effective clearance of mouse hepatitis virus from the central nervous system requires both CD4+ and CD8+ T-cells. *J Virol* 1990; 64:4589–4592.

77. Fleming JO, Ting JY, Stohlman SA, Weiner LP. Improvements in obtaining and characterizing mouse cerebrospinal fluid. Application to mouse hepatitis virus-induced encephalomyelitis. *J Neuroimmunol* 1983; 4:129–140.

78. Rodriguez M, Lucchinetti CF, Clark RJ, Yakash TL, Markowitz H, Lennon VA. Immunoglobulins and complement in demyelination induced in mice by Theiler's virus. *J Immunol* 1988; 140:800–806.

79. Drescher KM, Murray PD, David CS, Pease LR, Rodriguez M. CNS cell populations are protected from virus-induced pathology by distinct arms of the immune system. *Brain Pathol* 1999; 9:21–31.

80. Rodriguez M, Kenny JJ, Thiemann RL, Woloschak GE. Theiler's virus-induced demyelination in mice immunosuppressed with anti-IgM and in mice expressing the xid gene. *Microb Pathog* 1990; 8:23–35.

81. Yamada M, Zurbriggen A, Fujinami RS. Monoclonal antibody to Theiler's murine encephalomyelitis virus defines a determinant on myelin and oligodendrocytes, and augments demyelination in experimental allergic encephalomyelitis. *J Exp Med* 1990; 171:1893–1907.

82. Flory E, Stuhler A, Barac-Latas V, Lassmann H, Wege H. Coronavirus-induced encephalomyelitis: balance between protection and immune pathology depends on the immunization schedule with spike protein S. *J Gen Virol* 1995; 76(pt 4):873–879.

83. Koo M, Bendahmane M, Lettieri GA, et al. Protective immunity against murine hepatitis virus (MHV) induced by intranasal or subcutaneous administration of hybrids of tobacco mosaic virus that carries an MHV epitope. *Proc Natl Acad Sci USA* 1999; 96:7774–7779.

84. Lin MT, Hinton DR, Marten NW, Bergmann CC, Stohlman SA. Antibody prevents virus reactivation within the central nervous system. *J Immunol* 1999; 162:7358–7368.

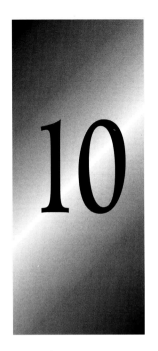

# 10 *Chlamydia pneumoniae* Infection and its Association with Multiple Sclerosis

*Harold Moses, Jr., M.D.*
*Subramaniam Sriram, M.D.*

Multiple sclerosis (MS) is the most common inflammatory disease of the central nervous system (CNS) in the Western world; although an infectious cause has been repeatedly proposed, identifying a specific infectious agent has been difficult (1). The interest in pursuing a viral etiology for MS is due to known viral associations with other CNS demyelinating disorders (2). These include progressive multifocal leukoencephalitis, human immunodeficiency virus, and human T-lymphotropic virus-1. These viruses also have known tropisms to the CNS white matter, periods of clinical latency, and at times a relapsing and remitting course. Despite the precedence of these agents and the clinical disorders they result in, the isolation of a virus has not met with success in MS, and this area of research has been one of many missteps and disappointment. We recently proposed that, even though an infectious theory of MS is the most likely explanation for the geographic distribution of the disease and the presence of epidemics in certain isolated regions of the world, other nonviral infectious agents need to be included in the search (3). In this chapter we describe the role of *Chlamydia pneumoniae* and other chlamydial species in various diseases, the association of *C. pneumoniae* infection and MS, and the underlying mechanisms of how *C. pneumoniae* may trigger MS.

## BIOLOGY OF CHLAMYDIAL INFECTION

*Chlamydia* belongs to a genus of intracellular organisms that are pathogenic to humans and other vertebrates (4). *Chlamydia* has a unique life cycle with multiple forms that are functionally and morphologically distinct (5,6). The extracellular form, the elementary body (EB), is infectious and metabolically inactive. After endocytosis, EBs differentiate into the reticulate body, which replicates by binary fission. Four species are known (*C. pneumoniae*, *C. psittacci*, *C. trachomatis*, and *C. pecorum*) and of these, *C. pneumoniae* is pathogenic to humans and are distributed worldwide (1).

In most instances, *C. pneumoniae* causes a self-limiting disease of the respiratory tract. More recently, *C. pneumoniae* infections have been thought to play a role in such diverse diseases as reactive arthritis, atherosclerosis, Alzheimer disease (AD), and MS (7–11). *Chlamydia pneumoniae* infects and replicates within macrophages and monocytes, endothelial cells, and vascular smooth muscle cells. Because these cell types are widely distributed, infection and disease ensuing from the infection may occur in many organ systems. *Chlamydia pneumoniae* is a ubiquitous respiratory agent, and seroconversion begins as early as age 4 years and by the sixth decade of life more than 70 percent of individuals show seropositivity (11). Dissemination of the organism after upper respiratory infections is common, and infection in circulating monocytes is seen in a large number of healthy individuals (12). Chlamydophila of all species are capable of entering a cryptic phase of quiescence and may live in "hibernation" for extended periods (13).

Mechanisms by which *Chlamydia* causes disease are not precisely known. The mechanism of tissue injury in all *Chlamydia*-related diseases appears to be immune mediated, and although the exact mechanisms remain unresolved it clearly involves a close interplay between the host and the pathogen. The recognition of an invading organism by the host leads to the initiation of immediate (innate) and late (adaptive) immune responses. Unlike other gram-negative bacteria, the ability of chlamydial lipopolysaccharide (LPS) to trigger the innate immune response and signal the danger of an invading host is weak (14). However, *Chlamydia* does possess a family of outer membrane proteins that are recognized by the host, leading to the activation of an immediate inflammatory response. It is believed that these signals are mediated by toll-like receptors (TLR) on macrophages and other antigen presenting cells. These receptors are phylogenetically conserved proteins and were first discovered as a host defense mechanism in *Drosophila* (15,16). As a consequence of TLR activation, rapid induction of proinflammatory cytokines occurs as a means to deter entry of the organism. This is the first line of defense but it is often insufficient to eradicate the organism. Once *Chlamydia* enters the confines of the host cell, it is beyond the reach of circulating antibodies. It is for these reasons that the development of an adaptive immune response (cellular immunity) is likely to play an important role in the long-term immune surveillance of the organism.

The development of an adaptive immune response depends on the activation and expansion of antigen-primed T-cells. In chlamydial infections these have involved priming of CD4$^+$ and CD8$^+$ T-cells (17). The mechanisms by which antigen-activated T-cells contain systemic infection with *C. pneumoniae* are unclear, but they are likely to involve the development of cytolytic T-cells. Studies in mice that lack CD8$^+$ or CD4$^+$ T-cells have shown that both cell types acting independently play a role in the clearance of the organism. Another potential mechanism to regulate *C. pneumoniae* is the induction of cytokines such as γ-interferon and tumor necrosis factor (TNF) by antigen-activated T-cells that impede the replication of the organism. γ-Interferon upregulates indoleamine 2,3-deoxygenase, leading to the depletion of tryptophan, an important nutrient for *Chlamydia*. In addition, γ-interferon induces nitric oxide synthase that also inhibits the replication of *Chlamydia* (18,19).

Because cellular immunity is an important means to contain chlamydial infections, the pathology of acute and chronic infections is inflammatory in nature. It is believed that tissue persistence of *Chlamydia* is responsible for many chronic infections in humans and animals, including chronic obstructive pulmonary disease, atherosclerosis and asthma (4,20). *Chlamydia* trachomatis infection of the eye causes trachoma, which is characterized clinically by periodic exacerbations and remissions, with progression of inflammation to eventual conjunctival and corneal scarring and, hence, blindness (4,20,21). During the quiescent phase of the disease, *C. trachomatis* can be demonstrated in tissues in the absence of inflammation. A similar process with *C. trachomatis* involving the genital tract is the most likely cause of chronic pelvic inflammatory disease and infertility. In cattle, *C. psittacci* can cause chronic infections of the lungs, mammary glands, and genital tract. Therefore, *C. pneumoniae* infection of the CNS could lead to a state of persistent infection and tissue injury resulting from the periodic activation of the intracellular pathogen. Because *C. pneumoniae* is a common respiratory pathogen, reactivation or reinfection can occur with subsequent dissemination of the organism. There is a well-known association of the development of an MS exacerbation after respiratory infections (22). Whether neurologic worsening is mediated in part by reactivation of chlamydial infection in these instances has not been studied.

Diseases mediated by intracellular pathogens such as *Chlamydia* result from shared accountability between the host and the organism as a result of immune interaction. The former responds to the invading organism by mediating a robust immune response, and the latter uses strategies to evade and elude immune surveillance. It is believed that tissue damage is the result of the interaction between the infected cell and the cellular immune response to contain and eradicate the infection (i.e., direct tropism) (5). A second and perhaps equally plausible disease mechanism is the development of an autoimmune response after infection.

## Acute Neurologic Syndromes Associated with *C. pneumoniae* Infection

Table 10.1, summarizes acute CNS disorders after *C. pneumoniae* infections. In most instances, involvement of the CNS and the peripheral nervous system occurs in the context of a recent respiratory infection, with serologic evidence pointing to infection with *C. pneumoniae*. Clinical and radiologic studies have shown cortical and subcortical involvement (gray and white matter) but detailed neuropathology is lacking. In all cases reported thus far, the acute neurologic disease has been monophasic. Direct evidence of CNS infection with *C. pneumoniae* has been difficult to demonstrate. It is possible that the neurologic involvement is due to an autoimmune process resulting from a systemic infection.

**TABLE 10.1**
*Acute Central Nervous System Manifestations Associated with* Chlamydia pneumonia *Infection*

| REFERENCE | YEAR OF REPORT | CLINICAL PRESENTATION | C. PNEUMONIA SEROLOGY |
|---|---|---|---|
| 50 | 1989 | Encephalitis (3 days after the onset of respiratory tract infection) | IgM < 1:16–1:64<br>IgG < 1:16–1:128 |
| 51 | 1993 | Meningitis (in addition, the patient had hepatitis, iritis, and atypical erythema nodosum; the symptoms of meningitis began 4 days after a high temperature) | IgM < 1:16<br>IgG: 1:1024 –1:4096 |
| 52 | 1994 | Meningoencephalitis (10 days after the onset of respiratory tract infection) | IgM:1:32, IgG: 1:512 on admission; 4 months later, IgM: (−), IgG: 1:64 |
| 53 | 1996 | Meningoencephalitis (5 patients), meningitis (4 patients), polyradiculoencephalitis (1 patient); (without other associated or causative infection) | 4-fold change in *C. pneumonia* IgG antibody titers or IgM antibodies |
| 54 | 2000 | Meningoencephalitis (6 days after the onset of respiratory tract infection) | Serum IgG: 2048, IgA: 515; blood SAA of IgG antibody to *C. pneumonia*: $100 \times 10^{-3}$, intrathecal SAA of IgG antibody to *C. pneumonia*: $1442 \times 10^{-3}$ |
| 55 | 1992 | Guillain-Barre syndrome (2 weeks after the onset of a respiratory infection) | IgM: 1:512 IgG: 1:16–1:512 |
| 56 | 1992 | Lumbosacral meningoradiculitis (10 days after the onset of respiratory infection) | Serum IgM: 1:64–<1:16,; serum:CSF antibody ratio for *C. pneumonia*: 1/8 |
| 57 | 1997 | Cerebellar dysfunction (with fever and pneumonia) | IgG: 1:16–1:128, IgM: (–), IgA: 1:64 |
| 58 | 2000 | ADEM (1 week after the onset of respiratory infection) | IgM: 1:32–1:64; *Chlamydia* complement binding test: positive; *C. pneumonia* DNA was positive on a tracheal swab |
| 59 | 2001 | Encephalitis (initial presentation with fever, lymphadenopathy, and sore throat; a few days later became drowsy and confused and had a generalized seizure) | IgM: none detected in serum or CSF, IgG: 317 U/l enzyme immunoassay in serum and 16 U/l in CSF 3 weeks after acute infection. |

ADEM, acute disseminatd encephalomyelitis; CSF, cerebrospinal fluid; IgA, immunoglobulin A; IgG, immunoglobulin G; IgM, immunoglobulin M; SAA, specific antibody activity.

## C. pneumoniae and Vascular Diseases

Atherosclerotic vascular disease is not mediated strictly through metabolic disease. It is clear that local and systemic inflammatory processes have a role in the progression of vascular lesions. Infectious agents may act in conjunction with metabolic and other risk factors to mediate systemic and cerebrovascular diseases. *Chlamydia pneumoniae* infection has been associated with cardiovascular disease. Serologic and seroepidemiologic studies have confirmed that *C. pneumoniae* antibodies are seen more frequently in individuals with coronary artery disease and myocardial infarctions (5,10,11).

The role of *C. pneumoniae* in cerebrovascular disease also has been evaluated. Grayston et al. found that 37 of 61 carotid endarterectomy specimens had evidence of *C. pneumoniae* infection by immunohistochemistry. Patients with cerebral infarction or transient ischemic attack were evaluated in another study (11,23); 46.6 percent of the patients had elevated immunoglobulin A (IgA) titers to *C. pneumoniae* versus 23.1 percent of control subjects. Immunoglobulin G (IgG) antibodies were elevated in 24.1 percent of the patients compared with 7.7 percent of the control individuals. It was concluded that chronic infection with *C. pneumoniae* is associated with an increased risk of cerebrovascular events. The serologic pattern of elevated IgA titers and IgG immune complexes supported the role of a chronic persistent infection with *C. pneumoniae* in these patients (24,25).

### C. pneumoniae and Giant Cell Arteritis

Temporal arteritis occurs as a result of an autoimmune process in medium-sized blood vessels. Lymphocytic infiltration is seen within the walls of the blood vessels and the clinical symptoms respond well to steroid therapy. A recent study used immunohistochemistry, polymerase chain reaction (PCR), or both and found that eight of nine patients with giant cell arteritis had C. pneumoniae (26). None of the nine control arterial sections had C. pneumoniae.

### C. pneumoniae and AD

AD is largely a chronic degenerative process resulting in neuronal death. However, cellular inflammation is seen in areas of neuronal loss. Activated microglial cells, formation of microglial nodules, and proinflammatory cytokines are seen in AD brains. However, the role of infections or immune processes has not been examined in AD until recently. The first report on the association of AD and C. pneumoniae found that 17 of 19 patients with late-onset AD were positive for C. pneumoniae by PCR, and only 1 was positive in 19 control brains (9). Tissue culture, electron and immunoelectron microscopic, immunohistochemical, and immunolabeling studies confirmed the presence of C. pneumoniae in the brains of the AD patients. Similar studies in non-AD brains were negative. Another group analyzed tissue samples of 20 AD patients with the use of nested PCR and immunocytochemistry with a panel of antichlamydial antibodies and found neither C. pneumoniae–specific DNA nor chlamydial antigens (27). In that study, protocols for the PCR, immunocytochemistry, and sample processing differed from those of the initial study. More recent studies have found evidence of C. pneumoniae in AD (28). The role that C. pneumoniae may play in the neuropathology of AD remains unclear.

## EVIDENCE OF CHRONIC PERSISTENT INFLAMMATION IN THE CNS OF PATIENTS WITH MS

Over the past few years, we have attempted to demonstrate the presence of C. pneumoniae by PCR and culture in the cerebrospinal fluid (CSF) of patients with MS. In addition, the presence of antibodies to C. pneumoniae in the CSF indicates that an immune response occurs within the CNS. After the identification of C. pneumoniae in the CSF of an individual with rapidly progressive MS and his improvement after antibiotic therapy, (29) we undertook a larger study of the association between C. pneumoniae and relapsing–remitting and progressive MS. Forty-seven percent of patients (8 of 17)

with relapsing-remitting MS (RRMS) were culture positive for C. pneumoniae (8). Among patients with progressive MS, 80 percent of patients (16 of 20) were culture positive. Chlamydia pneumoniae was isolated from CSF in three other neurologic disease (OND) control patients. One of these three patients was diagnosed with postinfectious encephalomyelitis. The presence of C. pneumoniae in the CNS was evaluated by PCR methods that assayed CSF for the major outer membrane protein (MOMP) gene of C. pneumoniae. The MOMP gene for C. pneumoniae was amplified and confirmed in all 17 (100 percent) relapsing-emitting MS patients and 19 of 20 (95 percent) progressive MS patients versus 5 of 27 (18 percent) OND controls. One of the major issues concerning the ability of other laboratories to validate our studies has been the difference in technique in performing the PCR. In our initial study we noted the PCR results in 33 of 37 MS patients with established MS. In a representative sample of other neurologic disease control patients, 25 percent of OND controls also were positive. To establish the specificity of this study and to show that these results did not exist only within our center, a collaborative study was initiated with the Carolinas Medical Center (under Dr. Kaufman, M.D.). In that study, 52 blinded samples were obtained from patients with MS and other neurologic diseases and sent to three different laboratories. Our laboratory identified C. pneumoniae in 22 of 28 MS patients and 5 of 22 patients with other neurologic diseases. The laboratories of Gaydos, Boman, and Tondilla did not find C. pneumoniae in the CSF of any of the 52 CSF samples (30). The inability of other laboratories, with established PCR techniques, to find the organism suggested significant differences in the handling of the CSF, the techniques used to extract bacterial DNA, the sensitivity of the PCR primer, and the PCR reactions. The laboratories of Gaydos, Boman, and Tondilla used different PCR conditions that were developed in their laboratories for their use. At least two other studies have shown that technical conditions may be responsible for the disparate results (30). Ikejima et al. found C. pneumoniae in 68 percent of MS patients when they used the Quiagen DNA extraction kit (Qiagen, Chatsworth, CA, USA) to extract bacterial DNA (31). Mahony et al. used replicate testing, and phenol chloroform replicate testing and with this method found that more than 60 percent of MS patients were positive for the presence of C. pneumoniae. A summary of results from different laboratories is shown in Table 10.2. Gieffers et al. found C. pneumoniae in the CSF of patients with MS and a number of other neurologic diseases (32). Unfortunately, whether PCR signal correlated with the underlying clinical diagnosis was not clear, so this group may have included patients with early signs of MS.

These different results show that the ability to find C. pneumoniae depends on the laboratory. These dis-

**TABLE 10.2**

**Results of Studies on Finding the C. pneumoniae Genome by Polymerase Chain Reaction in the Cerebrospinal Fluid in Patients with Multiple Sclerosis and Control Subjects**

| POSITIVE STUDIES | MS PATIENTS | CONTROL SUBJECTS | METHOD† | NEGATIVE STUDIES | MS PATIENTS | CONTROL SUBJECTS | METHOD† |
|---|---|---|---|---|---|---|---|
| 60 | 7/30 | 0/56 | B | 61 | 0/48 | 0/51 | B |
| 62 | 21/103 | 0/47 | B | 63 | 0/19 | 0/20 | B |
| 65 | 9/41 | 0/41 | B | 66 | 0/20 | 0/7 | Not reported |
| 30 | 22/28 | 5/22 | P/C | 30 | 0/28 | 0/24 | B |
| 67 | 12/18 | 4/21 | P/C | | | | |
| 68 | 18/34 | 4/25 | P/C | | | | |
| 31 | 9/9 | Not done | M | | | | |
| 8 | 33/37 | 5/28 | P/C | — | — | — | |

†B, blood DNA extraction kit (Qiagen, Chatsworth, CA, USA); M, bacterial DNA extraction kit (Qiagen, Chatsworth, CA, USA); P/C, phelon chloroform extraction.

crepancies might be related to the different strategies used by the different laboratories for the extraction procedure and the running conditions of the PCR. In addition, methods of handling CSF from the moment it is obtained and the conditions of its subsequent storage conditions are important factors that have not been formally addressed.

## SEROLOGIC EVIDENCE FOR C. PNEUMONIAE ANTIBODIES IN THE CSF ADSORPTION OF OLIGOCLONAL BANDS WITH EB ANTIGENS OF C. PNEUMONIAE

Elevated IgG indices and oligoclonal bands in the CSF are well-established features of MS (33). The restricted amplification of antibodies in the CSF is a consistent feature of MS, but the specificity of the response to antigens has remained a mystery. After isoelectric focusing gel (IEF), the CSF antibodies migrate to the cathodal region of the gel and are seen as specific bands between isoelectric points 7.0 and 9.6. These bands can be identified by immunostaining. When agarose gels using equal amounts of antibody from CSF and serum are used in the isoelectric focusing experiments, immunoglobulins found mainly in the CSF and not in serum are visible. These bands of immunoglobulins are often termed *oligoclonal bands*. In many chronic infectious diseases, oligoclonal bands represent antibodies to the infectious pathogen, although not exclusively so. One method is to establish the reactivity of the antibodies with adsorption techniques. If oligoclonal bands represent the dominant CNS humoral response to C. pneumoniae infection, antigens of C. pneumoniae should adsorb these bands. We per-

formed solid-phase adsorption assays with a 25-fold excess of antigen over antibody. In parallel experiments, CSF samples containing 0.8 μg of IgG were added to wells coated with 25-fold excess of myelin basic protein (MBP), measles, or herpes simplex virus-1 (HSV-1) antigens, which served as antigen specificity controls. In 13 of 17 MS patients, the adsorption by C. pneumoniae EB antigens was partly or fully removed by the incubation of CSF IgG with excess antigen. Among CSF samples obtained from those with other neurologic diseases, no changes in the signal on the gel of the oligoclonal bands were seen after adsorption with C. pneumoniae antigens in OND controls. Oligoclonal bands were adsorbed with excess measles antigen but not with HSV-1 or EB antigens in all three patients with subacute sclerosing panencephalitis, suggesting that the anti-measles antibody response in the CSF constituted the major antibody response in these patients. These results suggest that most oligoclonal bands in CSF of MS patients represent antibodies to C. pneumoniae antigens (34).

## INFECTION, IMMUNITY, AND AUTOIMMUNITY: A SYNTHESIS OF MECHANISMS INVOLVED IN CHLAMYDIAL-ASSOCIATED CNS INFECTIOUS DISEASE

It is clear that the infectious hypothesis of MS must reconcile the large amount of data on the role of autoantigens and autoimmunity in MS (35). Considerable evidence has suggested that autoantigens are involved in the disease process, and to a large degree this is substantiated by the prevalent autoimmune animal models of CNS demyelination. The most commonly used model is experimental allergic encephalitis (EAE) (36,37). This disease can be induced in a number of experimental laboratory animals, including primates, by the injection of whole brain homogenate or a purified preparation of MBP or proteolipid protein (PLP) in adjuvant. Passive transfer of MBP or PLP reactive T-cells is sufficient to induce disease in naive hosts, and the antigenic peptides for MBP and PLP that cause disease are known. The peptides that induce disease differ within and between species; e.g., in SJL/J mice the encephalitogenic peptides reside between residues 89 and 103 of MBP, and in PL/J mice the predominant epitope is at the N' terminus (residues 1 to 14). Altering the immunization protocols results in a chronic form of EAE, referred to as chronic relapsing EAE. In the chronic relapsing model, animals go through multiple episodes of relapses and remissions, a clinical picture that closely mimics that of MS. To develop animal models that more closely resemble the human disease, a number of transgenic mice models of spontaneous EAE have been generated. The most ambitious of these models is the triple transgenic model of human MS, in which mice are made to express human HLA class II, human CD4, and T-cell receptor that express the genes that recognize human MBP p84-102 (38–40). These mice develop spontaneous relapses that are reminiscent of clinical MS. All experimental systems that involve the induction of EAE involve the use of immunogens in adjuvant or transgenic mice in which all T-cells express the receptor for myelin antigens to induce disease. In these situations, the experimental system favors the activation and expansion of a large population of autoreactive lymphocytes. It is apparent that the spontaneous development of autoimmune diseases remains rare in animals as it is in humans. Infectious agents may activate a population of autoreactive T-cells and continue to be the most plausible trigger in the development of autoimmunity.

## MOLECULAR MIMICRY

Since the early report of cross-reactivity between self and bacterial antigens, there has been a great deal of interest in showing the development of autoimmune responses after infection. Many studies have examined the role of molecular mimicry in CNS inflammatory disease. With the understanding that the T-cell receptor is degenerate in its recognition of peptide antigens, the development of autoimmunity despite similarity between self and autoantigens is unpredictable. PLJ mice infected with *Vaccinia* virus containing the MBP epitope 1-11 resulted in the development of tolerance to EAE. In addition, when the PLP epitope was transfected into *Vaccinia* virus and PLJ mice were subsequently infected, no paralytic disease was noted. However, mice infected with the PLP encephalitogenic gene showed enhanced EAE after immu-

nization with PLP in adjuvant in contrast to the MBP epitope. These studies confirmed the difficulty in the development of spontaneous EAE in outbred animals after immunization with epitopes that cross-react with autoantigens (41,42).

There has been considerable interest in the development of autoimmune diseases caused by chlamydial antigens. In view of the link between chlamydial antigens and heart disease, sequence homology between heart myosin and *C. pneumoniae* antigens was screened for and the peptides were immunized into mice. Although chlamydial antigens are not known to cause myocarditis, the cross-reactive peptide induced active inflammation of myocardial tissue (43). In another study, Lenz et al. showed the development of inflammatory CNS disease in rats after immunization with chlamydial peptides having homology with MBP. Rats developed EAE after immunization with the peptide. Interestingly, the same group showed that immunization with *C. pneumoniae*–infected cells alone resulted in disease, suggesting that *C. pneumoniae* infection can induce autoimmunity (44). Although several infectious agents have been described as inducing autoimmune disease, Rose and McKay urged caution: "in spite of great interest no firm evidence of molecular mimicry has been proved for human disease" (41).

Infectious agents amplify immune responses including those that are autoreactive. In most instances, this results in the amplification of a large number of T-cells specific for the initiating agent. Expansion of other clonal population of T-cells also may occur through the secretion of cytokines, superantigens, or epitope spreading. In most instances, such as that seen with lymphocyte choriomeningitis virus (LCMV) infection, the specific immune response is dominant; however, expansion of T-cells not specific for the inciting pathogen does occur, but whether the expansion is sufficient to expand an autoreactive pool of cells remains controversial. In at least two instances, nonspecific activation has been sufficient to cause disease. BDC2.5 mice harbor the transgene encoding the T-cell receptor specific for a diabetogenic islet cell granule antigen that is separate and distinct from the GAD65 antigen, and the receptor shows no cross-reactivity with Coxsackie-B virus antigens. However, after infection with the Coxsackie virus, these mice rapidly developed diabetes. This may be due to the nonspecific activation of T-cells that recognize autoantigens on the granule cells, leading to pancreatic destruction and diabetes (45). Bystander activation also has been seen in mice after intracerebral infection with Theiler murine encephalomyelitis virus (TMEV). In early TMEV infection, the disease appears to result from an active viral infection. The later demyelinating portion of the disease results from an autoimmune response to neural antigens (46). Induction of tolerance to self-antigens reduces the severity of the disease. However, the relative contribution of infection versus immunity (in this case, autoimmunity) remains unknown because there are no antiviral agents that can treat TMEV; further, demyelination is seen in nude mice, suggesting that development of autoimmunity alone is unlikely to fully explain the pathology of demyelination.

## POSSIBLE INTERACTIONS BETWEEN INFECTIONS AND AUTOIMMUNITY IN CNS DEMYELINATING DISEASE

Although T-cells are critical in the development of an autoimmune response, neither myelin nor oligodendrocytes express major histocompatibility complex (MHC) class II antigens and both express only very low levels of MHC class I antigens, thereby precluding any direct T-cell involvement in the demyelinating process (47). Hence, the mechanism of tissue injury is very likely to be indirect and mediated by a concerted action of macrophages, cytokines, antibody, and complement (48). Because chlamydial infections are inflammatory in nature and therefore likely to activate proinflammatory cytokines and the complement pathway, it may facilitate antibody-dependant cell-mediated cytotoxicity (ADCC). Proinflammatory cytokines such as tumor necrosis factor may act as a two-edged sword. Although tumor necrosis factor may be necessary to limit bacterial replication, high levels of the cytokine may cause injury to the myelin oligodendrocyte unit. Antibodies to chlamydial antigens may cross-react with myelin or oligodendrocyte surface proteins, resulting in the development of ADCC. Such a process has been proposed in acute inflammatory polyneuropathy after *Campylobacter* infections (42). In many microbial diseases, tissue damage follows the colonization of the organism, development of an immune response, and the antigenic clearance. Disease is not necessarily the "fault of the pathogen" but in many instances is a shared responsibility between the host and the organism. The inflammatory immune response to the pathogen and the resultant disease often is the result of "friendly fire." The immune response may be acute (innate) or delayed (adaptive). In this scenario the pathologic feature of MS is a direct sequela of infection (chronic) in the white matter of the CNS (49).

## CONCLUSION

The concept that an infectious agent may in part trigger MS has been well known for over a century. Relapses in MS are preceded by the development of upper respiratory infections in a substantial number of individuals. *Chlamydia pneumoniae* fits the epidemiologic profile of an infectious agent in MS, but the data to substantiate this idea needs validation from other laboratories. The underpin-

nings of a common etiology for diseases as diverse as MS, cerebrovascular disease, and reactive arthritis are also seen in other systemic diseases mediated by chlaymdophylia organisms. Different biovars of *C. trachomatis* cause distinctively different diseases such as lymphogranuloma venorum and trachoma. Further, differences in the pathology of primary and tertiary syphilis is persuasive in thinking of unified infectious etiologies in the array of immunopathologic processes (38). Defining the mechanism(s) of disease pathogenesis will be critical in establishing a causal role of *C. pneumoniae* in MS. It will be particularly important to determine which immunologic processes take place that enable *C. pneumonia* to cause or worsen MS. Development of an animal model would be very useful to analyze immune mechanisms of disease. Further, host factors, in particular genetic susceptibility, need further study with regard to the role of *C. pneumoniae* and MS. MHC is clearly important in MS and other immune-mediated disorders; however, other genes are involved and have not been identified. The interaction of various gene products likely confers susceptibility to MS and other autoimmune diseases. Therefore, only a small subset of individuals will develop an autoimmune disease, despite the potential ubiquity of a triggering infectious agent. We feel that our results thus far are persuasive in implicating *C. pneumoniae* in MS.

## References

1. Noseworthy JH, et al. Multiple sclerosis. *New Eng J Med*, 2000; 343:938–946.
2. Johnson RT. *Viral Infections of the Nervous System*. New York: Raven Press; 1982.
3. Yucasan C, Sriram S. *Chlamydophila pneumoniae* infection of the central nervous system. *Curr Opin Neurol* 2001.
4. Stevens RS. Challenge of *Chlamydia* research. *Infect Agents Dis* 1993; 279–293.
5. Ward ME. The immunobilogy and immunopathology of chlamydial infections. *APMIS* 1995; 769–796.
6. Beatty WL, Morrison RP, Byrne GI. Persistent *Chlamydiae* from cell culture to a paradigm for chlamydial pathogenesis. *Microbiol Rev* 1994; 686–699.
7. Kuo CC, et al. Demonstration of *Chlamydia pneumoniae* in atherosclerotic lesions of coronary arteries. *J Infect Dis* 1993; 167:841–849.
8. Sriram S, et al. *C. pneumoniae* infection of the CNS in MS. *Ann Neurol* 1999; 46:6–14.
9. Balin BJ, et al. Identification and localization of *Chlamydia pneumoniae* in the Alzheimer's brain. *Med Microbiol Immunol (Berl)* 1998; 187:23–42.
10. Siscovick DS, et al. *Chlamydia pneumoniae* and atherosclerotic risk in populations: the role of seroepidemiology. *J Infect Dis* 2000; 181(suppl 3):S417–S420.
11. Grayston, J.T., Background and current knowledge of *Chlamydia pneumoniae* and atherosclerosis. *J Infect Dis*, 2000. 181 Suppl 3: p. S402-10.
12. Boman J, Gaydos CA. Polymerase chain reaction detection of *Chlamydia pneumoniae* in circulating white blood cells. *J Infect Dis* 2000; 181(suppl 3):S452–S454.
13. Gerard HC, et al. Expression of *Chlamydia* trachomatis genes encoding products required for DNA synthesis and cell division during active versus persistent infection. *Mol Microbiol* 2001; 41(3):731–741.

14. Kosma P. Chlamydial LPS—a review. *Biochim Biophys Acta* 1999; 1455:387–402.

15. Imler JL, Hoffmann JA. Toll receptors in innate immunity. *Trends Cell Biol* 2001; 11(7):304–311.

16. Thoma-Uszynski S, et al. Induction of direct antimicrobial activity through mammalian toll-like receptors. *Science* 2001; 291(5508):1544–1547.

17. Rottenberg ME, et al. Role of innate and adaptive immunity in the outcome of primary infection with *Chlamydia pneumoniae*, as analyzed in genetically modified mice. *J Immunol* 1999; 162:2829–2836.

18. Chan J, et al. Effect of nitric oxide synthase inhibitors on murine infection with mycobacterium tuberculosis. *Infect Immun* 1995; 63:736–740.

19. Pantoja LG, et al. Inhibition of *Chlamydia pneumoniae* replication in human aortic smooth muscle cells by gamma interferon-induced indoleamine 2, 3-dioxygenase activity. *Infect Immun* 2000; 68:6478–6481.

20. Schachter J,Dawson CR. The epidemiology of Trachoma. *Scand J Infec Dis* 1990; 69(suppl):S55–S62.

21. Washington AE, et al. Assessing risk of PID and its sequelae. *JAMA* 1991; 266:2581–2586.

22. Sibley WA, Bamford CR, Clark K. Clinical viral infections and multiple sclerosis. *Lancet* 1985; 1(8441):1313–1315.

23. Elkind MS, et al. *Chlamydia pneumoniae* and the risk of first ischemic stroke: The Northern Manhattan Stroke Study. *Stroke* 2000; 31(7):1521–1525.

24. Shor A, Phillips JI. *Chlamydia pneumoniae* and atherosclerosis. *JAMA* 1999; 282(21):2071–2073.

25. Shor A, Phillips JI. Histological and ultrastructural findings suggesting an initiating role for *Chlamydia pneumoniae* in the pathogenesis of atherosclerosis. *Cardiovasc J S Afr* 2000; 11(1):16–23.

26. Wagner AD, et al. Detection of *Chlamydia pneumoniae* in giant cell vasculitis and correlation with the topographic arrangement of tissue-infiltrating dendritic cells. *Arthritis Rheum* 2000; 43(7): 1543–1551.

27. Gieffers J, et al. Failure to detect *Chlamydia pneumoniae* in brain sections of Alzheimer disease patients. *J Clin Microbiol* 2000; 38(2):881–882.

28. Mahony J, Woulfel J, Munoz D. *C. pneumoniae* in the Alzheimer brain. *Proceedings of the Fourth European Society for Chlamydia Research* 2000; 20–23.

29. Sriram S, Mitchell W, Stratton C. Multiple sclerosis associated with *Chlamydia pneumoniae* infection of the CNS. *Neurology* 1998; 50:571–572.

30. Kaufman M, et al. Is *C. pneumoniae* found in spinal fluid of MS patients? *Mult Scler* 2002; 8:289–294.

31. Ikejima H, et al. PCR-based method for isolation and detection of *Chlamydia pneumoniae* DNA in cerebrospinal fluids. *Clin Diagn Lab Immunol* 2001; 8(3):499–502.

32. Gieffers J, et al. Presence of *Chlamydia pneumoniae* DNA in the cerebral spinal fluid is a common phenomenon in a variety of neurological diseases and not restricted to multiple sclerosis. *Ann Neurol* 2001; 49(5):585–589.

33. Andersson M, et al. Cerebrospinal fluid in the diagnosis of multiple sclerosis: a consensus report. *J Neurol Neurosurg Psychiatry* 1994; 57(8):897–902.

34. Yao SY, et al. CSF oligoclonal bands in MS include antibodies against Chlamydophila antigens. *Neurology* 2001; 56(9):1168–1176.

35. Noseworthy JH. Progress in determining the causes and treatment of multiple sclerosis. *Nature* 1999; 399(6738, suppl):S40–S47.

36. Owens T, Sriram S. The immunology of MS and of its animal model, EAE. *Neurol Clin of North Am* 1995; 13:51–73.

37. Owens T, Wekerle H, Antel J. Genetic models of CNS inflammation. *Nature Medicine* 2001; 7:161–166.

38. Antel JP, Owens T. Immune regulation and CNS autoimmune disease. *J Neuroimmunol* 1999; 100(1–2):181–189.

39. Madsen LS, et al. A humanized model for multiple sclerosis using HLA-DR2 and a human T-cell receptor. *Nat Genet* 1999; 23(3):343–347.

40. Martin R, McFarland HF, McFarlin DE. Immunology of demyelinating disease. *Annu Rev Immunol* 1992; 10:153–169.

41. Rose NR, Mackay IR. Molecular mimicry: a critical look at exemplary instances in human diseases. *Cell Mol Life Sci* 2000; 57(4):542–551.

42. Rose NR. Infection, mimics, and autoimmune disease. *J Clin Invest* 2001; 107(8):943–944.

43. Bachmaier K, et al. *Chlamydia* infections and heart disease linked through antigenic mimicry. *Science* 1999; 283(5406):1335–1339.

44. Lenz DC, et al. A *Chlamydia pneumoniae*-Specific Peptide Induces Experimental Autoimmune Encephalomyelitis in Rats. *J Immunol* 2001; 167(3):1803–1808.

45. Horwitz MS, et al. Diabetes induced by Coxsackie virus: initiation by bystander damage and not molecular mimicry. *Nat Med* 1998; 4(7):781–785.

46. Katz-Levy Y, Miller SD. Endogenous presentation of self myelin epitopes tby CNS resident APC's in TMEV infected mice. *J Clin Invest* 1999; 104:599–610.

47. Scolding NJ, Zajicek JP. Compston DAS The pathogenesis of demyelinating disease. *Prog Neurobiol* 1994; 43:143–173.

48. Lucchinetti CF, et al. Distinct patterns of MS pathology indicated heterogeneity in pathogenesis. *Brain Pathology* 1996; 6:259–274.

49. Bachmann MF, Kopf M. On the role of the innate immunit in autoimmune disease. *J Exp Med* 2001; 193:47–51.

50. Fryden A, Kihlstrom E, Mallet R. A clinical and epidemiologic study or ornithosis caused by *C. pneumoniae* and *C. psittacci*. *Scand J Infect* 1989; 21:681–691.

51. Sundelof B, Gnarpe H, Gnarpe J. An unusual manifestation of *C. pneumoniae* meningitis. *Scand J Infect Dis* 1993; 25:259–261.

52. Socan M, Beovic B, Kesse D. *C. pneumoniae* associated meningoencephalitis. *N Engl J Med* 1994; 331:406.

53. Koskiniemi M, et al. *C. pneumoniae* associated with CNS infections. *Eur J Neurol* 1996; 36:160–163.

54. Guiglelminotti J, Lellouche N, Maury E. Severe meningoencephalitis an unusual manifestation of *C. pneumoniae* infection. *Clin Infect Dis* 2000; 30:209–210.

55. Haidl S, et al. Guillain Barre syndrome after *C. pneumoniae* infection. *N Engl J Med* 1992; 326:576–577.

56. Michel D, Antoinne JC, Pozetto B. Lumbosacral radiculopathy associated with *C. pneumoniae* infection. *J Neurol Neurosurg Psychiatry* 1992; 55:511.

57. Korman TM, Turnidge J D, Grayston ML. Neurologic complications of chlamydial infections:case report and review of the literature. *Clin Infect Dis* 1997; 25:847–851.

58. Heick A. *C. pneumoniae* associated ADEM. *Eur J Neurol* 2000; 7:435–438.

59. Airas L, et al. Encephalitis associated with *Chlamydia pneumoniae*. *Neurology* 2001; 56(12):1778–1779.

60. Layh-Schmitt G, et al. Evidence for infection with *Chlamydia pneumoniae* in a subgroup of patients with multiple sclerosis. *Ann Neurol* 2000; 47:652–655.

61. Boman J. et al. Failure to detect *Chlamydia pneumoniae* in the central nervous system of patients with MS. *Neurology* 2000; 54(1):265.

62. Grimaldi L, Blasi F, Pincherle A, et al. Association between *C. pneumoniae* infection and clinical activity in MS. Unpublished observations.

63. Marcos MA, Sanz A, Vidal J, et al. Lack of detection of *C. pneumoniae* in CSF from patients with MS. *Proceedings of the Fourth Meeting of the European Society for Chlamydia Research*. 2000; 301–302.

64. Zuzak KB, Theodore M, Kaufman M, et al. Lack of detection of *C. pneumoniae* by PCR and tissue cultures in CSF of MS patients and controls. Proceeding of 10th meeting of European Society of Chlamydia. *Res* 2000; 401–402.

65. Geiffers J, Maas M. *C. pneumoniae* infection in patients with MS and related pathologies. Paper presented at: Interscience Conference on Antimicrobial Agents and Chemotherapy; 1999.

66. Pucci E, Tauas C, Cartechini E. Lack of infection with *Chlamydia* in CSF of MS patients. *Ann Neurol* 2000; 48:399–400.

67. Tuan DS, et al. *C. pneumoniae* is found frequently in CSF of patients with MS. *Ann Neurol* 2000; 48(448).

68. Contini C, Fainardi E. Pathogenic link between *C. pneumoniae* and MS. Paper presented at: ICAAC Abstracts; 2001.

# III

# CYTOKINES, CHEMOKINES, AND INTERFERONS

# 11

# Role of Cytokines in Multiple Sclerosis and Experimental Autoimmune Encephalomyelitis

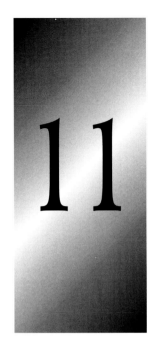

*Tanuja Chitnis, M.D.*
*Samia J. Khoury, M.D.*

ytokines are soluble proteins that mediate and regulate interactions between cells of the immune system. The term *cytokine* encompasses those factors previously referred to as *monokines* (cytokines produced by mononuclear phagocytes), *lymphokines* (cytokines produced by lymphocytes), and colony-stimulating factors (CSFs). *Interleukin* (IL) is a broad term referring to factors produced by T cells or monocytes that act on other lymphocytes. This term has gained a much broader usage, and many cytokines are denoted with the prefix IL.

## CELLS PRODUCING CYTOKINES

Cytokines are produced by a variety of cells, including T cells, B cells, monocytes, macrophages, natural killer (NK) cells, eosinophils, basophils, and mast cells. Although the primary producers of cytokines are cells of the immune system, other cells in the body produce and are affected by cytokines. These include cells of the central nervous system (CNS), neurons, astrocytes, and microglia.

## CYTOKINE FUNCTIONS

Cytokines perform a multitude of tasks and may be broadly categorized into the following, nonmutually exclusive, categories based on function (1):

1. Growth factors: IL-1, IL-2, IL-3, and IL-4 and CSF
2. Factors involved in the initiation of immune responses: interferon-α (IFN-α), IFN-β, and IFN-γ, all of which also have antiviral effects
3. Regulatory or cytotoxic factors: IL-10, IL-12, transforming growth factor-β (TGF-β), lymphotoxin (LT), and tumor necrosis factor-α (TNF-α)
4. Chemokines, which are chemotactic inflammatory factors: IL-8, monocyte inflammatory protein-1a (MIP-1a) and MIP-1b. These are discussed in detail in Chapter 12
5. Cytokines that activate inflammatory cells: IFN-γ, LT, and IL-5

Alternatively, cytokines may be classified according to the roles they play in the immune response. Innate immunity targets foreign pathogens nonspecifically and is mediated primarily by mononuclear phagocytes. Specific immunity requires the participation of antigen-

**TABLE 11.1**
*Cytokines and Their Effects*

| CYTOKINE | PRODUCING CELLS | TARGET | EFFECTS |
|---|---|---|---|
| IL-1 | Monocytes, macrophages, astroglia, microglia | Many cells | Fever, cachexia, potentiates tissue injury caused by TNF-α |
| IL-2 | T-cells, lymphocytes, astrocytes, macrophages | T-cells, NK cells | T- and B-cell growth factor activation of NK cells, proapoptotic factor |
| IL-3 | T-cell | Immature progenitors | Growth and differentiation |
| IL-4 | T-cells, macrophages, cells, basophils, B cells | Mast cells, eosinophils, T-cells, B-cells | IgE production, mast cell growth, mast expression of adhesion molecules, Th2 growth factor, inhibits IgG2a and IgG3, class switching |
| IL-5 | T-cell | Eosinophil B-cells | Eosinophil activation and cytokine production, B-cell growth factor |
| IL-6 | Mononuclear phagocytes, fibroblasts, EC | B-cells, hepatocytes | Growth factor for B-cells, synthesis of acute-phase reactants |
| IL-7 | Fibroblast, bone marrow, stromal cells | Immature progenitors | Lymphocyte growth and differentiation |
| IL-9 | | T-cells | T-cell growth |
| IL-10 | Monocytes, T- and B-cells, cytes, microglia | Macrophages | Inhibits cytokine production by macrophages, reduces MHC II and costimulatory molecule expression |
| IL-11 | Bone marrow stromal cells | Platelets, Megakaryopoiesis | |
| IL-12 | p35 subunit, many cells; P40 subunit—monocytes and dendritic cells | NK, T-, and B-cells | IFN-γ secretion by T and NK cells, Th1 differentiation, cytolytic function of NK and CD8+ cells |
| IL-13 | Macrophages, EC | EC | Induction of adhesion molecules and chemokines |
| IL-15 | Mononuclear phagocytes | NK cells | Proliferation of NK cells |
| IL-16 | T-cells | Eosinophils | Eosinophil chemoattractant |
| IL-17 | T-cells | Many | Similar to TNF-α and LT |
| IL-18 | Macrophages | T and NK cells | Th1 cytokine production, NK cell activation |
| IFN-α | Mononuclear phagocyte | All | Antiviral state, increases MHC I expression, inhibits MHC II expression, inhibits cell proliferation |
| IFN-β | Fibroblast | NK cell | Antiviral state, increases MHC I expression, inhibits MHC II expression, inhibits cell proliferation |
| IFN-γ | T-cells, NK cells, astrocytes | Many | Activator of mononuclear phagocytes, NK cells, neutrophils; increases MHC I and II expression; differentiation of T-cells; B-cell class switching to IgG2a and IgG3; adhesion molecule expression on EC apoptosis |
| TNF-α | LPS-activated mononuclear phagocytes, mast cells, NK cells, activated T cells, astrocytes, microglia, EC | Many, monocytes | Adhesion molecule expression on EC; activation of neutrophils, monocytes, Cytokines and chemokine secretion by tissue remodeling, endogenous pyrogen; production of acute phase reactants; activation of coagulation; suppression of stem cell division; apoptosis |
| LT | T-cell | Neutrophils, EC | Activation |
| TGF-β | T-cells, LPS-activated mononuclear phagocytes, astrocytes, microglia | T-cell, others | Inhibitor of T-cell activation and proliferation, inhibitor of inflammation, synthesis of extracellular matrix proteins |

EC, endothelial cells; Ig, immunoglobulin; IL, interleukin; LPS, lipopolysaccharide; LT, lymphotoxin; MHC, major histocompatibility complex; NK, natural killer; TGF, transforming growth factor; Th, T helper cell; TNF, tumor necrosis factor.

specific T and B cells that intensify a focused immune response. Stimulators of hematopoiesis act on bone marrow progenitor cells (1).

1. Mediators of innate immunity: type I IFN (IFN-α and IFN-β), IL-15, IL-12, TNF-α, IL-1, IL-6, IL-10, and chemokines
2. Mediators of specific immunity: IL-2, IL-4, TGF-β, IFN-γ, LT, and IL-5 (IL-16, IL-17, and macrophage migration inhibitory factor [MIF])
3. Stimulators of hematopoiesis: IL-7, IL-3, IL-9, IL-11, and granulocyte-monocyte CSF (GM-CSF)

Table 11.1 details each cytokine, the cells that are the primary producers, the cell targets, and the principal effects of the cytokine on its target.

## CYTOKINE RECEPTORS

All cytokine receptors are transmembrane proteins and therefore have extracellular and intracellular portions. The cytokine receptor translates the extracellular cytokine signal into an intracellular signal that may lead to a cellular response. The cytokine binding to its receptor initiates this process by triggering a cascade of signaling events that lead to effector responses of the cell.

Cytokine receptors are grouped into six families based on the presence of conserved folding motifs or sequence homologies.

1. Immunoglobulin (Ig) superfamily receptors: Several cytokine receptors contain domains that belong to the Ig superfamily. These include the type I and type II IL-1 receptors and several growth factor receptors.
2. Type I family of cytokine receptors: A conserved sequence containing five amino acids of trytophan-serine-X-trytophan-serine linked to two cysteine residues is present in the receptors for the following cytokines: IL-2, IL-3, IL-4, IL-5, IL-6, IL-7, IL-9, IL-11, IL-13, IL-15, and GM-CSF.
3. Type II family of receptors: These receptors have a definitive nucleotide sequence and include receptors for the type I (IFN-α and IFN-β) and type II (IFN-γ) interferons.
4. Type III cytokine receptors: The TNF receptors I and II (TNF-RI and TNF-RII) are defined by the cysteine-rich domains contained within their structure. TNF-RI and Fas share a conserved sequence motif that delivers proapoptotic signals to the cell nucleus. TNF-RII and CD40 share a common protein-association domain that is termed TNF-receptor-associated factors (TRAFs). There are six TRAF members that are differentially linked to protein kinases, or transcription factors, including nuclear factor-κB (NF-κB).
5. Transmembrane α-helical receptors: A series of seven transmembrane α-helical receptors is found in a large family of cytokine receptors that includes the chemokine family.
6. Multichain receptor complexes: Several cytokine receptors consist of two or more separate transmembrane polypeptide chains that function as a complex. These include the IL-2 receptor, which contains α, β, and γ chains. Different chains mediate different functions.

Intracellular signaling mechanisms provide the link between the binding of the cytokine with its receptor and the effect of the cytokine on cellular function. The Janus kinase (Jak) and signal transducer and activator of transcription (STAT) families of transducer and transcription activating factors play a critical role in the signaling of many cytokine receptors. There are four main Jak molecules and six major STAT proteins, and typically one or two of each are associated with a particular cytokine receptor. Cytokine binding to the specific receptor activates the Jak molecule associated with the receptor, causing phosphorylation of tyrosine residues, and binding of the Jak molecules to its receptor. Phosphorylation of the tyrosine residues on the receptor also facilitates binding of STAT proteins to the phosphorylated receptor. The phosphorylated STAT protein then dissociates from the receptor, dimerizes, and activates transcription of genes containing specific cis-regulatory STAT-binding sequences. Different cytokine receptors are associated with different Jak/STAT proteins. For example, the IL-4 receptor is associated with Jak-1,3 and STAT6 (2,3). The IL-12 receptor is associated with Jak-2 and STAT3,4, (4). The IFN-γ receptor is associated with Jak1,2 and STAT1α.

The activation of transcription factors mediates many of the actions of cytokines on the cell. Binding of STAT1α, otherwise known as γ-activating factor (GAF), to the regulatory DNA sequence, called γ-activating sequences (GAS), on cells results in the transcription of γ-related genes.

Several transcription factors are critical for the transcription of cytokines. Here are a few examples: C-Maf is a transcription factor that controls the transcription of the IL-4 gene in vivo (5). GATA-3 is transcription factor involved in the production of IL-4 (6), and T-bet controls the production of IFN-γ (7).

Signaling and transcription factors are potential targets for immunologic intervention.

## REGULATION OF THE CYTOKINE RESPONSE IN T-CELLS

T-cells play a central role in adaptive immunity. Because autoimmune or immune-mediated disorders are thought to be antigen specific, much effort has gone into studying the role of the T-cell and in particular the CD4$^+$ T helper (Th) cell. Many of the effects of the Th cell in modulating the immune response depend on the cytokines it produces. Two major types of Th cell responses have been described: Th1 cells produce IL-2, TNF-$\alpha$, and IFN-$\gamma$; and Th2 cells produce IL-4, IL-5, IL-10, and IL-13. These cytokines mediate different functions, as described previously in Table 11.1. A Th3 cell that secretes primarily TGF-$\beta$ has been described in the context of oral tolerance to myelin antigens (8,9) and in other immune-mediated settings (10). Effector cells in experimental autoimmune encephalomyelitis (EAE) express predominantly Th1 cytokines and mediate inflammatory disease (11,12); the expression of Th2 cytokines is associated with disease recovery (13–15). The evidence for multiple sclerosis (MS) being a Th1-mediated disease is less clearcut. A similar division of CD8 effector cells has been demonstrated, with Tc1 type CD8 cells secreting IL-2 and IFN-$\gamma$ and Tc2 cells secreting IL-4, IL-5, and IL-10 (16).

## METHODS FOR STUDYING CYTOKINES

Much of the information currently available on the function of cytokines in EAE and MS is derived from laboratory studies in experimental models and human patients, respectively. Understanding the methodology used in collecting the data is critical for interpreting the results. Different studies often yield conflicting results that may be related to differences in methodologies, sampling times, or patient populations. Because of the redundancy of function, single cytokine knockout or transgenic animals may not point definitively to the role of a cytokine in vivo.

## GENERAL RESPONSE OF CYTOKINES IN EAE AND MS

### Cytokines Involved in EAE

#### EAE versus TMEV

Two models of MS exist: EAE and Theiler murine encephalomyelitis virus (TMEV) infection. Each model has unique characteristics in terms of its pathology and immunology that resemble the variants seen in MS (17). Different strains of mice or rats may experience different forms of EAE: e.g., SJL mice experience a relapsing remitting form of EAE when immunized with proteolipid protein, whereas C57BL/6 mice have a chronic form of EAE when immunized with myelin oligodendrocyte peptide 35-55. This further delineates the importance of genetic background and response to immunizing pep-

tide. These variants help us in understanding different aspects of the heterogeneous disease MS.

### Th1 versus Th2 Paradigm in EAE

INTERFERON-$\gamma$.    IFN-$\gamma$ plays a central role in EAE. Expression in the CNS, as shown by immunohistochemical staining, starts at onset of disease, increases during the peak of disease, and decreases during disease remission (18,19). Overexpression of IFN-$\gamma$ in the CNS of mice results in progressive demyelinating disease (20,21). Contrary to expected results, studies using IFN-$\gamma$ knockout mice demonstrated that these mice are still susceptible to EAE, have massive inflammatory infiltrates into the CNS, and experience a more progressive form of EAEthan wildtype mice (22). Moreover, IFN-$\gamma$ receptor-deficient mice developed severe EAE with a morbidity and mortality higher than those in control animals (23). Interestingly, BALB/c mice that are normally resistant to EAE become susceptible and develop severe EAE when the IFN-$\gamma$ gene is knocked out (24). In addition, studies using an anti–IFN-$\gamma$ antibody in SJL mice, which have a relapsing-remitting form of EAE, showed that treatment with the antibody during the afferent limb of the immune response enhances EAE (25). Although IFN-$\gamma$ is clearly a Th1 cytokine, these paradoxical results concerning its role in EAE may be explained by its dual role as an inflammatory cytokine and a mediator of apoptosis, thereby regulating the T-cell response. Experiments showed that IFN-$\gamma$–deficient mice have lower rates of apoptosis of CD4$^+$ cells in the CNS and spleen (26). Therefore, IFN-$\gamma$'s antiinflammatory effects may be explained by its anti-proliferative effect on T-cells (27,28) and induction of T-cell apoptosis, (26,29,30) possibly mediated through expression of nitric oxide (28,29). More evidence has emerged for the role of chemokines in inflammation in initiating the immune response and clearing cells from the target organ, thereby aiding termination of inflammation. IFN-$\gamma$ is a potent regulator of chemokine expression (31,32). Recent studies showed that IFN-$\gamma$–deficient mice and IFN-$\gamma$ receptor deficient–mice display a lack of RANTES and MCP-1 and have excess MIP-2 and TAG-3 compared with controls (33). MIP-2 and T-cell activation gene-3 (TAG-3) are neutrophil-attracting chemokines, which correlate with a high neutrophil invasion in the CNS of the IFN-$\gamma$ receptor–deficient mice (33). Therefore, changes in the profiles of IFN-$\gamma$–dependent chemokines may have profound effects on cellular trafficking and inflammatory responses in EAE.

In summary, the expression of IFN-$\gamma$ correlates with the course of EAE disease. However, this cytokine plays dual roles as a proinflammatory and anti-inflammatory factor. Therefore, complete elimination of this cytokine worsens EAE by abrogating the termination of the immune response. Theoretically, partial elimination of this cytokine reduces its proinflammatory effects. This has been shown in STAT4-deficient mice, which lack a major pathway for the production of IFN-γ, but can produce small amounts of the cytokine and experience very mild EAE (34).

**TUMOR NECROSIS FACTOR-α.** The TNF family of cytokines is composed of TNF-α, LT, and LT-β. LTα refers to the secreted form of LT. Most studies have found little difference between the biologic effects of soluble TNF and LT; however, LT is synthesized by T-cells, whereas TNF is derived predominantly from mononuclear phagocytes. LT-β is a type II membrane protein that can merge with LT to form a receptor related to TNF-RI and TNF-RII. As with IFN-γ, the expression of TNF-α in the CNS parallels the disease course of EAE (15,19,35). Injections of TNF-α resulted in a significant prolongation of clinical EAE and more severe cellular infiltration in the spinal cords of TNF-α injected mice than in controls (36). Intraperitoneal injections of anti–TNF-α abrogated clinical EAE in an SJL/J adoptive transfer model, and CNS tissue from these mice showed no pathologic infiltrates or demyelination (37). Monoclonal antibodies to TNF-α and LT injected into recipient SJL/J mice prevented the passive transfer of EAE with myelin basic protein (MBP)–reactive T-cells (38).

Mice transgenic for TNF-α expression in the CNS develop a spontaneous chronic inflammatory demyelinating disease characterized by infiltration of CD4+, CD8+ T-cells, astrogliosis, and demyelination, which was completely reversed by peripheral administration of a neutralizing murine anti–TNF-α antibody (39). Local production of TNF in the CNS induced oligodendrocyte apoptosis (40). Mice transgenic for CNS expression of TNF had more oligodendrocyte apoptosis and demyelination (41). These results point to an inflammatory role for TNF and suggest that absence of TNF should ameliorate EAE. In contrast to the expected findings, EAE induced with whole mouse spinal cord homogenate in TNF-α and LT-α double knockout mice on SJL/J and 129 × C57BL/6 backgrounds was as severe as in control animals (42). However, EAE induced with myelin aligodendrocyte glycoprotein (MOG) peptide in 129 × C57BL/6 TNF-α and LT-α double knockout mice resulted in a significant delay in disease onset and a reduction in disease severity (43). This was paralleled by a drastic reduction in demyelination but an increase in inflammatory infiltrates. TNF-α single knockout mice on a C57BL/6 background or 129 background developed a more severe form of EAE than did controls (44). This was characterized by significantly more inflammation and demyelination. An interesting finding was a decreased anti-MOG peptide antibody response in C57BL/6 TNF knockout mice compared with controls. These results suggest that TNF-α and

LT-α play significant proinflammatory roles in some forms of EAE and that this depends on the myelin components used for immunization and the genetic backgrounds of the animals.

The incongruous results regarding the role of TNF in EAE may be explained by understanding the many roles of TNF and TNF receptors in inflammation. There are two types of TNF receptors, TNF-RI (p55) and TNF-RII (p75). TNF-RI–deficient mice developed a significantly milder course of EAE than did wild-type mice. In contrast, TNF-RII knockout mice had a more severe course of EAE (43). Injection of a soluble TNF-RI molecule prevented the induction of EAE and subsequent relapses in SJL/J mice (45). There was an absence of pathologic changes in the CNS, including demyelination and inflammatory cell infiltration. Similarly, injection of TNF-RI–IgG into Lewis rats dramatically reduced the EAE disease score (46). Therefore, the inflammatory actions of TNF in the CNS are mediated primarily by TNF-RI. TNF-RI plays a significant role in the apoptosis of T-cells (47,48) and, hence, may play an important role in regulating the immune response.

In summary, TNF has an important homeostatic role in initiating and limiting the extent and duration of immune-mediated inflammatory processes and mediating end organ damage through apoptosis, inflammation, and demyelination.

**INTERLEUKIN-12.** IL-12 is produced principally by monocytes and dendritic cells and is critical for the differentiation of Th1 cells. IL-12 mRNA is elevated immediately before the onset of disease in a monophasic EAE rat model (15,35) and a relapsing murine model (14,49). IL-12 is a disulfide-linked heterodimer p70 complex composed of 1 p40 and 1 p35 subunit. The p35 component is synthesized by most cell types, whereas the p40 component is synthesized only by mononuclear phagocytes and dendritic cells. In a Lewis rat EAE model, IL-12 p40 mRNA levels as measured by semiquantitative reverse transcriptase–polymerase chain reaction (RT-PCR), increased a few days after the peak of T-cell infiltration into the CNS, as did IFN-γ synthesis. In contrast, IL-12 p35 expression remained unchanged during the course of disease (50). Systemic administration of recombinant (r) IL-12 to rats exacerbated the clinical symptoms of EAE and induced relapse in animals that had recovered from the initial clinical attack (51). Similarly, adoptive transfer of proteolipid protein (PLP)–primed lymph node cells resulted in a more severe course of EAE when the cells were pretreated with rIL-12 (52). This was associated with a 10-fold increase in IFN-γ production and a 2-fold increase in TNF-α production. B10.S mice are classically resistant to the induction of EAE but may be induced to develop EAE by adoptive transfer of MBP-reactive lymphocytes treated with IL-12 in vitro before transfer

(53). In this model, the restoration of defective IFN-γ production was concomitant with an attenuation in clinical disease. A similar model using PLP as the immunizing peptide showed an increase in macrophages staining positively for inducible nitric oxide synthase (iNOS) within perivascular lesions and a restoration of IFN-γ production (54,55). Treatment of mice with anti–IL-12 antibody after cell transfer significantly reduced the severity of EAE (52). Overexpression of IL-12 in the CNS resulted in increased inflammation and cellular infiltrate (56). IL-12–deficient mice were resistant to developing EAE (57).

In summary, IL-12 is consistently associated with the induction of EAE and consistently plays a proinflammatory role, unlike other Th1 cytokines such as IFN-γ and TNF-α.

**INTERLEUKIN-6.** The Th1 cytokine IL-6 is synthesized by mononuclear phagocytes, vascular endothelial cells, fibroblasts, and other cells in response to IL-1 and, to a lesser extent, TNF. It is also synthesized by some activated T-cells, astrocytes, and microglia in the CNS. It is important for the growth and differentiation of B cells. IL-6 was upregulated in the CNS during the induction phase of EAE in murine MBP (58,59), MOG-induced models of EAE (60,61), and a Lewis rat model (62). Overexpression of IL-6 in the CNS resulted in neurodegenerative pathology (56). Administration of an anti–IL-6 neutralizing antibody reduced the incidence of actively induced and adoptively transferred EAE (63). IL-6–deficient mice were resistant to the induction of EAE whereas in a MOG-induced model (64–66). Treatment of those mice with IL-6 during the preclinical phase caused typical EAE (64–66). Cytokine profiles in the CNS of IL-6–deficient mice were similar for other Th1 cytokines; in peripheral lymphoid organs, one study showed an increase in Th2 cytokines (64), whereas another showed a deficiency of Th1 and Th2 cytokines (66). A third study found a reduction of anti-MOG antibody titres in IL-6–deficient compared with control mice and a reduction in vascular cell-adhesion molecule-1 (VCAM-1) and intercellular cell-adhesion molecule-1 (ICAM-1) expression on the CNS endothelium, which may affect the entry of Th1 cells into the CNS (65). IL-6 is a known activator of B cells; therefore, the absence of IL-6 might result in the suppression of anti-MOG antibody production. The role of IL-6 in EAE is consistently a proinflammatory one. Its absence suppresses both cellular and humorally mediated immunity.

**INTERLEUKIN-1.** The major producer of IL-1 is the activated mononuclear phagocyte. There are two principal forms of IL-1, IL-1α and IL-1β. Both members bind the same cell surface receptors, and their mechanisms of action are identical. IL-1α is biologically active, but IL-1β must be processed by IL-1 converting enzyme (ICE) before it can exert a biological effect. The biologic functions of IL-1 are similar to those of TNF and may involve a TFNα receptor associated factor (TRAF) signaling pathway.

IL-1 expression was upregulated in the CNS during the induction of EAE, and its expression paralleled that of other Th1 cytokines (58,60,67,68). Administration of IL-1α exacerbated EAE (69), whereas soluble(s) IL-1 receptor suppressed disease (69–71). IL-1 activated astrocytes to release cytokines such as TNF-α and IL-6 (72) and induced synthesis of nitric oxide (73–75) in culture. Expression of ICE, also known as caspase 1, increased during the acute stages of EAE as measured by semiquantitative RT-PCR (50). Caspase 1–deficient mice experienced a milder course of EAE, correlating with reduced IFN-γ levels (76). There has been little work on the direct role of IL-1β in EAE.

**INTERLEUKIN-18.** IL-18 has only recently been described as an IFN-γ–inducing factor (77,78). It is synthesized as an inactive precursor protein that exhibits structural homology to that of IL-1 and, similarly, must be processed by caspase 1 for functional activation (78,79). IL-12 and IL-18 enhanced the production of IFN-γ by Th1 cells but likely used different intracellular signaling pathways (4,80). IL-12 may affect the IL-18–dependent IFN-γ production and vice versa by other mechanisms (81–84). IL-18 mRNA expression as determined by semiquantitative RT-PCR, EAE correlated with disease course and lymphocytic infiltration of the CNS (50). Th1 and NK activity were impaired in IL-18–deficient mice after Bacillus Calmette-Guerin (BCG) infection, but the effect of EAE in IL-18–deficient mice has yet to be explored.

**INTERLEUKIN-4.** IL-4 is a classical Th$_2$ cytokine and acts through the STAT6 pathway. However, few cells expressing IL-4 mRNA were found in the spinal cord of Lewis rats with EAE, and there was no clear relation to clinical symptoms or histopathology (18). In DA rats there was no expression of IL-4, IL-10, or TGF-β throughout the course of EAE (35). In SJL mice immunized with PLP, IL-4 mRNA was undetectable until disease remission (19). In contrast, TMEV-infected SJL/J mice expressed IFN-γ, TNF-α, IL-4, and IL-10 throughout the clinical course, with increasing levels as the disease proceeded (19). IL-4 has been implicated as a suppressor cytokine in EAE. Resistance to EAE mediated by a self-antigen–induced Th2 response was attributed to IL-4–secreting CD4 cells (85,86). Cells grown in IL-4 have a reduced encephalitogenic potential when transferred, and intraperitoneal injections of IL-4 after adoptive transfer of MBP-reactive cells reduced the clinical severity of EAE (72).

Studies in IL-4 knockout mice have led to unexpected and often conflicting results. Contrary to expected results, IL-4–deficient PLJ mice immunized with mouse spinal cord homogenate had a similar incidence of EAE, as well as a similar mean maximal score, or fatality rate, as wild-type mice (87). Similar results were found in IL-4–deficient C57BL/6 mice immunized with MOG (88). There was a slight prolongation of disease in IL-4–deficient PLJ mice, signifying that IL-4 may play a role in the termination of disease (87). One group reported more severe disease in IL-4–deficient mice on C57BL/6 and BALB/c backgrounds (89). Neutralizing anti–IL-4 antibody did not exacerbate the clinical severity of passively transferred EAE (38). There have been no reports on the in vivo treatment with the anti–IL-4 antibody during the induction phase of actively induced EAE.

Transgenic expression of IL-4 in T-cells does not protect from EAE (88); however, encephalitogenic T-cells, transduced with a retroviral gene construct expressing IL-4, can delay the onset and reduce the severity of EAE when adoptively transferred to MBP immunized mice (90). A number of therapeutic strategies have increased IL-4 production (85), including induction of oral tolerance using myelin proteins (91) to protect against EAE. In summary, it seems that the presence of IL-4 reduces the severity of EAE, whereas the absence of IL-4 may not alter the course of EAE. This implies that other Th2 cytokines may substitute for IL-4 in the regulation of EAE.

## INTERLEUKIN-10.

IL-10 is another classical Th$_2$ cytokine. In contrast to IL-4, IL-10 does not exert its effects throught the STAT6 pathway, but instead through the STAT3 pathway. Its main function is to inhibit IL-12 production by macrophages.

In SJL mice immunized with PLP, IL-10 mRNA was continuously expressed throughout the course of EAE (19). Likewise, TMEV-infected SJL/J mice expressed IFN-γ, TNF-α, IL-4, and IL-10 throughout the clinical course, with increasing levels as the disease proceeded (19). Systemic administration of human IL-10 suppressed IFN-γ–induced major histocompatibility complex (MHC) class II upregulation in rat peritoneal macrophages and reduced the incidence and severity of EAE in Lewis rats (92). In a murine EAE model, IL-10 worsened disease when administered just before the onset of clinical signs or had no effect when administered early after sensitization (93). Mice overexpressing human IL-10, but not murine IL-10, under the MHC class II promoter were resistant to developing EAE (94). IL-10–deficient mice on a C57BL/6 background, were more susceptible and developed a more severe form of EAE than did IL-4–deficient or wild-type mice. T-cells from IL-10–deficient mice exhibited stronger antigen-specific proliferation, produced more proinflammatory cytokines

(IFN-γ and TNF-α) when stimulated with an encephalitogenic peptide, and induced very severe EAE with transfer into wild-type mice (88). Spontaneous recovery occurred in wild-type and IL-4–deficient mice but not IL-10–deficient mice, suggesting that IL-10 plays an important role in recovery from EAE (95).

In contrast to the other Th2 cytokine, IL-4, absence of IL-10 consistently results in a more severe form of EAE, suggesting that its function is unique and cannot be replaced by other Th2 cytokines. However, exogenous administration of IL-10 in vivo may worsen disease, raising the possibility that the addition of Th2 cytokines when disease is already in progress may worsen disease. This is a concept that requires further investigation.

## TRANSFORMING GROWTH FACTOR-β.

The TGF family of molecules has the general property of allowing normal cells to grow in soft agar, a characteristic of malignant cells. TGF-α is a polypeptide growth factor for epithelial and mesenchymal cells. A second factor required for cell survival is TGF-β. The TGF-β family of molecules consists of TGF-β1, TGF-β2, and TGF-β3 which interacts with three types of TGF-β receptors, I to III. The actions of TGF-β are highly pleiotropic. TGF-β inhibits proliferation of T-cells, maturation of cytotoxic lymphocytes and NK cells (96), and activation of macrophages. It also acts on other cells to counteract the activities of proinflammatory cytokines. Mice deficient for TGF-β1 developed uncontrolled inflammatory reactions (97). Therefore TGF-β is an attractive target for immunoregulation in EAE.

In the Lewis rat model of EAE, expression of mRNA for TGF-β in the CNS increased at the peak of disease and shortly preceding recovery (18); however, in the DA rat model of EAE, expression of TGF-β was almost absent (35). TGF-β1,2,3 were found in inflammatory perivascular brain lesions of SJL mice immunized for EAE (98). Daily injections of TGF-β1 from the time of immunization protected against the development of relapsing EAE, (98,99) whereas injections administered during peak of disease only delayed the onset of further relapses by 2 to 3 days (99). In the same model, when TGF-β was administered during disease remission, it prevented the occurrence of further relapses. Data from another group demonstrated that administration of TGF-β1 or TGF-β2 to SJL mice immunized with spinal cord homogenate on days 5–9 after immunization, just before the onset of disease, can be protective, whereas administration before or after this time point was not (100). Histologic studies in similarly treated mice demonstrated a reduction in inflammatory infiltrates and reduced demyelination in the CNS (98,101).

Anti–TGF-β1 antibody worsened EAE when administered in vivo and inhibited myelin antigen T-cell proliferative responses in vitro (102). MBP-reactive clones genetically engineered to produce TGF-β, protected against EAE (103). Similarly MBP-reactive Th1 clones when transduced to express TGF-β1 were protective in EAE in an antigen-specific fashion (104). Overexpression of TGF-β1 in the CNS resulted in enhanced EAE, with an earlier onset compared with controls (105). These mice also showed increased β-amyloid deposition, which may enhance glial reactivity and therefore exacerbate EAE (106,107).

Investigators further examined the mechanisms whereby TGF-β modulates EAE. TGF-β1 and -2 have similar effects in vitro because both factors strongly inhibited in vitro activation of autoimmune T-cells, suppressed the accumulation of IL-2 mRNA, and decreased the expression of T-cell activation antigens (108). Other investigators found that TGF-β2 decreases migration of lymphocytes in vitro and homing of cells into the CNS in vivo (109). The cytokine, TGF-β1 also inhibited TNF-α production (110).

TGF-β played a regulatory role in EAE, as shown by oral tolerance–induced suppression of disease. MBP orally tolerized animals displayed a marked reduction of the perivascular infiltrate and downregulation of all inflammatory cytokines, with an upregulation of the inhibitory cytokine TGF-β (91). T-cell clones isolated from mesenteric lymph nodes of these orally tolerized animals demonstrated an increased production of TGF-β, IL-4, and IL-10 and suppressed EAE induced with MBP or PLP (91).

Taken together, these data demonstrate that TGF-β plays an important regulatory role in EAE; however, within the CNS, it also may play a deleterious role by enhancing glial reactivity.

**INTERLEUKIN-13.** IL-13 is a Th2 cytokine that resembles IL-4 in that it signals through the STAT6 pathway. However, it does not replace IL-4 as a differentiation or growth factor for T or B cells. IL-13 can induce expression of VCAM-1 and production of several C-C chemokines and may play an important role in lymphocyte trafficking. IL-13 is increased during remission of EAE (13).

In vivo administration of human IL-13–secreting vector cells into MBP-immunized animals markedly suppressed the development of EAE. This suppression of disease coincided with only a minimal reduction of MBP-directed T-cell autoreactivity and no alteration in MBP-specific autoantibody production. IL-13 may primarily target cells of the macrophage/monocyte lineage rather than suppress T-cell or B-cell immunoreactivity in vivo (111).

**INTERLEUKIN-5.** IL-5 is an important Th2 cytokine. Its primary role is as an activator of eosinophils, and it also functions as a costimulator for B-cell growth.

As with IL-13, IL-5 is now being used as a marker for Th2 cells in EAE studies, but little information is available on its specific role in the disease.

## Cytokines In Multiple Sclerosis

Unlike in the animal model, the study of the role of cytokines in MS is limited to indirect measurement of cytokines produced by peripheral blood cells or measurement of serum or cerebrospinal fluid levels. Some information also can be obtained from postmortem tissue. Other approaches have relied on measuring cytokine production by myelin-specific T-cell clones and lines isolated from MS patients and control individuals. Myelin-specific clones can be isolated from MS patients and normal individuals, but the clones isolated from MS patients are activated in vivo (112).

### Studies of Cytokines in the CNS

Immunohistochemical studies have been used to examine the expression of cytokines in the CNS. In addition to lymphocytes and macrophages, resident CNS cells, astrocytes, and microglia are capable of producing the cytokines IL-1β, IL-2, IL-4, IL-10, TNF-α, and TGF-β, whereas only astrocytes are capable of producing IFN-γ. Significantly increased expressions of TNF-α and IL-4 were found in brains of MS patients compared with controls (113). Low levels of reactivity of TGF-β and IL-10 were also found in those samples. In that study, IL-4 was expressed in high levels in acute and chronic active MS lesions, with no obvious correlation to the resolution of the lesion. IL-10 immunoreactivity was associated with astrocytes in chronic active lesions. TGF-β1 was associated with endothelial cells and the extracellular matrix around blood vessels. This and other studies using confocal microscopy demonstrated that the highest expression of TNF-α was in macrophages, microglia, and astrocytes (113–115) in chronic active lesions. Another study examining acute MS lesions found that IL-2 was expressed predominantly in association with perivascular inflammatory cells (116). IL-6, IFN-γ, and TNF-α were expressed by cells in the perivascular cuffs, suggesting that inflammatory cells are the most important source of these cytokines in acute MS lesions (117).

Semiquantitative RT-PCR and immunocytochemistry were used to quantify expression of IL-12 p40 in vascular CNS infarcts compared with inflammatory MS plaques from the same brain. The investigators observed increased expressions of B7-1 and IL12 p40 in acute MS plaques compared with samples isolated from inflammatory infarcts (118). Another study using RT-PCR examined samples obtained from inflammatory plaques in MS brains compared with samples isolated from noninflammatory white matter regions in control patients. Analysis of RNA transcripts showed upregulations of IL-2R, IL-1b, TNFR1, IL-15, IL-18, TGF-β, IL-3, IL-5, and IL-6/IL-6R in samples from MS patients compared with controls.

INTERFERON-γ.     IFN-γ is a hallmark Th1 cytokine and appears to play an important role in disease pathogenesis, because increased production of IFN-γ in a whole blood mitogen assay precede clinical attacks (119), and administration of IFN-γ to patients resulted in clinical attacks (120). Peripheral blood mononuclear cells (PBMCs) activated with the nonspecific stimulant concavalin A produced significantly higher levels of IFN-γ in progressive MS (121). Another study similarly found increased IFN-γ expression in patients with secondary progressive (SP) MS compared with controls, whereas the levels in patients with untreated relapsing-remitting (RR) MS were reduced compared with those of controls (122). In the same study, relapsing-remitting patients treated with IFN-β had an even greater reduction in the percentage of IFN-γ–secreting cells.

T-cell receptor–mediated IFN-γ secretion in SPMS patients, as determined by anti-CD3 stimulation, was mediated by increased IL-12 secretion produced via CD40–CD40 ligand interaction (123). Cytokine production by PBMCs from SPMS patients is dysregulated compared with that from RR or control patients. Anti-CD3–stimulated PBMCs from RRMS and SPMS patients demonstrated increased levels of IFN-γ in both groups compared with controls (124). In addition, in vitro studies using anti-cytokine neutralizing antibodies demonstrated that endogenous IL-10 downregulates IFN-γ production by anti-CD3–activated PBMCs in control and RRMS patients but not in SPMS patients. Seasonal variations in IFN-γ secretion have been observed in chronic progressive MS patients, with significantly increased IFN-γ production in the autumn and winter months compared with the spring and summer months, and this increase was linked to endogenous IL-12 production (125). Increased seasonal IFN-γ was not observed in normal control subjects, and there were no seasonal changes in IL-10 in progressive MS (125).

As is seen in the EAE model, IFN-γ may play dual roles, but it clearly plays a significant proinflammatory role in MS. Control of IFN-γ production appears to be dysregulated in SPMS patients and may be an important factor in understanding the immunologic differences between RRMS and SPMS.

TUMOR NECROSIS FACTOR-α.     Several studies found a correlation between TNF-α levels in the serum or culture supernatants and the clinical course of MS (119,126). One study found that increased levels of IFN-γ and TNF-α levels can precede the onset of a relapse by approximately 2 weeks (119). In contrast, another study found that TNF-α is a weak predictor of disease activity and found no correlation of IFN-γ levels with disease activity (127).

Levels of sTNF-R p55 were higher in patients with stable MS than in those with actively relapsing MS, and levels increased several weeks after the onset of a relapse (128). A study examining TNF and sTNF-R p55 levels in serum and cerebrospinal fluid (CSF) found no significant correlations with enhancing lesions on magnetic resonance imaging (MRI) (129).

We used frequent sampling at weekly and biweekly intervals, examined serum levels of sTNF-RI (p55) and sTNF-RII (p75), and compared levels with clinical and MRI measures of disease activity (130). We found increased levels of sTNF-R p55 in chronic progressive patients compared with controls. These increases correlated with increases in the Expanded Disability Status Scale (EDSS) and Ambulation Index (AI) in chronic progressive patients. In addition, the change in TNF-R p55 correlated with the appearance of new gadolinium-enhancing lesions on MRI (130).

A clinical trial of a TNF antagonist had the unexpected result of increasing enhancing lesions on MRI (131). This unexpected result may be due to prolongation of TNF half-life in the serum by binding to the antagonist. Decreasing TNF in the serum may be unrelated to TNF level in the lesions; alternatively, TNF may play a protective role.

In summary, TNF-α and TNF-RI levels show correlations with disease relapse, but these correlations may not be of sufficient magnitude to allow prediction of clinical or MRI disease activity. As in the EAE model, TNF-α and its receptors play multiple roles; thus, systemic immunotherapy may not have the desired effect.

INTERLEUKIN-12.     In a longitudinal study, IL-12 production was measured by competitive PCR of unstimulated PBMCs from controls, RRMS, and SPMS patients (132). IL-12 p40 levels were increased in SPMS and RRMS patients compared with controls, and IL-12 p40 correlated with the development of active lesions on MRI but not with disease relapse. In contrast, IL-12 p35 levels were decreased in both groups compared with controls, and there was a significant decline in the IL-12 p35 mRNA levels during the development of active lesions in SPMS patients. Serum levels of IL-12 p70 were elevated in chronic progressive MS patients (133). Production of IL-12 p70 by PBMCs stimulated with a T-cell–independent mitogen was higher in secondary progressive patients compared with controls or patients with acute MS (134). IL-12 p70 also was increased in cultures of PBMCs from SPMS as compared with cultures from RRMS patients or normal controls. The increase in IL-12 was found to be mediated via CD40–CD40L interactions (123). The percentage of IL-12–expressing monocytes was increased in chronic progressive-MS patients, and this increase was reversed in patients treated with cyclophosphamide (135).

INTERLEUKIN-10. Semiquantitative PCR of cytokines in PBMCs demonstrated that IL-10 levels are decreased before the onset of an exacerbation in RRMS patients (128). The same study showed decreased levels of IL-10 and TGF-β in MS patients compared with controls. Levels of IL-10 were significantly lower in SPMS patients than in RRMS patients or controls (132). Decreases in IL-10 levels were noted only in RRMS patients 4 weeks before the occurrence of MRI activity and 6 weeks before clinical relapses. Increase of IL-10 message to normal levels occurred at the time of MRI activity (132).

INTERLEUKIN-4. IL-4 is the prototypic Th2 cytokine. Studies of IL-4 in MS patients have been limited. Increased IL-4 secretion by CD3-stimulated PBMCs was demonstrated in SPMS patients treated with cyclophosphamide/methylprednisolone compared with untreated patients, suggesting that the mechanism of action of this drug is to increase the Th2/Th1 cytokine ratio. Eosinophilia was observed concomitant with increases in IL-4 levels (136).

### Studies of Cytokines in Myelin-Specific T-Cell Clones

Analysis of PLP-reactive clones isolated from patients during acute relapses and remission and from normal controls demonstrated PLP-specific skewing toward Th1 cytokine production (IFN-γ and TNF-α) in clones isolated from MS patients during acute relapse. Those isolated during remission showed increased production of IL-10 and TGF-β compared with controls or clones isolated during acute relapse (137).

Elispot analysis of PLP-reactive memory cells isolated from MS patients versus controls demonstrated increased levels of IFN-γ-producing cells in MS patients and negligible numbers of IL-5–producing T-cells in either group (138).

MS patients orally tolerized with daily treatments of bovine myelin showed increased frequencies of TGF-β1 secreting short-term T-cell lines in response to MBP or PLP (8). Cytoxan/methylprednisolone-treated MS patients had increased frequencies of MBP- and PLP-specific IL-4–secreting T-cells compared with untreated MS patients (139).

### Cytokine Immunotherapy

Absence of IFN-γ in EAE led to worsened disease, suggesting that IFN-γ plays a predominantly anti-inflammatory role (22). These and other studies led to the administration of IFN-γ to MS patients (120). Eighteen patients with clinically definite RRMS received 1-, 30-, or 1000-μg doses of IFN-γ given by intravenous infusion twice a week for 4 weeks. Seven patients had exacerbations during treatment. This exacerbation rate, compared retrospectively with the pretreatment rate and prospectively with the post-treatment rate, was significantly greater than expected. Exacerbations were not precipitated by fever or other dose-dependent side effects. A concomitant increase in circulating monocytes bearing class II (HLA-DR) surface antigen suggested that the attacks induced during treatment were immunologically mediated (120). Although IFN-γ may play a dual role, as seen in EAE studies, the negative effects far outweigh its positive effects, making it an unsuitable candidate for immunotherapy of MS.

INF-α and INF-β are currently used to treat MS. This topic is covered in Chapter 13.

Lenercept, or TNF-R IgG p55, is a dimeric recombinant protein molecule built from two copies of the 55-kd TNF-R extracellular domain fused to a fragment of the human IgG1 heavy chain. This molecule therefore binds TNF-α and neutralizes it in vitro. Studies using a murine equivalent protein showed a protective effect in EAE (140). Patients treated with Lenercept experienced a larger number of exacerbations that was dose dependent (131). There was no significant change in EDSS or the number of new gadolinium-enhancing lesions on MRI in treated or untreated patients. The paradoxical effect of Lenercept may be related to the dual roles of TNF-α in disease induction and termination of the immune response, as observed in EAE. In addition, the role of the TNF-α p55 receptor in humans may differ from that observed in EAE (131).

TGF-β is an attractive candidate for the immunotherapy of MS. A safety clinical trial was done with 12 chronic progressive MS patients treated with TGF-β2 2 times a week for 4 weeks. There was a significant decline in renal glomerular filtration rate, with no change on EDSS or MRI (141). Glomerular nephrotoxicity was observed in a TGF-β1 transgenic murine model and associated with an accumulation of glomerular extracellular matrix protein (142). Thus, high doses of TGF-β are considered unsuitable treatment choices for MS.

In summary, studies of cytokines in humans indicate that many cytokines, in particular IFN-γ and TNF-α, may play pro- and anti-inflammatory roles, and understanding these mechanisms is critical before immunotherapy targeting these or other cytokines is considered. We require further study of cytokines in EAE and MS to determine whether immune deviation will ultimately be a viable treatment option for MS.

## CONCLUSION

Cytokines play an integral role in the immunopathogenesis of MS. Studies of cytokines in the EAE model and in MS patients will help us better understand the pathogenesis of the disease and may lead to novel therapeutic options.

# References

1. Abbas A, Lichtman A, Pober J. *Cellular and Molecular Immunology*, fourth edition Philadelphia: W.B. Saunders Company, 2000, 553.

2. Kaplan MH, Schindler U, Smiley ST, and Grusby MJ. Stat6 is required for mediating responses to IL-4 and for development of Th2 cells. *Immunity* 1996; 4:313–319.

3. Takeda K, Tanaka T, Shi W, Matsumoto M, Minami M, Kashiwamura S, et al. Essential role of Stat6 in IL-4 signalling. *Nature* 1996; 380:627–630.

4. Jacobson NG, Szabo SJ, Weber-Nordt RM, Zhong Z, Schreiber RD, Darnell JE Jr, Murphy KM. Interleukin 12 signaling in T helper type 1 (Th1) cells involves tyrosine phosphorylation of signal transducer and activator of transcription (Stat)3 and Stat4. *J Exp Med* 1995; 181:1755–1762.

5. Ho IC, Hodge MR, Rooney JW, Glimcher LH. The proto-oncogene c-maf is responsible for tissue-specific expression of interleukin-4. *Cell* 1996; 85:973–983.

6. Zheng W Flavell RA. The transcription factor GATA-3 is necessary and sufficient for Th2 cytokine gene expression in CD4 T cells. *Cell* 1997; 89:587–596.

7. Szabo SJ, Kim ST, Costa GL, Zhang X, Fathman CG, Glimcher LH. A novel transcription factor, T-bet, directs Th1 lineage commitment. *Cell* 2000; 100:655–669.

8. Hafler DA, Kent SC, Pietrusewicz MJ, Khoury SJ, Weiner HL, Fukaura H. Oral administration of myelin induces antigen-specific TGF-beta 1 secreting T cells in patients with multiple sclerosis. *Ann N Y Acad Sci* 1997; 835:120–131.

9. Fukaura H, Kent SC, Pietrusewicz MJ, Khoury SJ, Weiner HL, Hafler DA. Induction of circulating myelin basic protein and proteolipid protein-specific transforming growth factor-beta1-secreting Th3 T cells by oral administration of myelin in multiple sclerosis patients. *J Clin Invest* 1996; 98:70–77.

10. Minguela A, Torio A, Marin L, Sanchez-Bueno F, Garcia-Alonso AM, Ontanon J, Parrilla P, Alvarez-Lopez MR. Implication of Th1, Th2, and Th3 cytokines in liver graft acceptance. *Transplant Proc* 1999; 31:519–520.

11. Powell MB, Mitchell D, Lederman J, Buckmeier J, Zamvil SS, Graham M, Ruddle NH, Steinman L. Lymphotoxin and tumor necrosis factor-alpha production by myelin basic protein-specific T cell clones correlates with encephalitogenicity. *Int Immunol* 1990; 2:539–544.

12. Zamvil SS, Nelson PA, Mitchell DJ, Knobler RL, Fritz RB, Steinman L. Encephalitogenic T cell clones specific for myelin basic protein. An unusual bias in antigen recognition. *J Exp Med* 1985; 162:2107–2124.

13. Khoury SJ, Hancock WW, Weiner HL. Oral tolerance to myelin basic protein and natural recovery from experimental autoimmune encephalomyelitis are associated with downregulation of inflammatory cytokines and differential upregulation of transforming growth factor beta, interleukin 4, and prostaglandin E expression in the brain. *J Exp Med* 1992; 176:1355–1364.

14. Issazadeh S, Navikas V, Schaub M, Sayegh M, Khoury S. Kinetics of expression of costimulatory molecules and their ligands in murine relapsing experimental autoimmune encephalomyelitis in vivo. *J Immunol* 1998; 161:1104–1112.

15. Issazadeh S, Ljungdahl A, Hojeberg B, Mustafa M, Olsson T. Cytokine production in the central nervous system of Lewis rats with experimental autoimmune encephalomyelitis: dynamics of mRNA expression for interleukin-10, interleukin-12, cytolysin, tumor necrosis factor alpha and tumor necrosis factor beta. *J Neuroimmunol* 1995; 61:205–212.

16. Li L, Sad S, Kagi D, Mosmann TR. CD8Tc1 and Tc2 cells secrete distinct cytokine patterns in vitro and in vivo but induce similar inflammatory reactions. *J Immunol* 1997; 158:4152–4161.

17. Dal Canto MC, Melvold RW, Kim BS, Miller SD. Two models

18. Issazadeh S, Mustafa M, Ljungdahl A, Hojeberg B, Dagerlind A, et al. Interferon gamma, interleukin 4 and transforming growth factor beta in experimental autoimmune encephalomyelitis in Lewis rats: dynamics of cellular mRNA expression in the central nervous system and lymphoid cells. *J Neurosci Res* 1995; 40:579–590.

19. Begolka WS, Vanderlugt CL, Rahbe SM, Miller SD. Differential expression of inflammatory cytokines parallels progression of central nervous system pathology in two clinically distinct models of multiple sclerosis. *J Immunol* 1998; 161:4437–4446.

20. Renno T, Taupin V, Bourbonniere L, Verge G, Tran E, et al. Interferon-gamma in progression to chronic demyelination and neurological deficit following acute EAE. *Mol Cell Neurosci* 1998; 12:376–389.

21. Horwitz MS, Evans CF, McGavern DB, Rodriguez M, Oldstone MB. Primary demyelination in transgenic mice expressing interferon-gamma. *Nat Med* 1997; 3:1037–1041.

22. Ferber IA, Brocke S, Taylor-Edwards C, Ridgway W, Dinisco C, et al. Mice with a disrupted IFN-gamma gene are susceptible to the induction of experimental autoimmune encephalomyelitis (EAE). *J Immunol* 1996; 156:5–7.

23. Willenborg DO, Fordham S, Bernard CC, Cowden WB, Ramshaw IA. IFN-gamma plays a critical down-regulatory role in the induction and effector phase of myelin oligodendrocyte glycoprotein-induced autoimmune encephalomyelitis. *J Immunol* 1996; 157:3223–3227.

24. Krakowski M, Owens T. Interferon-gamma confers resistance to experimental allergic encephalomyelitis. *Eur J Immunol* 1996; 26:1641–1646.

25. Lublin FD, Knobler RL, Kalman B, Goldhaber M, Marini J. et al. Monoclonal anti-gamma interferon antibodies enhance experimental allergic encephalomyelitis. *Autoimmunity* 1993; 16:267–274.

26. Chu CQ, Wittmer S, Dalton DK. Failure to suppress the expansion of the activated CD4 T cell population in interferon gamma-deficient mice leads to exacerbation of experimental autoimmune encephalomyelitis. *J Exp Med* 2000; 192:123–128.

27. Duong TT, Finkelman FD, Strejan GH. Effect of interferon-gamma on myelin basic protein-specific T cell line proliferation in response to antigen-pulsed accessory cells. *Cell Immunol* 1992; 145:311-323.

28. van der Veen RC, Dietlin TA, Dixon Gray J, Gilmore W. Macrophage-derived nitric oxide inhibits the proliferation of activated T helper cells and is induced during antigenic stimulation of resting T cells. *Cell Immunol* 2000; 199:43–49.

29. Willenborg DO, Fordham SA, Staykova MA, Ramshaw IA, Cowden WB. IFN-gamma is critical to the control of murine autoimmune encephalomyelitis and regulates both in the periphery and in the target tissue: a possible role for nitric oxide. *J Immunol* 1999; 163:5278–5286.

30. Liu Y, Janeway CA, Jr. Interferon gamma plays a critical role in induced cell death of effector T cell: a possible third mechanism of self-tolerance. *J Exp Med* 1990; 172:1735–1739.

31. Sallusto F, Lenig D, Mackay CR, Lanzavecchia A. Flexible programs of chemokine receptor expression on human polarized T helper 1 and 2 lymphocytes. *J Exp Med* 1998; 187:875–883.

32. Vanguri P, Farber JM. IFN and virus-inducible expression of an immediate early gene, crg-2/IP-10, and a delayed gene, I-A alpha in astrocytes and microglia. *J Immunol* 1994; 152:1411–1418.

33. Tran EH, Prince EN, Owens T. IFN-gamma shapes immune invasion of the central nervous system via regulation of chemokines. *J Immunol* 2000; 164:2759–2768.

34. Chitnis T, Najafian N, Grusby M, Sayegh MH. Effect of targeted disruption of STAT4 and STAT6 genes on the induction of experimental autoimmune encephalomyelitis. submitted; 2001.

35. Issazadeh S, Lorentzen JC, Mustafa MI, Hojeberg B, Mussener A, Olsson T. Cytokines in relapsing experimental autoimmune encephalomyelitis in DA rats: persistent mRNA expression of proinflammatory cytokines and absent expression of interleukin-

10 and transforming growth factor-beta. *J Neuroimmunol* 1996; 69:103-115.

36. Kuroda Y, Shimamoto Y. Human tumor necrosis factor-alpha augments experimental allergic encephalomyelitis in rats. *J Neuroimmunol* 1991; 34:159–164.

37. Selmaj K, Raine CS, Cross AH. Anti-tumor necrosis factor therapy abrogates autoimmune demyelination. *Ann Neurol* 1991; 30:694–700.

38. Ruddle NH, Bergman CM, McGrath KM, Lingenheld EG, Grunnet ML, Padula SJ, Clark RB. An antibody to lymphotoxin and tumor necrosis factor prevents transfer of experimental allergic encephalomyelitis. *J Exp Med* 1990; 172:1193–1200.

39. Probert L, Akassoglou K, Pasparakis M, Kontogeorgos G, Kollias G. Spontaneous inflammatory demyelinating disease in transgenic mice showing central nervous system-specific expression of tumor necrosis factor alpha. *Proc Natl Acad Sci USA* 1995; 92:11294–11298.

40. Selmaj KW, Raine CS. Tumor necrosis factor mediates myelin and oligodendrocyte damage in vitro. *Ann Neurol* 1988; 23:339–346.

41. Akassoglou K, Bauer J, Kassiotis G, Pasparakis M, Lassmann H, Kollias G, Probert L. Oligodendrocyte apoptosis and primary demyelination induced by local TNF/p55TNF receptor signaling in the central nervous system of transgenic mice: models for multiple sclerosis with primary oligodendrogliopathy. *Am J Pathol* 1998; 153:801–813.

42. Frei K, Eugster HP, Bopst M, Constantinescu CS, Lavi E, Fontana A. Tumor necrosis factor alpha and lymphotoxin alpha are not required for induction of acute experimental autoimmune encephalomyelitis. *J Exp Med* 1997; 185:2177–2182.

43. Eugster HP, Frei K, Bachmann R, Bluethmann H, Lassmann H, Fontana A. Severity of symptoms and demyelination in MOG-induced EAE depends on TNFR1. *Eur J Immunol* 1999; 29:626–632.

44. Liu J, Marino MW, Wong G, Grail D, Dunn A, et al. TNF is a potent anti-inflammatory cytokine in autoimmune-mediated demyelination. *Nat Med* 1998; 4:78–83.

45. Selmaj K, Papierz W, Glabinski A, Kohno T. Prevention of chronic relapsing experimental autoimmune encephalomyelitis by soluble tumor necrosis factor receptor I. *J Neuroimmunol* 1995; 56:135–141.

46. Korner H, Lemckert FA, Chaudhri G, Etteldorf S, Sedgwick JD. Tumor necrosis factor blockade in actively induced experimental autoimmune encephalomyelitis prevents clinical disease despite activated T cell infiltration to the central nervous system. *Eur J Immunol* 1997; 27:1973–1981.

47. Bachmann R, Eugster HP, Frei K, Fontana A, Lassmann H. Impairment of TNF-receptor-1 signaling but not fas signaling diminishes T-cell apoptosis in myelin oligodendrocyte glycoprotein peptide-induced chronic demyelinating autoimmune encephalomyelitis in mice. *Am J Pathol* 1999; 154:1417–1422.

48. Speiser DE, Sebzda E, Ohteki T, Bachmann,MF, Pfeffer K, et al. Tumor necrosis factor receptor p55 mediates deletion of peripheral cytotoxic T lymphocytes in vivo. *Eur J Immunol* 1996; 26:3055–3060.

49. Bright JJ, Musuro BF, Du S, Sriram S. Expression of IL-12 in CNS and lymphoid organs of mice with experimental allergic encephalitis. *J Neuroimmunol* 1998; 82:22–30.

50. Jander S, Stoll G. Differential induction of interleukin-12, interleukin-18, and interleukin-1beta converting enzyme mRNA in experimental autoimmune encephalomyelitis of the Lewis rat. *J Neuroimmunol* 1998; 91:93–99.

51. Smith T, Hewson AK, Kingsley CI, Leonard JP, Cuzner ML. Interleukin-12 induces relapse in experimental allergic encephalomyelitis in the Lewis rat. *Am J Pathol* 1997; 150:1909–1917.

52. Leonard JP, Waldburger KE, Goldman SJ. Prevention of experimental autoimmune encephalomyelitis by antibodies against interleukin 12. *J Exp Med* 1995; 181:381–386.

53. Segal BM, Shevach EM. IL-12 unmasks latent autoimmune disease in resistant mice. *J Exp Med* 1996; 184:771–775.

54. Waldburger KE, Hastings RC, Schaub RG, Goldman SJ, Leonard JP. Adoptive transfer of experimental allergic encephalomyelitis after in vitro treatment with recombinant murine interleukin-12. Preferential expansion of interferon-gamma-producing cells

and increased expression of macrophage-associated inducible nitric oxide synthase as immunomodulatory mechanisms. *Am J Pathol* 1996; 148:375–382.

55. Leonard JP, Waldburger KE, Goldman SJ. Regulation of experimental autoimmune encephalomyelitis by interleukin-12. *Ann N Y Acad Sci* 1996; 795:216–226.

56. Campbell IL, Stalder AK, Akwa Y, Pagenstecher A, Asensio VC. Transgenic models to study the actions of cytokines in the central nervous system. *Neuroimmunomodulation* 1998; 5:126–135.

57. Segal BM, Dwyer BK, Shevach EM. An interleukin (IL)-10/IL-12 immunoregulatory circuit controls susceptibility to autoimmune disease. *J Exp Med* 1998; 187:537–546.

58. Kennedy MK, Torrance DS, Picha KS, Mohler KM. Analysis of cytokine mRNA expression in the central nervous system of mice with experimental autoimmune encephalomyelitis reveals that IL-10 mRNA expression correlates with recovery. *J Immunol* 1992; 149:2496–2505.

59. Okuda Y, Sakoda S, Yanagihara T. The pattern of cytokine gene expression in lymphoid organs and peripheral blood mononuclear cells of mice with experimental allergic encephalomyelitis. *J Neuroimmunol* 1998; 87:147–155.

60. Okuda Y, Sakoda S, Bernard CC, Yanagihara T. The development of autoimmune encephalomyelitis provoked by myelin oligodendrocyte glycoprotein is associated with an upregulation of both proinflammatory and immunoregulatory cytokines in the central nervous system. *J Interferon Cytokine Res* 1998; 18:415–421.

61. Mendel I, Katz A, Kozak N, Ben-Nun A, Revel M. Interleukin-6 functions in autoimmune encephalomyelitis: a study in gene-targeted mice. *Eur J Immunol* 1998; 28:1727–1737.

62. Diab A, Zhu J, Xiao BG, Mustafa M, Link H. High IL-6 and low IL-10 in the central nervous system are associated with protracted relapsing EAE in DA rats. *J Neuropathol Exp Neurol* 1997; 56:641–650.

63. Gijbels K, Brocke S, Abrams JS, Steinman L. Administration of neutralizing antibodies to interleukin-6 (IL-6) reduces experimental autoimmune encephalomyelitis and is associated with elevated levels of IL-6 bioactivity in central nervous system and circulation. *Mol Med* 1995; 1:795–805.

64. Okuda Y, Sakoda S, Fujimura H, Saeki Y, Kishimoto T, Yanagihara T. IL-6 plays a crucial role in the induction phase of myelin oligodendrocyte glucoprotein 35-55 induced experimental autoimmune encephalomyelitis. *J Neuroimmunol* 1999; 101:188–196.

65. Eugster HP, Frei K, Kopf M, Lassmann H, Fontana A. IL-6-deficient mice resist myelin oligodendrocyte glycoprotein-induced autoimmune encephalomyelitis. *Eur J Immunol* 1998; 28:2178–2187.

66. Samoilova EB, Horton JL, Hilliard B, Liu TS, Chen Y. IL-6-deficient mice are resistant to experimental autoimmune encephalomyelitis: roles of IL-6 in the activation and differentiation of autoreactive T cells. *J Immunol* 1998; 161:6480–6486.

67. Okuda Y, Sakoda S, Bernard CC, Fujimura H, Saeki Y, Kishimoto T, Yanagihara T. IL-6-deficient mice are resistant to the induction of experimental autoimmune encephalomyelitis provoked by myelin oligodendrocyte glycoprotein. *Int Immunol* 1998; 10:703–708.

68. Bauer J, Berkenbosch F, Van Dam AM, Dijkstra CD. Demonstration of interleukin-1 beta in Lewis rat brain during experimental allergic encephalomyelitis by immunocytochemistry at the light and ultrastructural level. *J Neuroimmunol* 1993; 48:13–21.

69. Jacobs CA, Baker PE, Roux ER, Picha KS, Toivola B, et al. Experimental autoimmune encephalomyelitis is exacerbated by IL-1 alpha and suppressed by soluble IL-1 receptor. *J Immunol* 1991; 146:2983–2989.

70. Martin D, Near SL. Protective effect of the interleukin-1 receptor antagonist (IL-1ra) on experimental allergic encephalomyelitis in rats. *J Neuroimmunol* 1995; 61:241–245.

71. Badovinac V, Mostarica-Stojkovic M, Dinarello CA, Stosic-Grujicic S. Interleukin-1 receptor antagonist suppresses experimental autoimmune encephalomyelitis (EAE) in rats by influencing the activation and proliferation of encephalitogenic cells. *J Neuroimmunol* 1998; 85:87–95.

72. Racke MK, Bonomo A, Scott DE, Cannella B, Levine A, et al. Cytokine-induced immune deviation as a therapy for inflammatory autoimmune disease. *J Exp Med* 1994; 180:1961–1966.

73. Beasley D, Eldridge M. Interleukin-1 beta and tumor necrosis factor-alpha synergistically induce NO synthase in rat vascular smooth muscle cells. *Am J Physiol* 1994; 266:R1197–1203.

74. Romero LI, Tatro JB, Field JA, Reichlin S. Roles of IL-1 and TNF-alpha in endotoxin-induced activation of nitric oxide synthase in cultured rat brain cells. *Am J Physiol* 1996; 270:R326–332.

75. Brosnan CF, Battistini L, Raine CS, Dickson DW, Casadevall A, Lee SC. Reactive nitrogen intermediates in human neuropathology: an overview. *Dev Neurosci* 1994; 16:152–161.

76. Furlan R. Martino G, Galbiati F, Poliani PL, Smiroldo S, et al. Caspase-1 regulates the inflammatory process leading to autoimmune demyelination. *J Immunol* 1999; 163:2403–2409.

77. Okamura H, Tsutsi H, Komatsu T, Yutsudo M, Hakura A, et al. Cloning of a new cytokine that induces IFN-gamma production by T cells [see comments]. *Nature* 1995; 378:88–91.

78. Ushio S, Namba M, Okura T, Hattori K, Nukada Y, Aet al. Cloning of the cDNA for human IFN-gamma-inducing factor, expression in Escherichia coli, and studies on the biologic activities of the protein. *J Immunol* 1996; 156:4274–4279.

79. Tone M, Thompson SA, Tone Y, Fairchild PJ, Waldmann H. Regulation of IL-18 (IFN-gamma-inducing factor) gene expression. *J Immunol* 1997; 159:6156–6163.

80. Matsumoto S, Tsuji-Takayama K, Aizawa Y, Koide K, Takeuchi M, et al. Interleukin-18 activates NF-kappaB in murine T helper type 1 cells. *Biochem Biophys Res Commun* 1997; 234:454–457.

81. Yoshimoto T, Takeda K, Tanaka T, Ohkusu K, Kashiwamura S, et al. IL-12 up-regulates IL-18 receptor expression on T cells, Th1 cells, and B cells: synergism with IL-18 for IFN-gamma production. *J Immunol* 1998; 161:3400–3407.

82. Xu D, Chan WL, Leung BP, Hunter D, Schulz K, et al. Selective expression and functions of interleukin 18 receptor on T helper (Th) type 1 but not Th2 cells. *J Exp Med* 1998; 188: 1485–1492.

83. Chang JT, Segal BM, Nakanishi K, Okamura H, Shevach EM. The costimulatory effect of IL-18 on the induction of antigen-specific IFN-gamma production by resting T cells is IL-12 dependent and is mediated by up-regulation of the IL-12 receptor beta2 subunit. *Eur J Immunol* 2000; 30:1113–1119.

84. Fantuzzi G, Reed DA, Dinarello CA. IL-12-induced IFN-gamma is dependent on caspase-1 processing of the IL-18 precursor. *J Clin Invest* 1999; 104:761–767.

85. Cua DJ, Hinton DR, Stohlman SA. Self-antigen-induced Th2 responses in experimental allergic encephalomyelitis (EAE)-resistant mice. Th2-mediated suppression of autoimmune disease. *J Immunol* 1995; 155:4052–4059.

86. Karpus WJ, Gould KE, Swanborg RH. CD4+ suppressor cells of autoimmune encephalomyelitis respond to T cell receptor-associated determinants on effector cells by interleukin-4 secretion. *Eur J Immunol* 1992; 22:1757–1763.

87. Liblau R, Steinman L, Brocke S. Experimental autoimmune encephalomyelitis in IL-4-deficient mice. *Int Immunol* 1997; 9:799-803.

88. Bettelli E, Das MP, Howard ED, Weiner HL, Sobel RA, Kuchroo VK. IL-10 is critical in the regulation of autoimmune encephalomyelitis as demonstrated by studies of IL-10- and IL-4-deficient and transgenic mice. *J Immunol* 1998; 161:3299–3306.

89. Falcone M, Rajan AJ, Bloom BR, Brosnan CF. A critical role for IL-4 in regulating disease severity in experimental allergic encephalomyelitis as demonstrated in IL-4-deficient C57BL/6 mice and BALB/c mice. *J Immunol* 1998; 160:4822–4830.

90. Shaw MK, Lorens JB, Dhawan A, DalCanto R, Tse HY, et al. Local delivery of interleukin 4 by retrovirus-transduced T lymphocytes ameliorates experimental autoimmune encephalomyelitis. *J Exp Med* 1997; 185:1711–1714.

91. Inobe J, Slavin AJ, Komagata Y, Chen Y, Liu L, Weiner HL. IL-4 is a differentiation factor for transforming growth factor-beta secreting Th3 cells and oral administration of IL-4 enhances oral tolerance in experimental allergic encephalomyelitis. *Eur J Immunol* 1998; 28:2780–2790.

92. Rott O, Fleischer B, Cash E. Interleukin-10 prevents experimental allergic encephalitis in rats. *Eur J Immunol* 1994; 24:1434–1440.

93. Cannella B, Gao YL, Brosnan C, Raine CS. IL-10 fails to abrogate experimental autoimmune encephalomyelitis. *J Neurosci Res* 1996; 45:735–746.

94. Cua DJ, Groux H, Hinton DR, Stohlman SA, Coffman RL. Transgenic interleukin 10 prevents induction of experimental autoimmune encephalomyelitis. *J Exp Med* 1999; 189:1005–1010.

95. Samoilova EB, Horton JL, Chen Y. Acceleration of experimental autoimmune encephalomyelitis in interleukin-10-deficient mice: roles of interleukin-10 in disease progression and recovery. *Cell Immunol* 1998; 188:118–124.

96. Koo GC, Manyak CL, Dasch J, Ellingsworth L, Shultz LD. Suppressive effects of monocytic cells and transforming growth factor-beta on natural killer cell differentiation in autoimmune viable motheaten mutant mice. *J Immunol* 1991; 147:1194–1200.

97. Shull MM, Ormsby I, Kier AB, Pawlowski S, Diebold RJ, Yin M, et al. Targeted disruption of the mouse transforming growth factor-beta 1 gene results in multifocal inflammatory disease. *Nature* 1992; 359:693–699.

98. Johns LD, Flanders KC, Ranges GE, Sriram S. Successful treatment of experimental allergic encephalomyelitis with transforming growth factor-beta 1. *J Immunol* 1991; 147:1792–1796.

99. Kuruvilla AP, Shah R, Hochwald GM, Liggitt HD, Palladino MA, Thorbecke GJ. Protective effect of transforming growth factor beta 1 on experimental autoimmune diseases in mice. *Proc Natl Acad Sci USA* 1991; 88:2918–2921.

100. Santambrogio L, Hochwald GM, Saxena B, Leu CH, Martz JE, et al. Studies on the mechanisms by which transforming growth factor-beta (TGF-beta) protects against allergic encephalomyelitis. Antagonism between TGF-beta and tumor necrosis factor. *J Immunol* 1993; 151:1116–1127.

101. Racke MK, Sriram S, Carlino J, Cannella B, Raine CS, McFarlin DE. Long-term treatment of chronic relapsing experimental allergic encephalomyelitis by transforming growth factor-beta 2. *J Neuroimmunol* 1993; 46:175–183.

102. Johns LD, Sriram S. Experimental allergic encephalomyelitis: neutralizing antibody to TGF beta 1 enhances the clinical severity of the disease. *J Neuroimmunol* 1993; 47:1–7.

103. Chen LZ, Hochwald GM, Huang C, Dakin G, Tao H, et al. Gene therapy in allergic encephalomyelitis using myelin basic protein-specific T cells engineered to express latent transforming growth factor-beta1. *Proc Natl Acad Sci USA* 1998; 95:12516–12521.

104. Thorbecke GJ, Umetsu DT, deKruyff RH, Hansen G, Chen LZ, Hochwald GM. When engineered to produce latent TGF-beta1, antigen specific T cells down regulate Th1 cell-mediated autoimmune and Th2 cell-mediated allergic inflammatory processes. *Cytokine Growth Factor Rev* 2000; 11:89–96.

105. Wyss-Coray T, Borrow P, Brooker MJ, Mucke L. Astroglial overproduction of TGF-beta 1 enhances inflammatory central nervous system disease in transgenic mice. *J Neuroimmunol* 1997; 77:45–50.

106. Wyss-Coray T, Masliah E, Mallory M, McConlogue L, Johnson-Wood K, Lin C, Mucke L. Amyloidogenic role of cytokine TGF-beta1 in transgenic mice and in Alzheimer's disease. *Nature* 1997; 389:603–606.

107. Wyss-Coray T, Lin C, Sanan DA, Mucke L, Masliah E. Chronic overproduction of transforming growth factor-beta1 by astrocytes promotes Alzheimer's disease-like microvascular degeneration in transgenic mice. *Am J Pathol* 2000; 156:139–150.

108. Schluesener HJ, Lider O. Transforming growth factors beta 1 and beta 2: cytokines with identical immunosuppressive effects and a potential role in the regulation of autoimmune T cell function. *J Neuroimmunol* 1989; 24:249–258.

109. Fabry Z, Topham DJ, Fee D, Herlein J, Carlino JA, Hart MN, Sriram S. TGF-beta 2 decreases migration of lymphocytes in vitro and homing of cells into the central nervous system in vivo. *J Immunol* 1995; 155:325–332.

110. Stevens DB, Gould KE, Swanborg RH. Transforming growth factor-beta 1 inhibits tumor necrosis factor-alpha/lymphotoxin production and adoptive transfer of disease by effector cells of autoimmune encephalomyelitis. *J Neuroimmunol* 1994; 51:77–83.

111. Cash E, Minty A, Ferrara P, Caput D, Fradelizi D, Rott O. Macrophage-inactivating IL-13 suppresses experimental autoimmune encephalomyelitis in rats. *J Immunol* 1994; 153:4258–4267.

112. Zhang J, Markovic-Plese S, Lacet B, Raus J, Weiner HL, Hafler DA. Increased frequency of interleukin 2-responsive T cells specific for myelin basic protein and proteolipid protein in peripheral blood and cerebrospinal fluid of patients with multiple sclerosis. *J Exp Med* 1994; 179:973–984.

113. Cannella B, Raine CS. The adhesion molecule and cytokine profile of multiple sclerosis lesions [see comments]. *Ann Neurol* 1995; 37:424-435.

114. Hofman, F.M., Hinton, D.R., Johnson, K., and Merrill, J.E. Tumor necrosis factor identified in multiple sclerosis brain. *J Exp Med* 1989; 170:607–612.

115. Selmaj K, Raine CS, Cannella B, Brosnan CF. Identification of lymphotoxin and tumor necrosis factor in multiple sclerosis lesions. *J Clin Invest* 1991; 87:949–954.

116. Hofman FM, von Hanwehr RI, Dinarello CA, Mizel SB, Hinton D, Merrill JE. Immunoregulatory molecules and IL 2 receptors identified in multiple sclerosis brain. *J Immunol* 1986; 136:3239–3245.

117. Woodroofe MN, Cuzner ML. Cytokine mRNA expression in inflammatory multiple sclerosis lesions: detection by non-radioactive in situ hybridization. *Cytokine* 1993; 5:583–588.

118. Windhagen A, Newcombe J, Dangond F, Strand C, Woodroofe MN, et al. Expression of costimulatory molecules B7-1 (CD80), B7-2 (CD86), and interleukin 12 cytokine in multiple sclerosis lesions. *J Exp Med* 1995; 182:1985–1996.

119. Beck J, Rondot P, Catinot L, Falcoff E, Kirchner H, Wietzerbin J. Increased production of interferon gamma and tumor necrosis factor precedes clinical manifestation in multiple sclerosis: do cytokines trigger off exacerbations? *Acta Neurol Scand* 1988; 78:318–323.

120. Panitch HS, Hirsch RL, Haley AS, Johnson KP. Exacerbations of multiple sclerosis in patients treated with gamma interferon. *Lancet* 1987; 1:893–895.

121. Noronha A, Toscas A, Jensen MA. Interferon beta decreases T cell activation and interferon gamma production in multiple sclerosis. *J Neuroimmunol* 1993; 46:145–153.

122. Becher B, Giacomini PS, Pelletier D, McCrea E, Prat A, Antel JP. Interferon-gamma secretion by peripheral blood T-cell subsets in multiple sclerosis: correlation with disease phase and interferon-beta therapy. *Ann Neurol* 1999; 45:247–250.

123. Balashov KE, Smith DR, Khoury SJ, Hafler DA, Weiner HL. Increased interleukin 12 production in progressive multiple sclerosis: induction by activated CD4+ T cells via CD40 ligand. *Proc Natl Acad Sci USA* 1997; 94:599–603.

124. Balashov KE, Comabella M, Ohashi T, Khoury SJ, Weiner HL. Defective regulation of IFNgamma and IL-12 by endogenous IL-10 in progressive MS. *Neurology* 2000; 55:192–198.

125. Balashov KE, Olek MJ, Smith DR, Khoury SJ, Weiner HL. Seasonal variation of interferon-gamma production in progressive multiple sclerosis. *Ann Neurol* 1998; 44:824–828.

126. Sharief MK, Thompson EJ. In vivo relationship of tumor necrosis factor-alpha to blood-brain barrier damage in patients with active multiple sclerosis. *J Neuroimmunol* 1992; 38:27–33.

127. van Oosten BW, Barkhof F, Scholten PE, von Blomberg BM, Ader HJ, Polman CH. Increased production of tumor necrosis factor alpha, and not of interferon gamma, preceding disease activity in patients with multiple sclerosis. *Arch Neurol* 1998; 55:793–798.

128. Rieckmann P, Albrecht M, Kitze B, Weber T, Tumani H, Broocks A, Luer W, Poser S. Cytokine mRNA levels in mononuclear blood cells from patients with multiple sclerosis. *Neurology* 1994; 44:1523–1526.

129. Spuler S, Yousry T, Scheller A, Voltz R, Holler E, Hartmann M, Wick M, Hohlfeld R. Multiple sclerosis: prospective analysis of TNF-alpha and 55 kDa TNF receptor in CSF and serum in correlation with clinical and MRI activity. *J Neuroimmunol* 1996; 66:57–64.

130. Khoury SJ, Orav EJ, Guttmann CR, Kikinis R, Jolesz FA, Weiner HL. Changes in serum levels of ICAM and TNF-R correlate with disease activity in multiple sclerosis. *Neurology* 1999; 53:758–764.

131. TNF neutralization in MS: results of a randomized, placebo-controlled multicenter study. The Lenercept Multiple Sclerosis Study Group and The University of British Columbia MS/MRI Analysis Group. *Neurology* 1999; 53:457–465.

132. van Boxel-Dezaire AH, Hoff SC, van Oosten BW, Verweij CL, Drager AM, et al. Decreased interleukin-10 and increased interleukin-12p40 mRNA are associated with disease activity and characterize different disease stages in multiple sclerosis. *Ann Neurol* 1999; 45:695–703.

133. Nicoletti F, Patti F, Cocuzza C, Zaccone P, Nicoletti A, Di Marco R, Reggio A. Elevated serum levels of interleukin-12 in chronic progressive multiple sclerosis. *J Neuroimmunol* 1996; 70:87–90.

134. Ferrante P, Fusi ML, Saresella M, Caputo D, Biasin M, et al. Cytokine production and surface marker expression in acute and stable multiple sclerosis: altered IL-12 production and augmented signaling lymphocytic activation molecule (SLAM)-expressing lymphocytes in acute multiple sclerosis. *J Immunol* 1998; 160:1514–1521.

135. Comabella M, Balashov K, Issazadeh S, Smith D, Weiner HL, Khoury SJ. Elevated interleukin-12 in progressive multiple sclerosis correlates with disease activity and is normalized by pulse cyclophosphamide therapy. *J Clin Invest* 1998; 102:671–678.

136. Smith DR, Balashov KE, Hafler DA, Khoury SJ, Weiner HL. Immune deviation following pulse cyclophosphamide/methylprednisolone treatment of multiple sclerosis: increased interleukin-4 production and associated eosinophilia. *Ann Neurol* 1997; 42:313–318.

137. Correale J, Gilmore W, McMillan M, Li S, McCarthy K, Le T, Weiner LP. Patterns of cytokine secretion by autoreactive proteolipid protein-specific T cell clones during the course of multiple sclerosis. *J Immunol* 1995; 154:2959–2968.

138. Pelfrey CM, Rudick RA, Cotleur AC, Lee JC, Tary-Lehmann M, Lehmann PV. Quantification of self-recognition in multiple sclerosis by single-cell analysis of cytokine production. *J Immunol* 2000; 165:1641–1651.

139. Takashima H, Smith DR, Fukaura H, Khoury SJ, Hafler DA, Weiner HL. Pulse cyclophosphamide plus methylprednisolone induces myelin-antigen-specific IL-4-secreting T cells in multiple sclerosis patients. *Clin Immunol Immunopathol* 1998; 88:28–34.

140. Klinkert WE, Kojima K, Lesslauer W, Rinner W, Lassmann H, Wekerle H. TNF-alpha receptor fusion protein prevents experimental auto-immune encephalomyelitis and demyelination in Lewis rats: an overview. *J Neuroimmunol* 1997; 72:163–168.

141. Calabresi PA, Fields NS, Maloni HW, Hanham A, Carlino J, et al. Phase 1 trial of transforming growth factor beta 2 in chronic progressive MS. *Neurology* 1998; 51:289–292.

142. Kopp JB, Factor VM, Mozes M, Nagy P, Sanderson N, et al. Transgenic mice with increased plasma levels of TGF-beta 1 develop progressive renal disease. *Lab Invest* 1996; 74:991–1003.

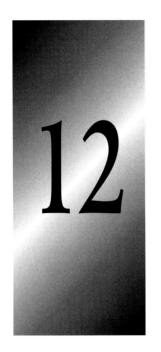

# 12 Chemokines and Their Receptors in Multiple Sclerosis

*Richard M. Ransohoff, M.D.*
*William J. Karpus, Ph.D.*

## INFLAMMATION, TISSUE INJURY, AND DISABILITY IN MULTIPLE SCLEROSIS

he natural history of neurologic disability in multiple sclerosis (MS) has been studied intensely (1,2). For most patients, the disease will have a significant impact on daily function. Most importantly, 50 percent of patients with the desease achieve an Extended Disability Status Score (EDSS) of at least 6.0 (indicating requirement of aids for ambulation) between 15 and 20 years. Given the peak age of onset at 30 years, this statistic translates into a population of individuals aged 45 to 50 years who require canes or walkers for routine ambulation. Although textbooks commonly indicate that as many as 30 percent of patients may experience "benign" nondisabling disease, contemporary follow-up studies have demonstrated that two-thirds of patients classified as having benign MS after 10 years of disease are disabled after 25 years (3).

One hypothesis of the origin of disability in MS is that the pathogenetic cascade begins with invasion of the nervous system by leukocytes and culminates with irreversible injury to myelin and axons (4). Recent studies have indicated that the disease is pathologically heterogeneous so that some cases feature a dissociation of inflammation and tissue injury (5,6). However, in most cases, the intensity of inflammation is directly related to the extent of tissue injury. This conclusion rests on several lines of evidence, from which representative studies are cited below:

1. Examination of autopsy MS brain sections has indicated that the destruction of myelin/axon units (7) and the death of oligodendrocytes (8) is directly correlated to numbers of inflammatory cells in tissue lesions.
2. Prospective analyses have suggested that cerebrospinal fluid (CSF) markers of inflammation, such as white cell count in the CSF, predict the severity of the neurologic course (9).
3. Investigations using magnetic resonance imaging (MRI) have shown that clinical deterioration is predicted by the number of inflammatory events, typified by disruption of the blood–brain barrier (BBB), as revealed by foci of gadolinium leakage into brain parenchymal lesions (10).

### MS Neuropathology and The Pathogenesis of Disability

The pathology of MS has been characterized with progressively more detail and specificity during the past 120 years (11). MS specifically and exclusively affects the central nervous system (CNS, brain, and spinal cord). Therefore, the evolution of MS studies has been entirely concurrent with the development of modern neuropathology (11). In turn, each advance in neuropathologic techniques has produced a new wave of insights into the pathogenesis of MS. The pathologic hallmarks of MS include primary demyelination, inflammation, gliosis, and axonal pathology (11). Primary demyelination is the most important single pathologic feature of the disease (12), which implies that the principal target of the pathologic process within the affected CNS is myelin (13). Myelin is a lipid-rich membrane made exclusively by oligodendroglia within the CNS. Myelin has the function of promoting rapid and efficient conduction in nerve fibers (axons). In addition, myelin provides trophic support and protection against toxic environmental exposures. Studies performed in pathologic material from very acute lesions have indicated clearly that the initial and primary injured component in the CNS of MS patients is myelin (14).

However, tissue injury in MS extends far beyond demyelination. Specifically, demyelinated nerve fibers exhibit physiologic abormalities and many undergo transection, an irreversible event. This fact has been known since the earliest pathologic descriptions of MS (15). Recently, with quantitative immunohistochemical techniques, it has become apparent that nerve fiber transection occurs frequently in acute lesions (7,15–19). Research to uncover the molecular bases of axon transection in MS lesions is embryonic but at present guided by the observation that the maximal density of transected axons is found in regions of highest concentration of activated macrophages, in zones of acute demyelination (7,14). Certainly, removal of the protective myelin sheath from the nerve fiber exposes the axon membrane to a toxic inflammatory microenvironment, but specific destructive components have not been identified. Hypotheses center around exposure to substances such as tumor necrosis factor (TNF) and products generated by nitric oxide (NO) and reactive oxygen species.

Axons also may suffer the consequences of chronic demyelination. It has been known for some years that diseases of the peripheral nervous system in which myelin is damaged or aberrantly formed (dysmyelination) bring about axonal pathology, which in turn is related to disability (20). This pathology appears to arise from loss of the trophic influences provided by myelin. Denial of myelin's trophic support is also deleterious to CNS fibers: mice engineered to produce abnormal CNS myelin by targeted deletion of the myelin proteolipid protein gene exhibited axonal pathology during adulthood (21,22). Therefore, chronically demyelinated MS lesions are plausible substrates for axon loss and likely to produce clinical progression (16,18,23).

## CHEMOKINES AND LEUKOCYTE TRAFFICKING IN THE CNS

### Chemokines and Leukocyte Trafficking

#### Understanding Leukocyte Extravasation

New information about the role of tissue inflammation in the pathogenesis of MS has driven a search for effective and specific therapeutics that address leukocyte trafficking. These developments in understanding MS are complemented by advances in clarifying the molecular mechanisms of leukocyte extravasation that provide the knowledge base needed to modulate tissue inflammation. These concepts have been applied with partial success through therapeutic trials of humanized monoclonal antibodies that block leukocyte adhesion molecule interactions with endothelial cells.

Additional targets for study and potential intervention in MS are the chemokines and their receptors. Chemokines constitute a large family of chemoattractant peptides that regulate the vast spectrum of leukocyte migration events. One attribute of chemokines that has led to intense interest is that their receptors, members of the superfamily of G-protein coupled receptors (GPCR), are among the most appealing drug targets of all immune-system components (24).

Considerable attention has recently been devoted to understanding leukocyte trafficking during inflammatory processes affecting the CNS and integrating chemokines into this process (25). The fundamental mechanisms underlying leukocyte extravasation during physiological migration and into sites of inflammation have been dissected in some detail during the past decade (26–33). The process relies on the sequential and overlapping interaction of three species of ligand–receptor pairs. Initial contact between the leukocyte and the endothelial cell is mediated by selectins and their carbohydrate counterreceptors. This interaction is termed *rolling* and reduces the velocity of the cell within the bloodstream sufficiently so that inflammatory parenchymal events can be monitored.

Chemokines are implicated in two subsequent steps of leukocyte extravasation. First, chemokine signals activate leukointegrins to bind avidly to their counterreceptors, the cell adhesion molecules (CAMs) on the endothelial lumenal surface (34). This binding is essential for the rolling leukocyte to arrest, achieve firm adhesion to the endothelial cell, and flatten. The final stage, diapedesis, is driven in part by gradient-dependent chemoattraction mediated by chemokines. It is not required that a single chemokine deliver the integrin-activating signals and the cues for directed migration (35).

Cells respond to chemokines by virtue of the expression (Table 12.1) of specific high-affinity receptors

## TABLE 12.1
### The Chemokine Superfamily

| SYSTEMATIC NAME | LIGAND HUMAN | LIGAND MOUSE | RECEPTOR(S) |
|---|---|---|---|
| **C family** | | | |
| XCL1;2 | Lymphotactin, SCM-1α ATAC; SCM-1β | Lymphotactin | XCR1 |
| **CC family** | | | |
| CCL1 | I309 | TCA-3, P500 | CCR8 |
| CCL2 | MCP-1, MCAF | JE, MCP-1 | CCR2 |
| CCL3 | MIP-1α, LD78α/β, AT 464.1/.2, GOS19-1/-2 | MIP-1α | CCR1, CCR5 |
| CCL4 | MIP-1β, AT744.1, AT744.2, Act-2, G-26, HC21, H400, LAG-1 | MIP-1β | CCR5 |
| CCL5 | RANTES | RANTES | CCR1, 3, 5, |
| CCL6 | ? | C10, MRP-1 | ? |
| CCL7 | MCP-3 | NC28, FIC, MARC | CCR1, 2, 3 |
| CCL8 | MCP-2, HC14 | MCP-2 | CCR2, 3 |
| CCL9,10 | ? | MRP-2, CCF18, MIP-1γ | ? |
| CCL11 | Eotaxin | Eotaxin | CCR3 |
| CCL12 | ? | MCP-5 | CCR2 |
| CCL13 | MCP-4, NCC-1, CKβ-10 | ? | CCR2,3 |
| CCL14 | HCC-1, HCC-3, NCC-2 | ? | CCR1 |
| CCL15 | HCC-2, MIP-1δ, NCC-3, MIP-5, Lkn-1 | ? | CCR1,3 |
| CCL16 | HCC-4, NCC-4, LEC, LMC | LCC-1 | CCR1 |
| CCL17 | TARC, dendrokine | TARC | CCR4 |
| CCL18 | DC-CK1, PARC, MIP-4, AMAC-1 | ? | ? |
| CCL19 | MIP-3β, ELC, exodus-3, CKβ-11 | MIP-3β | CCR7, CCR11 |
| CCL20 | MIP-3α, LARC, exodus-1 | MIP-3α | CCR6 |
| CCL21 | TCA4, exodus-2, SLC, 6Ckine | 6Ckine | CCR7, CCR11 |
| CCL22 | MDC, STCP-1, DCtactinβ | ABCD-1 | CCR4, ? |
| CCL23 | MPIF-1, MIP-3, CKβ-8, CKβ-8-1 | ? | CCR1 |
| CCL24 | Eotaxin-2, MPIF-2, CKβ-6 | ? | CCR3 |
| CCL25 | TECK | TECK | CCR9a,b;CCR11 |
| CCL26 | Eotaxin-3 | ? | CCR3 |
| CCL27 | CTACK/ALP | CTAK, ALP | CCR10 |
| **CXC family** | | | |
| CXCL1 | GRO-1, GRO-α, MGSA-α | GRO (KC) | CXCR2, 1 |
| CXCL2 | GRO-2, GRO-β, MIP-2α, MGSA-β | GRO (KC) | CXCR2 |
| CXCL3 | GRO-3, GRO-γ, MIP-2β | GRO (KC) | CXCR2 |
| CXCL4 | PF4 | PF4var1, PF4alt | ? |
| CXCL5 | ENA-78 | LIX | CXCR2 |
| CXCL6 | GCP-2 | Ckα-3 | CXCR1, 2 |
| CXCL7 | NAP-2 | ? | CXCR2 |
| CXCL8 | IL-8, MDNCF, NAP-1, NCF | ? | CXCR1,2 |
| CXCL9 | MIG, HuMIG | MIG | CXCR3 |
| CXCL10 | IP-10 | crg-2, mob-1 | CXCR3 |
| CXCL11 | b-R1, I-TAC, H174, | ? | CXCR3 |
| CXCL12 | SDF-1α, SDF-1β, PBSF | SDF-1α/β | CXCR4 |
| CXCL13 | BLC, BCA-1 | BLR1L, Angie | CXCR5 |
| CXCL14 | BRAK, bolekine | BRAK | ? |
| CXCL15 | ? | Lungkine | ? |
| **CX3C family** | | | |
| CX3CL1 | Fractalkine | Fractalkine | CX3CR1 |

BLC, B-lymphocyte chemokine; BLRIL, DCtactin; ENA-78, epithelial cell–derived neutrophil activating protein of 78 amino acids; GCP, G-coupled protein; GRO, growth regulated oncogene; HuMIG, human monokine induced by interferon-γ; IL, interleukin; IP-10, interferon-γ–induced peptide of 10 kd; I-TAC, interferon-inducible T-cell α-chemoattractant; MCP, monocyte chemoattractant protein; MCP, monocyte chemoattractant protein; MIG, monokine induced by interferon-γ; MIP, macrophage inflammatory protein; NAP, neutrophil-activating peptide; PF4, platelet factor-4; RANTES, regulated upon activation, normal T-cell, expressed and secreted.

(36–41). This overall scheme of leukocyte extravasation has been applied with great success to events as diverse as inflammation, developmental and recirculatory leukocyte trafficking, and colonization of gut and skin with resident populations of leukocytes; recent reviews have lucidly explicated these lines of research (42–44). Therefore, variants of this general scheme appear to underlie all leukocyte trafficking. Combinatorial diversity is cited to account for the enormous variety of leukocyte extravasation and migration events explained by the paradigm.

## Chemokines and Their Receptors: Background and Nomenclature

Chemokines comprise a large superfamily of approximately 50 peptides constituting a discrete subset of the general class of polypeptide mediators designated as cytokines. Distinct from peptide hormones such as insulin, cytokines typically act in a restricted microenvironment in paracrine or autocrine fashion. The only chemokine that is commonly included in lists of traditional cytokines is interleukin (IL)–8, which was assigned an interleukin designator before the defining characteristics of the superfamily of chemokines were recognized. The chemokines are at present considered a unique subclass of cytokines, for several reasons: 1) chemokines exhibit a highly-conserved structure (see below), 2) most chemokines are encoded in definable multigene arrays at specific chromosomal loci, and 3) the chemokine receptors constitute a specific class of cytokine receptors by virtue of belonging to the superfamily of heptahelical GPCRs.

Although they are involved in diverse processes, their "eponymous" role (as "chemotactic cytokines") appears to be chemoattraction of subpopulations of leukocytes (33). In this regard, chemokines differ from the classical chemoattractants, such as complement component C5a, which act toward a larger spectrum of leukocytes. Specificity of chemokine action is mediated by selective expression of chemokine receptors, the heptahelical G-protein–coupled membrane molecules. With time and further study, chemokines have been implicated in developmental organogenesis, angiogenesis, neoplasia, differentiation, and a host of other physiologic and pathologic processes (45,46). Considerable interest has been sparked by the discovery that several chemokine receptors are essential invasion coreceptors for human immunodeficiency virus (HIV)–1 and HIV-2 infection of human cells (47,48).

Given the size and complexity of the chemokine family, organizing principles are essential for initiating focused meaningful study of their biology in health and disease (Table 12.1). Fortunately, some such principles are readily apparent. All elements with chemokine activity are small (10–15 kd) and exhibit a conserved structure that features a core globular β-barrel established by three antiparallel β-strands. This core is flanked by a highly basic C-terminal α-helix and a short, relatively disordered, N-terminal segment (49). The N-terminal segment contains most or all of the structural information required for receptor specificity (50). Therefore, naturally occurring proteolytic modifications of the N-terminal segments of chemokine peptides can dramatically change receptor affinity or specificity (51–53). Further, engineered modifications of the chemokine N-terminus can give rise to peptides with potent receptor-blocking activity (54).

The core structures of chemokines are maintained in part by disulfide bonds between positionally conserved cysteine resides (49). For most chemokine peptides, a discernible structural characteristic is the distribution of four cysteines within the molecule. A convenient informal terminology for the chemokines has been derived from the observation that subfamilies of chemokine peptides are distinguished by the organization of the cysteines near the N-terminus of the molecule. With the use of this algorithm, four chemokine peptide families have been described. In the first, or α-chemokine family, the initial two cysteines are separated by a single residue. Thus, the α-chemokines are also known as *CXC chemokines*. In the β-chemokine family, the first two cysteines are adjacent, giving rise to the term *CC chemokines*. Lymphotactin, a peptide with all the characteristic features of a chemokine, has a single C residue near the N-terminus and defines the family of γ or *C chemokines*. The fourth family of chemokine elements is defined by a molecule termed *fractalkine*, which is a unique component of the chemokine superfamily. Fractalkine is expressed as a typical chemokine motif tethered to the cell membrane by a transmembrane anchor and "presented" by a long mucinlike stalk. The N-terminal cysteines of fractalkine are separated by three residues, and fractalkine defines the family of δ or *CX3C chemokines*. Beyond their structural similarities, the chemokine subfamilies exhibit genetic association. Many CXC chemokines are encoded in a multigene array on human chromosome 4. Most, but not all, CC chemokines are encoded in a similar large array on human chromosome 17. Lymphotactin and fractalkine are encoded elsewhere in the genome. A substantial, current, and practical chemokine Web site is maintained at http://cytokine.medic.kumamoto-u.jp/CFC/CK/chemokine.html.

A simplifying nomenclature for the chemokines and receptors has been proposed and a current version is shown in Table 12.1 (55). This scheme takes the chemokine subfamily name (e.g., CC or CX3C), adds the designator *L* for ligand or *R* for receptor, and appends a unique number. For ligands, the number corresponds to the order in which the genes were assigned an *SCY* (small cytokine family) designation, which usually follows the order of characterization by molecular cloning. The SCY designators can be found at the Web site mentioned earlier.

The new ligand designations are provided in this review, with traditional jargon names, although the nomenclature is not widely employed at present. The receptor nomenclature is more firmly established. For the receptors, the order of numeration includes demonstration of molecular uniqueness, characterizing specific binding of ligand(s), and documenting biologic function (calcium flux, chemotactic response, or other signaling).

## Chemokine Receptors

### Structure

Chemokine receptors belong to the superfamily of GPCRs. The GCPRs are a large family of biologically important receptors with conserved structure and signaling properties. Perhaps the best characterized family members are the retinal rhodopsins. GPCRs exhibit a heptahelical disposition in the plasma membrane, with residues in the intramembrane helices being highly conserved within families. The N-terminal segments and extracellular loops 1 to 3 constitute the ligand-binding domains of the receptors and vary to impart ligand specificity. The intracellular loops and C-terminal tails of GPCR provide sites of association with signaling components and vary consistently with different signaling outputs of the various receptors. The GPCRs are believed to be the largest superfamily of human genes and constitute important targets for small-molecule therapeutics. Chemokine receptors belong to the family of group A GPCRs, and to the subfamily of peptide-specific GPCRs, thus being closely related to the receptors for C5a anaphylotoxin and the bacterial N-formylated peptides, such as N-formylmethionine-leucine-proline (fMLP). Useful information about GPCR can be obtained at the Web site http://www.gpcr.org/7tm/html.

The juxtamembrane portion of the second intracellular loop of chemokine receptors contains a conserved DRYLAIV motif (using the single-letter code for amino acids) that has been found in all signaling chemokine receptors to date and is a variant of the acidic residue–arginine aromatic residue motif at this position in all GPCRs. Exceptions to this rule are the nonsignaling "promiscuous" chemokine receptorlike molecules, Duffy antigen receptor for chemokines (DARC) and D6 (56–58). Both D6 and DARC bind many CC and CXC chemokines with low nanomolar efficiency, despite their lack of signaling competence. D6 and DARC have provisionally been termed *chemokine-binding molecules* in preference to *chemokine receptors*. These observations document the functional significance of the conserved DRYLAIV motif.

DARC and D6 may exert nonsignaling functions such as immobilization of chemokines on endothelial surfaces for "presentation" to passing leukocytes. DARC is differentially expressed on erythrocytes and endothelia,

probably because of its adventitious function as the invasion receptor for *Plasmodium vivax*, a major human pathogen (59,60). DARC is accordingly downregulated on erythrocytes of individuals from malaria-endemic areas but is expressed on postcapillary venules even in people who are DARC-negative on erythrocytes (61,62). Interestingly, DARC is expressed in the CNS on a population of cerebellar Purkinje cell neurons and is upregulated at the mRNA level in brain tissue of MS patients (63–65).

### Nomenclature

A useful nomenclature of the chemokine receptors has been established. Molecular entities are assigned status as chemokine receptors with the demonstration that they represent specific species, that selective high-affinity ligand binding can be demonstrated, and that signaling (preferentially with biological response) can be documented. Using this approach, there are 18 currently defined chemokine receptors (CCR1-10, CXCR1-6, XCR1, and CX3CR1). Chemokine receptors are assigned to families by virtue of binding ligands from the structurally defined chemokine families. This nomenclature implies (which is indeed the case) that receptors preferentially bind ligands from individual families. Thus, CXCRs preferentially bind CXC chemokines, CCRs prefer to bind CC chemokines, and so forth. Individual reports indicated that CC chemokine bind CXC receptors, generally with high nanomolar affinity and occasionally with effects that suggest antagonist function (66). Despite these exceptions, the chemokine receptor nomenclature has been highly effective and useful.

### Ligand–Receptor Relationships

Ligand–receptor relationships in the chemokine superfamily are complex. The receptors have been operationally subdivided according to the complexity of their relationships to ligands into various groups (31). Thus, the private receptors (e.g., CXCR1) bind only a single ligand, in this case IL-8 (although it was recently reported that GCP-2/CXCL6 is also a full ligand at CXCR1). The public receptors (e.g., CXCR2) bind multiple ligands (all seven glutamateleucine orginine (ELR)-positive CXC chemokines: IL-8, three growth-regulated oncogene [GRO] peptides, neutrophil-activating peptide-2 [NAP-2], granulocyte chemotactic protein-2 [GCP-2], and epithelial cell–derived neutropil-activating protein-2 [ENA-78]). The promiscuous receptors (DARC and D-6) that bind multiple chemokines of several families do not signal or transduce biological effects. A substantial population of orphan receptors to which ligands have not yet been assigned but for which structural analysis indicates likely membership in the chemokine receptor family.

The fact that most chemokine receptors can respond to a diversity of ligands in vitro can lead to a confusing impression of redundancy in the chemokine system. Experiments in gene-targeted animals have indicated that functional redundancy in vivo is not the rule. These disparate results of experiments in vitro and in vivo suggest that the apparent overabundance of chemokines and receptors is a reflection of intricate biological complexity and specificity (67–69). At present, the most intellectually satisfying interpretation of chemokine ligand–receptor interactions holds that different combinations of ligands and receptors can produce precisely tuned responses to a wide variety of environmental challenges (70).

### Virus-Encoded Chemokine Receptors and Ligands

A fascinating group of functionally competent chemokine receptors and chemokines is encoded by viruses (primarily the herpesviridae) (71,72). These virus-encoded chemokines and receptors probably play important roles in the pathogenesis of primary viral infection (73,74). Mechanisms of action include expression of receptors that bind and sequester chemokines within cells, thereby limiting inflammatory responses. In some cases, these molecules may mediate unanticipated consequences of virus infection such as the development of Kaposi sarcoma (KS) in individuals infected with human herpes virus-8 (HHV8), likely resulting from expression of the chemokine receptor encoded by open recording frame (ORF)-74 (75,76). Assignment of ligands for the virus-encoded chemokine receptors is clearly complicated because biologic readouts are not always readily available (72,77,78). However, these receptors frequently bind multiple ligands from various chemokine families.

### Regulation of Chemokine Receptor Expression

Target cells respond to chemokines only by virtue of expressing cognate receptors. Therefore, the regulation of the receptor expression is a critical checkpoint in defining how cells respond to chemokines in the environment. Leukocytes express chemokines receptors according to their lineage, their stage of differentiation, and their state of activation. One example comes from studies of T-cells during activation and differentiation (79,80). Naive, resting T-cells express CXCR4 and CCR7. With activation, T-cells rapidly upregulate CCR5 and CXCR3, with the latter receptor exhibiting sustained expression only in cells that are polarized toward T-helper 1 (Th1) phenotypic commitment (79,81). T-cells exposed to chronic activating stimuli will gradually upregulate CCR2. T-cells that are polarized in a T-helper 2 (Th2) environment will express CCR3, CCR4, and CCR8 (79,81,82).

Perhaps the most intricate and well-defined program of regulated chemokine expression is exhibited by dendritic cells (42,43,80,83,84). Immature dentritic cells migrate from the blood stream into tissue under the influence of high expressions of CCR1, CCR2, and CCR5, receptors that respond to "inflammatory" chemokines. Such cells are competent for antigen ingestion and processing but not for presentation. After antigen uptake, immature dentritic cells prepare to undergo reverse transmigration from tissue into blood and eventually to lymphoid organs. In addition to other changes that indicate acquisition of the mature dentritic cell phenotype, these cells downregulate CCR1 and CCR5 to permit exit from the inflammatory site (where high concentrations of the ligands for these receptors are found). Mature dentritic cells upregulate CCR7, ligands that are highly expressed in lymphoid organs. These cells pass from tissue into the blood stream and advance to afferent vessels from secondary lymphoid organs. This program of regulated chemokine receptor expression has been termed *weigh the anchor* (indicating the decrease in CCR1 and CCR5) followed by *hoist the sail* (alluding to increased CCR7 expression). These concepts have been elegantly explicated (67), and the role of this chemokine receptor program in the adaptive immune response is described below.

### Signaling

As might be expected from the diversity of biologic responses mediated by chemokines, postreceptor signaling is complex, and this topic has been recently and ably reviewed (85). Signals from chemokine receptors generate outputs that direct two cardinal biological responses: integrin activation and directional migration (35). Integrin activation depends on calcium flux and mitogen-activated protein (MAP) kinase activation through inside-out signaling (86). Cytoskeletal reorganization, uropod formation, and directional migration depend on calcium entry, G-protein–coupled events, cytoplasmic GTPases including RhoA, and phospholipases C and D. Other functional responses (including proliferation and restraint of proliferation) appear to depend on these events but require a variety of protein tyrosine kinases and phosphoinositol-3 kinase (PI3K) (87,88).

One outstanding question in the chemokine receptor field is related to the G-protein–coupling for diverse responses in different cells. It is clear that such diversity exists: although early studies demonstrated that many consequences of chemokine receptor signaling are pertusis-toxin–sensitive (suggesting obligatory coupling to $G_i$), pertusis-toxin–insensitive responses to chemokine receptor stimulation have been unambiguously described (89). Differential use of $G_\alpha$ components by CXC and CC receptors has also been clearly demonstrated (90). Further, variation in G-protein coupling for individual receptors in different cellular backgrounds has been described.

## Chemokines, Their Receptors, and Immune Responses

### Chemokines and Their Receptors Control Migration in Secondary Lymphoid Organs During the Generation of Adaptive Immune Responses

Findings from gene-targeted mice, in vitro studies, cell transfer studies, and a large variety of descriptive analyses of gene expression have culminated in satisfying accounts of the roles of several chemokines and chemokine receptors in the generation of adaptive immune responses within secondary lymphoid organs (SLC) such as lymph nodes. These concepts and the data that underlie them have been extensively and elegantly reviewed (42,67,91–94).

In lymph nodes, dendritic cells charged with antigen must encounter naive T-cells with cognate receptors. Naive T-cells arrive in the T-cell zones of lymph nodes through the action of CCR7. CCR7 initially engages SLC (CCL21 in the new nomenclature), which is highly expressed by high endothelial venules (HEVs), the distinctive vascular component of lymph nodes. Subsequently, after extravasation, naive T cells enter T-cell zones and are retained there under the influence of high local concentrations of ELC/CCL19 and SLC/CCL21 acting on CCR7.

Immature dendritic cells in tissue express high levels of CCR1 and CCR5. After uptake of antigen and achievement of the mature dendritic cell phenotype, these cells rapidly downmodulate all chemokine receptors, in part through engagement of CD40 (43,83,84). Elimination of signaling from these receptors allows reverse transmigration from tissue into blood and is succeeded by gradual upregulation of CCR7. These dendritic cells, which are now fully competent antigen presenting cells (APCs), migrate through the lymph (which contains CCR7 ligands on endothelial surfaces) into the T-cell zones of lymph nodes under the influence of local high-level SLC/CCL21 and ELC/CCL19 concentrations. Therefore, through the action of CCR7 and its ligands, mature antigen-charged dendritic cells and naive T-cells are brought into apposition in the T-cell zones of lymph nodes. Dendritic cells promote even closer contact, specifically with activated T-cells, by producing macrophage-derived chemokine (MDC)/CCL22, which acts on CCR4, expressed on activated but not on naive T-cells (95,96). Upon activation by antigen, T-cells downregulate CCR7 and acutely upregulate CXCR3. However, CXCR3 expression is sustained only on those T-cells destined to become committed to the Th1 functional phenotype.

T-cells activated in T-cell zones but destined to provide help for immunoglobulin synthesis also may upregulate CXCR5, which could render these T cells able to draw close to the B-cell follicles of lymph nodes (under the influence of B-lymphocyte chemokine [BLC]/CXCL13 (97), there to provide help for B-cell immunoglobin synthesis (42). T-cells determined to persist as Th2-committed helpers will persistently upregulate CCR3, CCR4, and CCR8. High levels of interferon-γ–induced 10-Kd peptide (IP-10) and monokine induced by interferon-g (MIG) in sites of TH1-biased inflammatory responses are driven by the expression of interferon-g (IFN-γ) and will serve to attract Th1-committed T-cells through action on CXCR3 (80,98). Complementary effects will promote the accumulation of Th2 cells through the action of eotaxin on CCR3, MDC on CCR4, and I309 on CCR8. Although (RANTES)/CCL5 engages Th1- and Th2-associated receptors, its dominant effects promote Th1 and inhibit Th2 properties of T-cells (99). Therefore, through the action of a small number of chemokines and receptors, intricate, precise, and efficient adaptive immune responses can be generated.

### Roles of Chemokines in Cytokine Expression and T-cell Differentiation

In addition to their roles as chemoattractants, it is now clear that chemokines participate critically in regulating T-cell activation, cytokine production, and differentiation (100). Subsets of T-cells are classified based on the cytokines they produce: Th1 cells produce IFN-γ, IL-2, and TNF-β, whereas Th2 cells produce IL-4, IL-5, and IL-10 (101–103). Th1, but not Th2, cells produce lymphotactin/XCL1, monocyte chemoattractant protein (MCP)–1/CCL2, and macrophage inflammatory protein (MIP)–1α/CCL3, whereas both subsets can synthesize MIP-1β/CCL4 in vitro (104).

In an experimental animal asthma model, transfer of Th1 and Th2 cells regulated chemokine expression differently: lungs from animals that received Th2 cells expressed mainly eotaxin, whereas lungs from animals that received Th1 cells expressed lymphotactin, IP-10/CXCL10, RANTES/CCL5, and MCP-1/CCL2 (105). Collectively, these data indicate that differences exist in cytokine production and chemokine regulation when one compares Th1 and Th2 cells.

The differentiation of Th0 into Th1 cells required IL-12, whereas differentiation into Th2 cells required IL-4 (102). MIP-1α/CCL3 was associated with Th1-type granuloma formation, whereas MCP-1/CCL2 was associated with Th2-type granuloma formation in a schistosomiasis model (106,107). Recently it was shown that naive T-cells from T-cell receptor (TCR) transgenic, RAG-1 deficient mice showed enhanced IFN-γ production when incubated with MIP-1α/CCL3 and enhanced IL-4 production when incubated with MCP-1/CCL2 (108).

Further, MCP-1/CCL2 was important in vivo for T-cells to express properties of the Th2 phenotype (100). In particular, MCP-1/CCL2 knockout mice failed to develop antigen-specific Th2 commitment. In addition to inducing T-cell differentiation, chemokines regulate inflammatory cytokine production. Specifically, MCP-1/CCL2 downregulated IL-12 expression in the mucosa during oral tolerance induction, thereby contributing to the T-cell nonresponsive state (109). Thus, chemokines are not only induce differentiation of Th cells, they also can participate in tissue-specific regulation of inflammatory cytokine expression.

### Chemokine Receptors in T-Cell Differentiation

Using in vitro polarized T-cell lines, RNase protection assays, and calcium mobilization assays, Sallusto et al. (79,80,82) identified a profile of chemokine receptors expressed on human Th1 and Th2 cells. CCR3, originally described as a receptor on eosinophils and basophils for the chemokines eotaxin, eotaxin-2, RANTES/CCL5, MCP-2/CCL8, MCP-3/CCL7, and MCP-4/CCL13, (110,111) was found selectively expressed on Th2 cells from human peripheral blood and also polarized TH2 lines expanded in vitro (82). CCR4 was found on Th2 cells but was also found on non–IL-4–producing cells (79,81,112). These observations suggest that CCR3 expression by T-cells correlates Th2 phenotype.

CXCR3, which is a receptor for MIG/CXCL9, IP-10/CXCL10, and interferon-inducible γ-chemoattractant (I-TAC)/CXCL11, was expressed at higher levels on human Th1 cells than on Th2 cells (79,81,113). CCR5 expression was found on highly polarized human Th1 but not on Th2 clones (81,114). However, Sallusto et al. showed that CCR5 expression is transiently expressed on T-cells with an activated phenotype (CD86$^+$, L-selectin$^-$, CD45RO$^+$, and CD45RA$^{low}$) and therefore is not exclusively a Th1 marker (79). These investigators showed that, with removal of the T-cell growth factor IL-2, CCR5 is decreased, whereas CXCR3 expression remains elevated, suggesting that CCR5 is a marker for activated human T-cells, whereas CXCR3 is a marker for Th1 cells.

## Unusual Character of CNS Inflammation

Clearly, the concept that molecular determinants of trafficking define how inflammatory infiltrates are composed has great appeal as one attempts to account for the distinct characteristics of inflammatory processes in the CNS. Because swelling rapidly produces fatal shifts of the cerebral contents, the CNS is intolerant of acute inflammation, with accompaniments of neutrophilia and edema. It seems apparent that rapid increases in intrathecal fluid volume, produced by inflammation, will invariably be accommodated by abruptly reduced blood volumes, which will generate ischemic damage. Apparently, the CNS has evolved mechanisms to avoid such catastrophes.

Inflammation in the CNS appears to be severely restricted and controlled by multiple mechanisms including the BBB, which excludes most macromolecules and inflammatory cells (115–122).

The distinct character of CNS inflammation has been shown elegantly by studies using intracerebral injections of kainic acid, which produce a necrotizing neuronal injury due to excitotoxic mechanisms (123). In peripheral tissues, abundant cellular necrosis would be expected to elicit neutrophilic inflammation, vasogenic edema, and tissue swelling (124). However, such injury within the CNS produces gradual recruitment of hematogenous macrophages and activation of the resident macrophage population, represented by microglia (124).

What mechanisms underlie this distinctly restricted pattern of inflammation? First, cerebrovascular endothelial cells express lower levels of adhesion molecules (compared with other vascular beds) under resting conditions. However, the activated cerebrovascular endothelium expresses very high levels of adhesion substrates for leukocyte recruitment (124). Therefore, the principal shaping force for CNS accumulation of subpopulations of leukocytes appears to be expression of specific chemokines. At a first level of approximation, this tenet holds that the CNS is specialized to produce chemokines that attract cells involved in chronic inflammation (mononuclear cells) from the circulation, and that neutrophil recruitment occurs only under unusual circumstances. This concept is supported by the fact that neutrophil-specific chemokines can be highly expressed in the circumstances (such as brain abscess) in which neutrophils accumulate at high levels within the CNS. As a unifying statement, it appears likely that selective production of specific chemokines underlies the propensity of the nervous system to develop features of chronic rather than of acute inflammation.

Second, percussion injury to the rodent spinal cord produces a very sparse neutrophilic reaction followed by recruitment of macrophages (125). This pattern is mirrored by the brief low-level expression of neutrophil-specific chemokines followed by robust expressions of MCP-1 and MCP-5/CCL12 (126).

## Transgenic and Knockout Models

The concept that chemokines are major determinants of leukocyte recruitment to the nervous system has been subjected to numerous proof-of-principle experiments in animal models. Much of this work has been performed in a model of MS, experimental autoimmune encephalomyelitis (EAE). These studies are described below. Other studies have used transgenic (127) or knockout mice. Fuentes and colleagues overexpressed MCP-1/CCL2 within the CNS under the control of an oligodendrocyte-specific myelin basic protein (MBP) promoter (128). These mice developed sparse monocytic infiltrates in the CNS perivascular space. Upon activation of endothelium by intraperitoneal injection of lipopolysaccharide (LPS), the mice developed abundant monocytic infiltrates of the nervous system. Complementary experiments came from Tani et al. and Bell et al. (129,130). In the first case, a neutrophil chemoattractant, GRO-α/CXCL1 was expressed under the control of the MBP promoter, and mice developed remarkably abundant infiltrates of neutrophils (129). These cells invaded the CNS without becoming activated and subsequently underwent apoptosis. Therefore, chemokine signals were sufficient to recruit but not to activate these cells within the nervous system. Bell and coworkers expressed a related neutrophil chemoattractant, MIP-2/CXCL2, through injection of a recombinant adenovirus (130). Injection of this construct produced flamboyant neutrophilic invasion of the nervous system. In both cases, BBB disruption was observed. Subsequently, Perry and coworkers showed that this disruption is consequent to the extent of the neutrophil traffic across the cerebrovascular endothelium (131).

Recent studies in CCR5-deficient mice (generated by gene targeting through homologous recombination in embryonic stem cells) have provided dramatic evidence for the importance of chemokines in specific leukocyte recruitment to the CNS in a relevant model of microbial pathogenesis. In these experiments, the human pathogen *Cryptococcus neoformans* was instilled into the tracheae of wild-type and CCR5 knockout mice (132). Both wild type and CCR5 −/− mice mounted a vigorous inflammatory response in the lung and cleared the organism. However, CCR5-deficient mice died because of overwhelming cryptococcal meningoencephalitis. Defective recruitment of inflammatory cells to the CNS appeared to be responsible for the susceptibility of CCR5 knockout mice to this pathogenic process.

## Inflammatory Disease Models

### Descriptive Studies of Chemokine Expression

EAE often has been used as an animal surrogate for MS (133–137). Further, a great deal of understanding of immune-mediated inflammation in the nervous system has resulted from studies in this model (13,138,139). In early work on chemokine expression in this system, three groups almost simultaneously reported high-level expression of multiple chemokines in the CNS of mice with EAE (140–142). Interestingly, these chemokines would be predicted to act almost exclusively on lymphocytes and macrophages, the cells that overwhelmingly constitute the inflammatory infiltrate in EAE.

### Interventional Studies of Chemokine Function in EAE

Workers in this field were strongly motivated to proceed with their efforts by the demonstration, shortly after the initial descriptive studies, that antibodies to one chemokine, MIP-1α/CCL3, could abrogate adoptive transfer of EAE in SJL mice (143). This report by Karpus and colleagues represented the first demonstration of a functional role for chemokines in EAE. Karpus and coworkers subsequently showed that relapses of adoptive-transfer EAE are significantly diminished by antibodies to another chemokine, MCP-1/CCL2 (144). These results were confirmed and extended in additional reports by using the novel technique of naked DNA vaccination: these studies showed that vaccination against MCP-1/CCL2 or MIP-1α/CCL3 protects mice against EAE, whereas similar approaches targeted to other chemokines had no effect (in the case of RANTES/CCL5) or made the disease more severe (MIP-1β/CCL4) (145). Further innovative studies by Vanguri and colleagues implicated IP-10/CXCL10, an astrocyte-derived, T-cell-specific chemokine, in the Lewis rat model of EAE (146). These investigators used chronic intrathecal infusion of antisense oligodeoxynucleotides to modify the pathologic process in the CNS of the experimental animals (146). Such disparate observations were integrated by the hypothesis that specific chemokines regulate the different processes that comprise EAE (147).

### Sources and Regulation of Chemokines in the CNS of Animals with EAE

The sources of chemokines in EAE nervous system have been addressed by several groups, with generally concordant findings. Several chemokines (MIP-1α/CCL3, MIP-1β/CCL4, and RANTES/CCL5) are made predominantly by infiltrating leukocytes (148–150). Other chemokines (IP-10/CXCL10 and MCP-1/CCL2) are produced mainly by the resident population of astrocytes (148,149,151). Further, time course studies indicated that chemokines are elaborated immediately after the earliest T-cell infiltrates enter the affected CNS (152,153). Using all available data, it has been proposed that initial invasion of the CNS by activated antigen-specific T-cells occurs independently of production of chemokines within the CNS tissue (154,155). However, immediately after T-cells become resident within the nervous system and produce inflammatory cytokines, large-scale expression of multiple chemokines ensues and contributes to the dramatic amplification of the inflammatory response (150).

Recent studies have shown that the responder cells (infiltrating inflammatory leukocytes) express chemokine receptors that are appropriate for binding the chemokines produced in the affected CNS tissue (156). It is widely anticipated that studies in chemokine receptor knockout mice will uncover specific roles for individual receptors in the generation and propagation of the inflammatory pathology of EAE (25,157).

What drives the expression of chemokines in EAE? Based on simple descriptive considerations, it appears likely that inflammatory cytokines produced by activated T-cells and macrophages are responsible. Tissue culture studies have shown that such cytokines (IFN-γ, TNF-α, and IL-1) stimulate cells to produce remarkably large quantities of chemokines (158,159). Further, the distribution of chemokine-expressing cells, around aggregates of inflammatory cells, suggests that products of the inflammatory cells stimulate chemokine expression (151). Finally, a recent study in IFN-γ knockout (GKO) mice provided data that support this hypothesis (160). Surprisingly, GKO mice are susceptible to EAE and exhibit typical inflammatory pathology. Further, there is high-level intrathecal production of several chemokines including MCP-1/CCL2. Strikingly absent from the array of chemokines produced during GKO-EAE is IP-10/CXCL10 (160). Of interest, IP-10/CXCL10 was initially cloned in a differential hybridization experiment using IFN-γ to stimulate U937 cells (161). In most, but not all circumstances, IFN-γ is essential for the production of IP-10/CXCL10. Therefore, the absence of IP-10/CXCL10 in the CNS of GKO mice with EAE suggested that inflammatory cytokines regulated the expression of chemokines during EAE.

## CHEMOKINES AND THEIR RECEPTORS IN MULTIPLE SCLEROSIS

The study of chemokines in MS has been, to date, descriptive. Gratifyingly, much of the information we have about chemokines in MS can be readily correlated to findings in animal models, including EAE.

### Genetic Studies

There are hints that chemokine and chemokine receptor genes are related to the likelihood of getting MS or the severity of the disease. Fiten and colleagues reported that the risk to develop MS is decreased in Swedish patients who possess specific microsatellite polymorphisms in the upstream region of the MCP-3/CCL7 gene (162). Different polymorphisms conferred protection for patients with high-risk HLA haplotypes as compared with those with low-risk HLA haplotypes.

Additional work has focused on the well-characterized Δ32 polymorphism of CCR5. This genetic lesion leads to expression of a nonfunctional CCR5 protein. Homozygotes for this allele (about 1 percent of the Western European population) are functional "knockouts" for CCR5. In a study of 120 unrelated patients in Australia,

Bennets and colleagues showed that the homozygous Δ32 CCR5 genotype does not protect against MS. In all, two patients in that small sample were CCR5 Δ32 homozygotes, a frequency that would be expected by chance given the background allele frequency and prevalence of MS (163). Sellebjerg and colleagues found an intriguing effect of the CCR5 Δ32 heterozygote state on MS severity. They identified patients at the time of first attack and performed genotyping studies for CCR5. In this cohort, Δ32 heterozygotes progressed to clinically definite MS (defined by the occurrence of a second attack) significantly more slowly than did patients with wild-type CCR5 genes (164). Oksenberg and coworkers showed, in a well-documented cohort of familial MS cases, that Δ32 heterozygotes exhibit a mean 3-year delay in the onset of their MS, as compared with patients possessing wild-type CCR5 alleles (165).

These results have correlates in experimental model systems. Teuscher and colleagues identified a locus termed *eae7*, one of several that control the pattern of EAE in congenic inbred mouse strains (166). This quantitative trait locus (QTL) proved to be coincident with the β-chemokine gene cluster. Sequence polymorphisms for three chemokines distinguished the two eae7 alleles and predicted significant structural alterations in two of the chemokine proteins involved. As noted above (132), CCR5-null mice failed to recruit leukocytes into the nervous system in response to challenge to *Cryptococcus neoformans*. Therefore, in spontaneous human disease and the mouse model, inflammatory demyelination is linked, in susceptibility and severity, to polymorphic genes in the chemokine system.

### Clinical Studies

Other studies of the involvement of chemokines in MS have used material from patients. For the most part, studies have focused on body fluids (blood or CSF) or autopsy brain tissue.

Interestingly, the first study of a chemokine-related product in MS was reported in 1987 by Cananzi et al. before the chemokine family was defined (167). In that study, platelet factor 4 (PF4/CXCL4) was significantly increased in the plasma of MS patients as compared with healthy controls. Aspirin treatment did not affect PF4 production by cells isolated from patients, suggesting that the product originated from mast cells. Because the function of PF4 remains undefined, this observation has not been extensively followed up.

There have been limited reports of chemokine levels in the CSF of MS patients (168). Our group compared chemokine levels by enzyme-linked immunosorbent assay in the CSF of 38 patients with active symptomatic MS with the CSF of 21 healthy individuals without neurologic disease (169). Several chemokines (IP-10/CXCL10,

MIG/CXCL9, and RANTES/CCL5) were significantly elevated, whereas levels of MCP-1 were significantly decreased in the MS patients' CSF. These observations were extended by analyzing chemokine receptor expression on T-cells in blood and CSF obtained simultaneously at the time of lumbar puncture/phlebotomy during diagnostic work-up. We found that T-cells in the CSF express the IP-10/MIG receptor CXCR3 on approximately 90 percent of cells. This frequency was significantly increased over that observed in blood, where fewer than 40 percent of T-cells were CXCR3 positive. In the case of the RANTES/CCL5 receptor CCR5, a small fraction (less than 10 percent) of circulating T-cells were CCR5 positive, and the percentage of positive cells in CSF was significantly larger but remained a minority of total CSF T-cells.

These results were extended by immunohistochemical studies of autopsy brain sections containing active MS lesions. CXCR3-positive cells were found in the perivascular space around more than 99 percent of inflamed vessels within MS lesions.

Balashov and colleagues performed studies that confirmed and extended these results and that were reported at virtually the same time (170). First, they found that CXCR3-positive circulating T-cells from MS patients make more IFN-γ than those from controls. This result suggested that CXCR3 expression on Th1-committed T-cells (previously described in vitro) might be pertinent for the pathogenesis of MS. Balashov and coworkers also detected large numbers of IP-10/CXCL10–immunoreactive cells in MS lesions. Taken together, the results suggested that interactions between CXCR3 and its ligands might mediate trafficking, retention, or activation of T-cells in MS lesions.

However, it is clear that most CNS-infiltrating lymphocytes in MS are not CXCR3/CCR5 double positive because only a minority of CD4$^+$ or CD8$^+$ T-cells in MS CSF was identified as expressing CCR5 by Sørensen et al. (169). The relative lack of CCR5 expression on CSF T-cells may not, however, exclude a pathogenic role for these cells: in particular, Strunk and colleagues found that circulating lymphocytes in MS patients are more likely than those from controls to express CCR5 and that these CCR5$^+$ T-cells express higher levels of IFN-γ and TNF-α than do cells from control individuals, arguing in favor of the pathogenic role of Th1-like cells in MS (171).

In the case of CCR5, immunohistochemistry of lesional material indicated that relatively few perivascular cells were CCR5 positive but that a large population of activated phagocytotic macrophages expressed CCR5. These results suggest that the interactions between RANTES and CCR5 on monocytes and macrophages might be implicated in recruitment and activation of effectors in MS.

Several groups have focused on the production of β-chemokines within MS lesions, with generally concordant findings. Simpson et al., MacManus et al., and Van Der Voorn et al. described MCP-1/CCL2–immunoreactive astrocytes within MS lesions (172–174). MacManus et al. also described the production of MCP-2/CCL8 and MCP-3/CCL7 by glial cells within these lesions, and Simpson et al. further analyzed the production of MIP-1α/CCL3 and MIP-1β/CCL4. Hvas et al. found that RANTES/CCL5 mRNA is localized to perivascular inflammatory cells in MS lesions (175). Kivisakk and colleagues provided support for CNS parenchymal cell production of these chemokines by demonstrating that CSF cells from MS cases are no more likely than those from controls to express RANTES/CCL5 or MCP-1/CCL2 mRNA (176).

Taken together, these studies appear to support, in a general sense, the cellular sources of chemokines as described in EAE. In that model, our group showed that IP-10/CXCL10 and MCP-1/CCL2 are produced by astrocytes (140), and Godiska et al. showed that RANTES/CCL5 is produced by perivascular inflammatory cells (177), a finding that we and others subsequently confirmed (148,149). Compatible results concerning the sources of other chemokines were provided by Berman and colleagues (141,178).

## CONCLUSION

It appears plausible that the conceptual scheme of leukocyte trafficking into inflammatory lesions, derived in part from studies using the EAE animal model, may be applicable to MS. This situation provides a favorable circumstance for the evaluation of experimental anti-inflammatory strategies that are targeted to production of chemokines or the function of chemokines (via blocking chemokine receptors). Many key pieces of information about chemokines and MS are lacking, however. In particular, one awaits the results of studies that address serial changes in CSF chemokine levels, effects of standard treatment (IFN-β and glatiramer acetate) on the expression of chemokines and their receptors, clear-cut relationships between expression of chemokine receptors and demyelinating or axonal pathology in MS lesions, and relationships of chemokines or chemokine receptor expression to disease activity as defined by MRI. The results of these and other studies will determine how and if the explosion of new information about chemokines and leukocyte trafficking can be applied to understanding and treating MS.

## References

1. Weinshenker BG, Sibley WA. Natural history and treatment of multiple sclerosis. *Curr Opin Neurol Neurosurg* 1992; 5(2):203–211.

## TABLE 12.2
### Glossary of Terms Found in the Chemokine Literature

**BLC (CXCL13):** B-lymphocyte chemokine, -2, an ELR-negative CXC chemokine.

**CC:** The subfamily of chemokines for which the initial two cysteines are adjacent; β-chemokines.

**CCR1-CCRn:** the receptors for CC chemokines.

**CXC:** the subfamily of chemokines for which the initial two cysteines are separated by a single amino acid; α-chemokines.

**CXCR1-CXCRn:** the receptors for CXC chemokines.

**D6:** another non-signaling promiscuous chemokine-binding molecule.

**DARC:** the Duffy antigen receptor for chemokines; a non-signaling promiscuous chemokine-binding molecule found on erythrocytes and postcapillary venules.

**ELC (CCL19):** Epstein Barr virus–induced molecule 1 ligand chemokine.

**ELR:** containing a glutamate-leucine-arginine motif near the N-terminus; defines a subset of approximately seven CXC chemokines that bind CXCR1 and CXCR2 and act towards neutrophils.

**ENA-78 (CXCL5):** epithelial cell–derived neutrophil activating protein of 78 amino acids, an ELR-positive CXC chemokine.

**GCP-2 (CXCL6):** granulocyte chemotactic protein-2, an ELR-positive CXC chemokine.

**GPCR:** G-protein coupled receptors.

**GRO:** growth regulated oncogene (e.g., GRO-α) a family of ELR-positive CXC chemokines.

**IL-8 (CXCL8):** interleukin-8, an ELR-positive CXC chemokine.

**IP-10 (CXCL10):** interferon-γ–induced peptide of 10 kDa, an ELR-negative CXC chemokine.

**I-TAC (CXCL11):** interferon inducible T-cell α-chemattractant, an ELR-negative CXC chemokine.

**MCP:** monocyte chemoattractant protein (e.g., MCP-1 through MCP-5).

**MDC (CCL22):** macrophage derived chemokine.

**MIG (CXCL9):** monokine induced by interferon-γ, an ELR-negative CXC chemokine.

**MIP:** macrophage inflammatory protein (includes CC chemokines such as MIP-1α, MIP-1β, MIP-3α; also CXC chemokines such as MIP-2.

**NAP-2 (CXCL7):** neutrophil activating peptide-2, an ELR-positive CXC chemokine.

**PF4 (CXCL4):** platelet factor-4, an ELR-negative CXC chemokine.

**RANTES (CCL5):** regulated upon activation, normal T-cell, expressed and secreted.

**SCY:** small cytokine; this designation is used to categorize genes that encode chemokines. The α-chemokines are designated members of the SCYB family and the β-chemokines are assigned to the SCYA family. The SCY assignments are used to define the ligand terminology under the new nomenclature; thus, SCYA1 is the gene that encodes CCL1.

**SLC (CCL21):** secondary lymphoid organ chemokine.

2. Weinshenker BG. Natural history of multiple sclerosis. *Ann Neurol* 1994; 36(suppl):S6–S11.
3. Hawkins SA, McDonnell GV. Benign multiple sclerosis? Clinical course, long term follow up, and assessment of prognostic factors. *J Neurol Neurosurg Psychiatry* 1999; 67(2):148–152.
4. Sørensen TL, Ransohoff RM. Etiology and pathogenesis of multiple sclerosis. *Semin Neurol* 1998; 18(3):287–294.
5. Lucchinetti CF, Bruck W, Rodriguez M, Lassmann H. Distinct patterns of multiple sclerosis pathology indicates heterogeneity in pathogenesis. *Brain Pathol* 1996; 6(3):259–274.
6. Tienari PJ. Multiple sclerosis: multiple etiologies, multiple genes? *Ann Med* 1994; 26(4):259–269.
7. Ferguson B, Matyszak MK, Esiri MM, Perry VH. Axonal damage in acute multiple sclerosis lesions. *Brain* 1997; 120(pt 3):393–399.
8. Lucchinetti C, Bruck W, Parisi J, et al. A quantitative analysis of oligodendrocytes in multiple sclerosis lesions. A study of 113 cases. *Brain* 1999; 122(pt 12):2279–2295.
9. Rudick R, Cookfair D, Simonian N, et al. Cerebrospinal fluid abnormalities in a phase III trial of avonex (IFNB-1a) for relapsing multiple sclerosis. *J Neurimmunol* 1999; 93:8–15.
10. Simon JH. From enhancing lesions to brain atrophy in relapsing MS. *J Neuroimmunol* 1999; 98(1):7–15.
11. Hickey WF. The pathology of multiple sclerosis: a historical perspective. *J Neuroimmunol* 1999; 98(1):37–44.
12. Lassmann H, Raine C, Antel J, Prineas J. Immunopathology of multiple sclerosis. *J Neuroimmunol* 1998; 86:213–218.
13. Steinman L. Multiple sclerosis: a coordinated immunological attack against myelin in the central nervous system. *Cell* 1996; 85(3):299–302.
14. Bitsch A, Wegener C, da Costa C, et al. Lesion development in Marburg's type of acute multiple sclerosis: From inflammation to demyelination. *Mult Scler* 1999; 5(3):138–146.
15. Kornek B, Lassmann H. Axonal pathology in multiple sclerosis. A historical note. *Brain Pathol* 1999; 9(4):651–656.
16. Mews I, Bergmann M, Bunkowski S, Gullotta F, Bruck W. Oligodendrocyte and axon pathology in clinically silent multiple sclerosis lesions. *Mult Scler* 1998; 4(2):55–62.
17. Trapp BD, Peterson J, Ransohoff RM, et al. Axonal transection in the lesions of multiple sclerosis. *N Engl J Med* 1998; 338(5):278–285.
18. Trapp BD, Ransohoff R, Rudick R. Axonal pathology in multiple sclerosis: Relationship to neurologic disability. *Curr Opin Neurol* 1999; 12(3):295–302.
19. Silber E, Sharief MK. Axonal degeneration in the pathogenesis of multiple sclerosis. *J Neurol Sci* 1999; 170(1):11–18.
20. Griffin JW, George EB, Chaudhry V. Wallerian degeneration in peripheral nerve disease. *Baillieres Clin Neurol* 1996; 5(1):65–75.
21. Griffiths I, Klugmann M, Anderson T, et al. Axonal swellings and degeneration in mice lacking the major proteolipid of myelin. *Science* 1998; 280(5369):1610–1613.
22. Werner H, Jung M, Klugmann M, et al. Mouse models of myelin diseases. *Brain Pathol* 1998; 8(4):771–793.
23. Waxman SG. Demyelinating diseases—new pathological insights, new therapeutic targets. *N Engl J Med* 1998; 338(5):323–325.
24. Ponath P. Chemokine receptor antagonists: novel therapeutics for inflammation and AIDS. *EIOD: Expert Opin Invest Drugs* 1998; 7:1–18.
25. Asensio VC, Campbell IL. Chemokines in the CNS: Plurifunctional mediators in diverse states. *Trends Neurosci* 1999; 22(11):504–512.
26. von Andrian UH, Chambers JD, McEnvoy LM, et al. Two-step model of leukocyte–endothelial cell interaction in inflammation: Distinct roles for LECAM-1 and the leukocyte beta 2 integrins in vivo. *Proc Natl Acad Sci USA* 1991; 88:7538–7542.
27. Butcher E. Leukocyte–endothelial cell recognition: three (or more) steps to specificty and diversity. *Cell* 1991; 67:1033–1036.
28. Schall TJ, Bacon KB. Chemokines, leukocyte trafficking, and inflammation. *Curr Opin Immunol* 1994; 6(6):865–873.
29. Springer TA. Traffic signals for lymphocyte recirculation and leukocyte eMIGration: the multistep paradigm. *Cell* 1994; 76:301–314.
30. Butcher EC, Picker LJ. Lymphocyte homing and homeostasis. *Science* 1996; 272(5258):60–66.

31. Premack BA, Schall TJ. Chemokine receptors: Gateways to inflammation and infection. *Nature Med* 1996; 2:1174–1178.
32. Foxman EF, Campbell JJ, Butcher EC. Multistep navigation and the combinatorial control of leukocyte chemotaxis. *J Cell Biol* 1997;139(5):1349-1360.
33. Baggiolini M. Chemokines and leukocyte traffic. *Nature* 1998; 392(6676):565–568.
34. Campbell JJ, Hedrick J, Zlotnik A, et al. Chemokines and the arrest of lymphocytes rolling under flow conditions. *Science* 1998; 279(5349):381–384.
35. Campbell JJ, Qin S, Bacon KB, Mackay CR, Butcher EC. Biology of chemokine and classical chemoattractant receptors: Differential requirements for adhesion-triggering versus chemotactic responses in lymphoid cells. *J Cell Biol* 1996; 134(1):255–266.
36. Murphy P. The molecular biology of leukocyte chemoattractant receptors. *Annu Rev Immunol* 1994; 12:593–633.
37. Kelvin D, Michiel D, Johnston J, et al. Chemokines and serpentines: the molecular biology of chemokine receptors. *J Leukocyte Biol* 1993; 54:604–612.
38. Horuk R. Molecular properties of the chemokine receptor family. *Trends Pharmacol Sci* 1994; 15:159–165.
39. Oppenheim JJ, Zachariae C, Mukaida N, Matsushima K. Properties of the novel proinflammatory supergene "intercrine" cytokine family. *Annu Rev Immunol* 1991; 9:617–648.
40. Taub DD, Oppenheim JJ. Chemokines, inflammation and the immune system. *Ther Immunol* 1994; 1(4):229–246.
41. Oppenheim JJ. Overview of chemokines. *Adv Exp Med Biol* 1993; 351:183–186.
42. Cyster JG. Chemokines and cell MIGration in secondary lymphoid organs. *Science* 1999; 286(5447):2098–2102.
43. Sallusto F, Palermo B, Lenig D, et al. Distinct patterns and kinetics of chemokine production regulate dendritic cell function. *Eur J Immunol* 1999; 29(5):1617–1625.
44. Bacon KB, Oppenheim JJ. Chemokines in disease models and pathogenesis. *Cytokine Growth Factor Rev* 1998; 9(2):167–173.
45. Rollins BJ. Chemokines. *Blood* 1997; 90(3):909–928.
46. Zlotnik A, Morales J, Hedrick JA. Recent advances in chemokines and chemokine receptors. *Crit Rev Immunol* 1999; 19(1):1–47.
47. Bates P. Chemokine receptors and HIV-1: an attractive pair? *Cell* 1996; 86:1–4.
48. Feng Y, Broder CC, Kennedy PE, Berger EA. HIV-1 entry cofactor: functional cDNA cloning of a seven-transmembrane G protein-coupled receptor. *Science* 1996; 272:872–877.
49. Clark-Lewis I, Kim KS, Rajarathnam K, et al. Structure-activity relationships of chemokines. *J Leukoc Biol* 1995; 5745(522):703–711.
50. Lusti-Narasimhan M, Power CA, Allet B, et al. Mutation of Leu25 and Val27 introduces CC chemokine activity into interleukin-8. *J Biol Chem* 1995; 270:2716–2721.
51. Van Damme J, Rampart M, Conings R, et al. The neutrophil-activating proteins interleukin 8 and ß-thromboglobulin: *in vitro* and *in vivo* comparison of NH2- terminally processed forms. *Eur J Immunol* 1990; 20:2113–2118.
52. Oravecz T, Pall M, Roderiquez G, et al. Regulation of the receptor specificity and function of the chemokine RANTES (regulated on activation, normal T-cell expressed and secreted) by dipeptidyl peptidase IV (CD26)-mediated cleavage. *J Exp Med* 1997; 186(11):1865–1872.
53. Struyf S, De Meester I, Scharpe S, et al. Natural truncation of RANTES abolishes signaling through the CC chemokine receptors CCR1 and CCR3, impairs its chemotactic potency and generates a CC chemokine inhibitor. *Eur J Immunol* 1998; 28(4):1262–1271.
54. Proudfoot AE, Power CA, Hoogewerf AJ, et al. Extension of recombinant human RANTES by the retention of the initiating methionine produces a potent antagonist. *J Biol Chem* 1996; 271(5):2599–2603.
55. Zlotnik A, Yoshie O. Chemokines: a new classification system and their role in immunity. *Immunity* 2000; 12:121.
56. Chaudhuri A, Zbrzezna V, Polyakova J, et al. Expression of the Duffy antigen in K562 cells: Evidence that it is the human chemokine erythrocyte receptor. *J Biol Chem* 1994; 269:7835–7838.
57. Lu ZH, Wang ZX, Horuk R, et al. The promiscuous chemokine binding profile of the Duffy antigen/receptor for chemokines is primarily localized to sequences in the amino-terminal domain. *J Biol Chem* 1995; 270(44):26239–26245.
58. Nibbs RJB, Wylie SM, Pragnell IB, Graham GJ. Cloning and characterization of a novel murine beta chemokine receptor, D6. Comparison to three other related macrophage inflammatory protein-1alpha receptors, CCR-1, CCR-3, and CCR-5. *J Biol Chem* 1997; 272(19):12495–12504.
59. Horuk R, Chitnis CE, Darbonne WC, et al. A receptor for the malarial parasite *Plasmodium vivax*: The erythrocyte chemokine receptor. *Science* 1993; 261(5125):1182–1184.
60. Mallinson G, Soo KS, Schall TJ, Pisacka M, Anstee DJ. Mutations in the erythrocyte chemokine receptor (Duffy) gene: The molecular basis of the Fya/Fyb antigens and identification of a deletion in the Duffy gene of an apparently healthy individual with the Fy(a-b-) phenotype. *Br J Haematol* 1995; 90(4):823–829.
61. Hadley TJ, Lu ZH, Wasniowska K, et al. Postcapillary venule endothelial cells in kidney express a multispecific chemokine receptor that is structurally and functionally identical to the erythroid isoform, which is the Duffy blood group antigen. *J Clin Invest* 1994; 94(3):985–991.
62. Peiper SC, Wang ZX, Neote K, et al. The Duffy antigen/receptor for chemokines (DARC) is expressed in endothelial cells of Duffy negative individuals who lack the erythrocyte receptor. *J Exp Med* 1995; 181(4):1311–1317.
63. Horuk R, Martin A, Hesselgesser J, et al. The Duffy antigen receptor for chemokines: Structural analysis and expression in the brain. *J Leukoc Biol* 1996; 59(1):29–38.
64. Horuk R, Martin AW, Wang Z, et al. Expression of chemokine receptors by subsets of neurons in the central nervous system. *J Immunol* 1997; 158(6):2882–2890.
65. Whitney LW, Becker KG, Tresser NJ, et al. Analysis of gene expression in mutiple sclerosis lesions using cDNA microarrays. *Ann Neurol* 1999; 46(3):425–428.
66. Soto H, Wang W, Strieter RM, et al. The CC chemokine 6Ckine binds the CXC chemokine receptor CXCR3. *Proc Natl Acad Sci USA* 1998; 95(14):8205–8210.
67. Mantovani A (ed.), *Chemokines*. Basel: Karger; 1999.
68. Mantovani A. The chemokine system: redundancy for robust outputs. *Immunol Today* 1999; 20(6):254–257.
69. Broxmeyer HE, Kim CH. Regulation of hematopoiesis in a sea of chemokine family members with a plethora of redundant activities. *Exp Hematol* 1999; 27(7):1113–1123.
70. Gerard C. Chemokine receptors and ligand specificity: Understanding the enigma. In: Rollins BJ (ed.), *Chemokines and Cancer*. Totowa, NJ: Humana Press; 1999; 21–31.
71. Murphy PM. Molecular piracy of chemokine receptors by herpesviruses. *Infect Agents Dis* 1994; 3(2-3):137–154.
72. Lalani AS, Barrett JW, McFadden G. Modulating chemokines: more lessons from viruses. *Immunol Today* 2000; 21(2): 100–106.
73. Bodaghi B, Jones TR, Zipeto D, et al. Chemokine sequestration by viral chemoreceptors as a novel viral escape strategy: Withdrawal of chemokines from the environment of cytomegalovirus-infected cells. *J Exp Med* 1998; 188(5):855–866.
74. Howard J, Justus DE, Totmenin AV, Shchelkunov S, Kotwal GJ. Molecular mimicry of the inflammation modulatory proteins (IMPs) of poxviruses: Evasion of the inflammatory response to preserve viral habitat. *J Leukoc Biol* 1998; 64(1):68–71.
75. Arvanitakis L, Geras-Raaka E, Varma A, Gershengorn MC, Cesarman E. Human herpesvirus KSHV encodes a constitutively active G-protein–coupled receptor linked to cell proliferation. *Nature* 1997; 385(6614):347–350.
76. Bais C, Santomasso B, Coso O, et al. G-protein–coupled receptor of Kaposi's sarcoma–associated herpesvirus is a viral oncogene and angiogenesis activator. *Nature* 1998; 391(6662):86–89.
77. Rosenkilde MM, Kledal TN, Brauner-Osborne H, Schwartz TW. Agonists and inverse agonists for the herpesvirus 8-encoded constitutively active seven-transmembrane oncogene product, ORF-74. *J Biol Chem* 1999; 274(2):956–961.
78. Gershengorn MC, Geras-Raaka E, Varma A, Clark-Lewis I. Chemokines activate Kaposi's sarcoma–associated herpesvirus G protein-coupled receptor in mammalian cells in culture. *J Clin Invest* 1998; 102(8):1469–1472.

79. Sallusto F, Lenig D, Mackay CR, Lanzavecchia A. Flexible programs of chemokine receptor expression on human polarized T helper 1 and 2 lymphocytes. *J Exp Med* 1998; 187(6):875–883.

80. Sallusto F, Lanzavecchia A, Mackay CR. Chemokines and chemokine receptors in T-cell priming and Th1/Th2-mediated responses. *Immunol Today* 1998; 19(12):568–574.

81. Bonecchi R, Bianchi G, Bordignon PP, et al. Differential expression of chemokine receptors and chemotactic responsiveness of type 1 T helper cells (Th1s) and Th2s. *J Exp Med* 1998; 187(1):129–134.

82. Sallusto F, Mackay CR, Lanzavecchia A. Selective expression of the eotaxin receptor CCR3 by human T helper 2 cells. *Science* 1997; 277(5334):2005–2007.

83. Sallusto F, Schaerli P, Loetscher P, et al. Rapid and coordinated switch in chemokine receptor expression during dendritic cell maturation. *Eur J Immunol* 1998; 28(9):2760–2769.

84. Sozzani S, Allavena P, D'Amico G, et al. Differential regulation of chemokine receptors during dendritic cell maturation: a model for their trafficking properties. *J Immunol* 1998; 161(3):1083–1086.

85. Bacon KB. Analysis of signal transduction following lymphocyte activation by chemokines. *Methods Enzymol* 1997; 288: 340–361.

86. Hynes RO. Integrins: versatility, modulation, and signaling in cell adhesion. *Cell* 1992; 69:11–25.

87. Wong M, Fish EN. RANTES and MIP-1alpha activate stats in T cells. *J Biol Chem* 1998; 273(1):309–314.

88. Ganju RK, Dutt P, Wu L, et al. Beta-chemokine receptor CCR5 signals via the novel tyrosine kinase RAFTK. *Blood* 1998; 91(3):791–797.

89. Kelly MD, Naif HM, Adams SL, Cunningham AL, Lloyd AR. Dichotomous effects of beta-chemokines on HIV replication in monocytes and monocyte-derived macrophages. *J Immunol* 1998; 160(7):3091–3095.

90. Bischoff SC, Krieger M, Brunner T, et al. RANTES and related chemokines activate human basophil granulocytes through different G protein–coupled receptors. *Eur J Immunol* 1993; 23(3):761–767.

91. Cyster JG, Ngo VN, Ekland EH, et al. Chemokines and B-cell homing to follicles. *Curr Top Microbiol Immunol* 1999; 246:87–92.

92. Melchers F, Rolink AG, Schaniel C. The role of chemokines in regulating cell Migration during humoral immune responses. *Cell* 1999; 99(4):351–354.

93. Sedgwick JD, Riminton DS, Cyster JG, Korner I. Tumor necrosis factor: A master-regulator of leukocyte movement. *Immunol Today* 2000; 21(3):110–113.

94. Cyster JG. Leukocyte Migration: Scent of the T zone. *Curr Biol* 2000; 10(1):R30–R33.

95. Imai T, Chantry D, Raport CJ, et al. Macrophage-derived chemokine is a functional ligand for the CC chemokine receptor 4. *J Biol Chem* 1998; 273(3):1764–1768.

96. Tang HL, Cyster JG. Chemokine up-regulation and activated T-cell attraction by maturing dendritic cells. *Science* 1999; 284(5415):819–822.

97. Gunn MD, Ngo VN, Ansel KM, et al. A B-cell-homing chemokine made in lymphoid follicles activates Burkitt's lymphoma receptor-1. *Nature* 1998; 391(6669):799–803.

98. Farber JM. MIG and IP-10: CXC chemokines that target lymphocytes. *J Leukoc Biol* 1997; 61(3):246–257.

99. Chensue SW, Warmington KS, Allenspach EJ, et al. Differential expression and cross-regulatory function of RANTES during mycobacterial (type 1) and schistosomal (type 2) antigen-elicited granulomatous inflammation. *J Immunol* 1999; 163(1):165–173.

100. Gu L, Tseng S, Horner RM, et al. Control of TH2 polarization by the chemokine monocyte chemoattractant protein-1. *Nature* 2000; 404(6776):407–411.

101. Mosmann TR, Sad S. The expanding universe of T-cell subsets: Th1, Th2 and more. *Immunol Today* 1996; 17(3):138–146.

102. Abbas AK, Murphy KM, Sher A. Functional diversity of helper T lymphocytes. *Nature* 1996; 383:787–793.

103. Mosmann TR, Coffman RL. Th1 and Th2 cells: Different patterns of lymphokine secretion lead to different functional properties. *Annu Rev Immunol* 1989; 7:145–174.

104. Bradley LM, Asensio VC, Schioetz LK, et al. Islet-specific Th1, but not Th2, cells secrete multiple chemokines and promote rapid induction of autoimmune diabetes. *J Immunol* 1999; 162(5):2511–2520.

105. Li L, Xia Y, Nguyen A, Feng L, Lo D. Th2-induced eotaxin expression and eosinophilia coexist with Th1 responses at the effector stage of lung inflammation. *J Immunol* 1998; 161(6):3128–3135.

106. Chensue SW, Warmington KS, Lukacs NW, et al. Monocyte chemotactic protein expression during schistosome egg granuloma formation. Sequence of production, localization, contribution, and regulation. *Am J Pathol* 1995; 146(1):130–138.

107. Chensue SW, Warmington KS, Ruth JH, et al. Role of monocyte chemoattractant protein-1 (MCP-1) in Th1 (mycobacterial) and Th2 (schistosomal) antigen-induced granuloma formation: Relationship to local inflammation, Th cell expression, and IL-12 production. *J Immunol* 1996; 157(10):4602–4608.

108. Karpus W, Lukacs N, Kennedy K, et al. Differential CC chemokine-induced enhancement of T helper cell cytokine production. *J Immunol* 1997; 158:4129–4136.

109. Karpus W, Kennedy K, Kunkel S, Lukacs N. Monocyte chemotactic protein 1 regulates oral tolerance induction by inhibition of T helper cell 1-related cytokines. *J Exp Med* 1998; 187:733–741.

110. Ponath PD, Qin S, Post TW, et al. Molecular cloning and characterization of a human eotaxin receptor expressed selectively on eosinophils. *J Exp Med* 1996; 183(6):2437–2448.

111. Uguccioni M, Mackay CR, Ochensberger B, et al. High expression of the chemokine receptor CCR3 in human blood basophiles. Role in activation by eotaxin, MCP-4, and other chemokines. *J Clin Invest* 1997; 100(5):1137–1143.

112. Imai T, Nagira M, Takagi S, et al. Selective recruitment of CCR4-bearing Th2 cells toward antigen- presenting cells by the CC chemokines thymus and activation-regulated chemokine and macrophage-derived chemokine. *International Immunol* 1999; 11(1):81–88.

113. Loetscher M, Gerber B, Loetscher P, et al. Chemokine receptor specific for IP10 and MIG: structure, function, and expression in activated T-lymphocytes. *J Exp Med* 1996; 184(3):963–969.

114. Loetscher P, Uguccioni M, Bordoli L, et al. CCR5 is characteristic of Th1 lymphocytes. *Nature* 1998; 391(6665):344–345.

115. Bolton SJ, Perry VH. Differential blood-brain barrier breakdown and leucocyte recruitment following excitotoxic lesions in juvenile and adult rats. *Exp Neurol* 1998; 154(1):231–240.

116. Perry VH, Bolton SJ, Anthony DC, Betmouni S. The contribution of inflammation to acute and chronic neurodegeneration. *Res Immunol* 1998; 149(7-8):721–725.

117. Perry VH. A revised view of the central nervous system microenvironment and major histocompatibility complex class II antigen presentation. *J Neuroimmunol* 1998; 90(2):113–121.

118. Perry VH, Anthony DC, Bolton SJ, Brown HC. The blood–brain barrier and the inflammatory response. *Mol Med Today* 1997; 3(8):335–341.

119. Castano A, Bell MD, Perry VH. Unusual aspects of inflammation in the nervous system: Wallerian degeneration. *Neurobiol Aging* 1996; 17(5):745–751.

120. Perry VH, Bell MD, Brown HC, Matyszak MK. Inflammation in the nervous system. *Curr Opin Neurobiol* 1995; 5(5): 636–641.

121. Lawson LJ, Perry VH. The unique characteristics of inflammatory responses in mouse brain are acquired during postnatal development. *Eur J Neurosci* 1995; 7(7):1584–1595.

122. Fabry Z, Raine C, Hart M. Nervous tissue as an immune compartment: The dialect of the immune response in the CNS. *Immunol Today* 1994; 15:218–224.

123. Sperk G, Lassmann H, Baran H, Kish S, Seitelberger F. Kainic acid induced seizures: Neurochemical and histopathological changes. *Neuroscience* 1983; 10:1301–1315.

124. Bell MD, Perry VH. Adhesion molecule expression on murine cerebral endothelium following the injection of a proinflammagen or during acute neuronal degeneration. *J Neurocytol* 1995; 24(9):695–710.

125. Popovich P, Wei P, Stokes B. Cellular inflammatory response after spinal cord injury in Sprague-Dawley and Lewis rats. *J Comp Neurol* 1997; 377:443–464.

126. McTigue D, Tani M, Kravacic K, et al. Selective chemokine mRNA accumulation in the rat spinal cord after contusion injury. *J Neurosci Res* 1998; 53:368–376.

127. Lira S, Fuentes M, Strieter R, Durham S. Transgenic methods to study chemokine function in lung and central nervous system. *Methods Enzymol* 1997; 287:304–318.

128. Fuentes M, Durham S, Swerdel M, et al. Controlled recruitment of monocytes/macrophages to specific organs via transgenic expression of MCP–1. *J Immunol* 1995; 155:5769–5776.

129. Tani M, Fuentes ME, Peterson JW, et al. Neutrophil infiltration, glial reaction and neurological disease in transgenic mice expressing the chemokine N51/KC in oligodendrocytes. *J Clin Invest* 1996; 98:529–539.

130. Bell MD, Taub DD, Kunkel SJ, et al. Recombinant human adenovirus with rat MIP-2 gene insertion causes prolonged PMN recruitment to the murine brain. *Eur J Neurosci* 1996; 8(9):1803–1811.

131. Bell MD, Taub DD, Perry VH. Overriding the brain's intrinsic resistance to leukocyte recruitment with intraparenchymal injections of recombinant chemokines. *Neuroscience* 1996; 74(1):283–292.

132. Huffnagle GB, McNeil LK. Dissemination of *C. neoformans* to the central nervous system: role of chemokines, Th1 immunity and leukocyte recruitment. *J Neurovirol* 1999; 5(1):76–81.

133. Dal Canto M, Melvold R, Kim B, Miller S. Two models of multiple sclerosis: Experimental allergic encephalomyelitis (EAE) and Theiler's murine encephalomyelitis virus (TMEV) infection. A pathological and immunological comparison. *Microsc Res Tech* 1995; 32:215–229.

134. Raine CS. Analysis of autoimmune demyelination: Its impact upon multiple sclerosis. *Lab Invest* 1984; 50:608–635.

135. Eng LF, Ghirnikar RS, Lee YL. Inflammation in EAE: Role of chemokine/cytokine expression by resident and infiltrating cells. *Neurochem Res* 1996; 21(4):511–525.

136. Brosnan CF, Raine CS. Mechanisms of immune injury in multiple sclerosis. *Brain Pathol* 1996; 6(3):243–257.

137. Tsunoda I, Fujinami RS. Two models for multiple sclerosis: Experimental allergic encephalomyelitis and Theiler murine encephalomyelitis virus. *J Neuropathol Exp Neurol* 1996; 55(6):673–686.

138. Steinman L. A few autoreactive cells in an autoimmune infiltrate control a vast population of nonspecific cells: a tale of smart bombs and the infantry. *Proc Natl Acad Sci USA* 1996; 93(6):2253–2256.

139. Steinman L, Miller A, Bernard CC, Oksenberg JR. The epigenetics of multiple sclerosis: Clues to etiology and a rationale for immune therapy. *Annu Rev Neurosci* 1994; 17:247–265.

140. Ransohoff RM, Hamilton TA, Tani M, et al. Astrocyte expression of mRNA encoding cytokines IP-10 and JE/MCP-1 in experimental autoimmune encephalomyelitis. *FASEB J* 1993; 7:592–602.

141. Hulkower K, Brosnan CF, Aquino DA, et al. Expression of CSF-1, c-fms, and MCP-1 in the central nervous system of rats with experimental allergic encephalomyelitis. *J Immunol* 1993; 150:2525–2533.

142. Godiska R, Chantry D, Dietsch GN, Gray PW. Chemokine expression in murine experimental allergic encephalomyelitis. *J Neuroimmunol* 1995; 58(2):167–176.

143. Karpus WJ, Lukacs NW, McRae BL, et al. An important role for the chemokine macrophage inflammatory protein–1a in the pathogenesis of the T-cell–mediated autoimmune disease, experimental autoimmune encephalomyelitis. *J Immunol* 1995; 155:5003–5010.

144. Kennedy KJ, Strieter RM, Kunkel SL, et al. Acute and relapsing experimental autoimmune encephalomyelitis are regulated by differential expression of the CC chemokines macrophage inflammatory protein-1alpha and monocyte chemotactic protein-1. *J Neuroimmunol* 1998; 92(1-2):98–108.

145. Youssef S, Wildbaum G, Maor G, et al. Long-lasting protective immunity to experimental autoimmune encephalomyelitis following vaccination with naked DNA encoding C-C chemokines. *J Immunol* 1998; 161(8):3870–3879.

146. Wojcik WJ, Swoveland P, Zhang X, Vanguri P. Chronic intrathecal infusion of phosphorothioate or phosphodiester antisense oligonucleotides against cytokine responsive gene-2/IP-10 in experimental allergic encephalomyelitis of Lewis rat. *J Pharmacol Exp Ther* 1996; 278(1):404–410.

147. Karpus WJ, Ransohoff RM. Chemokine regulation of experimental autoimmune encephalomyelitis: Temporal and spatial expression patterns govern disease pathogenesis. *J Immunol* 1998; 161(6):2667–2671.

148. Miyagishi R, Kikuchi S, Takayama C, Inoue Y, Tashiro K. Identification of cell types producing RANTES, MIP-1α and MIP-1β in rat experimental autoimmune encephalomyelitis by in situ hybridization. *J Neuroimmunol* 1997; 77:17–26.

149. Glabinski A, Tani M, Strieter R, Tuohy V, Ransohoff R. Synchronous synthesis of α- and β-chemokines by cells of diverse lineage in the central nervous system of mice with relapses of experimental autoimmune encephalomyelitis. *Am J Pathol* 1997; 150:617–630.

150. Ransohoff RM, Glabinski A, Tani M. Chemokines in immune-mediated inflammation of the central nervous system. *Cytokine Growth Factor Rev* 1996; 7(1):35–46.

151. Tani M, Glabinski AR, Tuohy VK, et al. In situ hybridization analysis of glial fibrillary acidic protein mRNA reveals evidence of biphasic astrocyte activation during acute experimental autoimmune encephalomyelitis. *Am J Pathol* 1996; 148:889–896.

152. Glabinski A, Tani M, Tuohy VK, Tuthill R, Ransohoff RM. Central nervous system chemokine gene expression follows leukocyte entry in acute murine experimental autoimmune encephalomyelitis. *Brain Behav Immun* 1996; 9:315–330.

153. Glabinski AR, Tuohy VK, Ransohoff RM. Expression of chemokines RANTES, MIP-1alpha and GRO-alpha correlates with inflammation in acute experimental autoimmune encephalomyelitis. *Neuroimmunomodulation* 1998; 5(3-4): 166–171.

154. Hickey WF. Migration of hematogenous cells through the blood–brain barrier and the initiation of CNS inflammation. *Brain Pathol* 1991; 1:97–105.

155. Hickey WF, Hsu BL, Kimura H. T-lymphocyte entry into the central nervous system. *J Neurosci Res* 1991; 28:254–260.

156. Jiang Y, Salafranca MN, Adhikari S, et al. Chemokine receptor expression in cultured glia and rat experimental allergic encephalomyelitis. *J Neuroimmunol* 1998; 86(1):1–12.

157. Mennicken F, Maki R, de Souza EB, Quirion R. Chemokines and chemokine receptors in the CNS: a possible role in neuroinflammation and patterning. *Trends Pharmacol Sci* 1999; 20(2):73–78.

158. Majumder S, Zhou Z-HL, Ransohoff R. Transcriptional regulation of chemokine gene expression in astrocytes. *J Neurosci Res* 1996; 45:758–769.

159. Hayashi M, Luo Y, Laning J, Strieter RM, Dorf ME. Production and function of monocyte chemoattractant protein-1 and other beta-chemokines in murine glial cells. *J Neuroimmunol* 1995; 60(1-2):143–150.

160. Glabinski AR, Krakowski M, Han Y, Owens T, Ransohoff RM. Chemokine expression in GKO mice (lacking interferon-gamma) with experimental autoimmune encephalomyelitis. *J Neurovirol* 1999; 5(1):95–101.

161. Luster AD, Unkeless JC, Ravetch JV. Gamma-interferon transcriptionally regulates an early-response gene containing homology to platelet proteins. *Nature* 1985; 315:672–676.

162. Fiten P, Vandenbroeck K, Dubois B, et al. Microsatellite polymorphisms in the gene promoter of monocyte chemotactic protein-3 and analysis of the association between monocyte chemotactic protein-3 alleles and multiple sclerosis development. *J Neuroimmunol* 1999; 95(1-2):195–201.

163. Bennetts BH, Teutsch SM, Buhler MM, Heard RN, Stewart GJ. The CCR5 deletion mutation fails to protect against multiple sclerosis. *Hum Immunol* 1997; 58(1):52–59.

164. Sellebjerg F. CCR5 delta32, matrix metalloproteinase-9 and disease activity in multiple sclerosis. *J Neuroimmunol* 2000; 102(1):98–106.

165. Barcellos L, Schito A, Rimmler J, et al. CC-chemokine receptor 5 polymorphism and age of onset in familial multiple sclerosis. *Immunogenetics* 2000; 51:281–288.

166. Teuscher C, Butterfield RJ, Ma RZ, et al. Sequence polymorphisms in the chemokines Scya1 (TCA-3), Scya2 (monocyte chemoattractant protein (MCP)-1), and Scya12 (MCP-5) are candidates for eae7, a locus controlling susceptibility to monophasic remitting/nonrelapsing experimental allergic encephalomyelitis. *J Immunol* 1999; 163(4):2262–2266.

167. Cananzi AR, Ferro-Milone F, Grigoletto F, et al. Relevance of platelet factor four (PF4) plasma levels in multiple sclerosis. *Acta Neurol Scand* 1987; 76(2):79–85.

168. Miyagishi R, Kikuchi S, Fukazawa T, Tashiro K. Macrophage inflammatory protein-1a in the cerebrospinal fluid of patients with multiple sclerosis and other inflammatory neurological diseases. *J Neurol Sci* 1995; 129:223–227.

169. Sørensen T, Tani M, Jensen J, et al. Expression of specific chemokines and chemokine receptors in the central nervous system of mutiple sclerosis patients. *J Clin Invest* 1999; 106:807–815.

170. Balashov KE, Rottman JB, Weiner HL, Hancock WW. CCR5(+) and CXCR3(+) T-cells are increased in multiple sclerosis and their ligands MIP-1alpha and IP-10 are expressed in demyelinating brain lesions. *Proc Natl Acad Sci USA* 1999; 96(12):6873–6878.

171. Strunk T, Bubel S, Mascher B, et al. Increased numbers of CCR5+ interferon-g- and tumor necrosis factor-a–secreting T lymphocytes in multiple sclerosis patients. *Ann Neurol* 2000; 47:269–273.

172. McManus C, Berman JW, Brett FM, et al. MCP-1, MCP-2 and MCP-3 expression in multiple sclerosis lesions: An immunohistochemical and in situ hybridization study. *J Neuroimmunol* 1998; 86(1):20–29.

173. Simpson JE, Newcombe J, Cuzner ML, Woodroofe MN. Expression of monocyte chemoattractant protein-1 and other beta-chemokines by resident glia and inflammatory cells in multiple sclerosis lesions. *J Neuroimmunol* 1998; 84(2):238–249.

174. Van Der Voorn P, Tekstra J, Beelen RH, et al. Expression of MCP-1 by reactive astrocytes in demyelinating multiple sclerosis lesions. *Am J Pathol* 1999; 154(1):45–51.

175. Kivisakk P, Teleshova N, Ozenci V, et al. No evidence for elevated numbers of mononuclear cells expressing MCP-1 and RANTES mRNA in blood and CSF in multiple sclerosis. *J Neuroimmunol* 1998; 91(1-2):108–112.

176. Godiska R, Chantry D, Dietsch G, Gray P. Chemokine expression in murine experimental autoimmune encephalomyelitis [abstract]. *J Leukoc Biol* 1994; suppl:17.

177. Berman J, Guida M, Warren J, Amat J, Brosnan C. Localization of monocyte chemoattractant peptide-1 expression in the central nervous system in experimental autoimmune encephalomyelitis and trauma in the rat. *J Immunol* 1996; 156:3017–3023.

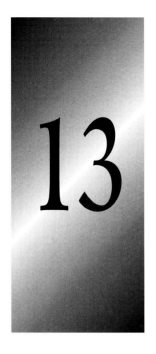

# 13 Interferons in Multiple Sclerosis

*Suhayl Dhib-Jalbut, M.D.*

nterferon-β (IFN-β) is an approved treatment for multiple sclerosis (MS) that results in relapse reduction and a slowdown in disease progression. The therapeutic mechanism of IFN-β in MS remains elusive, although several lines of experimental evidence and ex vivo findings in cells from MS patients receiving such treatment suggest a pleotropic effect on the immune system. This chapter reviews the evidence that IFN-β's therapeutic effect in MS involves several systemic effects, including inhibition of antigen presentation and T-cell activation, induction of immune deviation, antagonism of interferon-γ (IFN-γ) effects, and an effect at the blood–brain barrier (BBB). The potential effects of IFN-β in the central nervous system (CNS), including immunomodulation and remyelination, are also discussed.

## SOURCES OF INTERFERON

Interferons are naturally occurring proteins that were discovered in 1957 as products of virus-infected cells whose function was to prevent infection of other cells, hence, the name interferons (1). Interferons occur in two natural forms: type 1 interferons include interferon-α (IFN-α), produced by leukocytes, and IFN-β produced by fibroblasts; type 2 interferon or immune interferon, better known as IFN-γ is produced by immune T-cells. IFN-α is produced by lymphocytes and macrophages in response to virus infection and microbial proteins. The major type 1 interferon-producing cells in human blood are believed to be CD4$^+$, CD11c type 2 dendritic cell precursors (2). At least 15 human gene sequences are naturally expressed in humans and code for several subtypes of IFN-α (3). In contrast, one type of IFN-β exists in humans and is produced primarily by virus-infected fibroblasts. IFN-β is also produced by other cell types, including glial cells in the CNS. IFN-α and IFN-β share 32 to 40 percent homology at the nucleic acid and amino acid sequence levels: both are encoded on chromosome 9, and both interact with a common cell surface receptor (4). Naturally occurring IFN-β is a 23-kd glycoprotein that consists of 166 amino acids and 20 percent carbohydrates. Two recombinant forms of IFN-β are currently available for the treatment of MS: IFN-β1b (Betaseron®) is a 165-amino acid protein produced in *Escherichia coli*. It differs from the natural protein in that it is not glycoylated and contains a serine residue substitution for cysteine at position 17 (5). IFN-β1a (Avonex®) is obtained in Chinese hamster ovary cells and has the same primary structure, glycosylation pattern, and molecular weight as that of naturally occurring in IFN-β. IFN-β1a is also available pharmacologically as Rebif® (6).

IFN-γ (type 2 interferon) is produced by activated T lymphocytes, primarily T helper (Th) cells. It is a glycoprotein that does not share significant homology with either IFN-α or IFN-β; its gene is localized on a different chromosome, and it binds to a different cellular receptor (7).

## STRUCTURE AND BIOLOGIC EFFECTS

Interferons mediate their biologic effects by binding to species-specific cell surface receptors (8,9). The type 1 IFN receptor consists of two subunits referred to as IFN-α-R1 and IFN-α-R2. Recent experimental evidence suggested that IFN-α-R2 is primarily responsible for stabilizing the bound IFN–receptor complex (10), whereas IFN-α-R1 is responsible for the activation state of the receptor and its antiviral activity (11). The IFN-β molecule consists of a framework of five helices (A–E) and contains three closely located functionally important segments (12). Although IFN-α and IFN-β share this receptor, mutational analysis suggested distinct centers of binding for IFN-α and IFN-β on IFN-α-R2 (13). Regions of

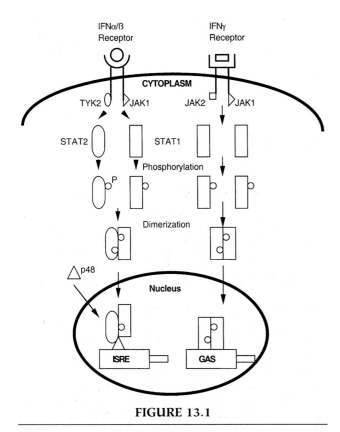

**FIGURE 13.1**

Type 1 (interferon-α/β) and type 2 (interferon-γ) signaling pathways. GAS, interferon-γ activated site; INF, interferon; ISRE, interferon-stimulated response element; STAT, signal transducer and activator of transcription.

the IFN-β molecule that are important for receptor binding and the topology of the ligand binding domain of the receptor are subjects of ongoing studies. In fact, recent evidence indicates that different domains of the IFN-α molecule bind to different receptor subunits (10). There is evidence that type 1 IFNs downregulate their receptors, which may have implications on the dosing frequency in clinical applications (14).

The IFN-α/β receptor lacks enzymatic activity but is associated with two cytoplasmic tyrosine kinases, Jak1 and Tyk2 (Figure 13.1) (15). These kinases phosphorylate latent cytoplasmic transcription factors known as STATs (signal transducers and activators of transcription). The STAT complex consists of STAT1a/β (p91/p84) and STAT2 (p113) and is designated ISGF3-α (interferon-stimulated gene factor 3), which enters the nucleus with a 48-kd DNA binding protein termed ISGF3-γ. The complex ISGF3-α/ISGF3-γ forms ISGF3, which binds a promoter region of IFN-inducible genes called ISRE (IFN-stimulated response element) and leads to the transcription of interferon-stimulated genes (ISGs) (16,17). A recent study reported that tyrosine phosphorylation of STAT1 and STAT2 and formation of ISFG3 complex are higher in response to IFN-β than to IFN-α in human myocardial fibroblasts, which correlated with the higher sensitivity of these cells to the antiviral effects of IFN-β (18).

Like other IFNs, IFN-β has antiviral, antiproliferative, and immunomodulatory effects (19). The mechanistic aspects of these effects are beginning to be understood at a molecular level. The antiviral effect of IFNs is thought to be due to the induction of cellular proteins that can inhibit viral replication at different steps in the virus replicative cycle. These proteins include 2',5'-oligoadenylate synthetase, Mx protein, double-stranded RNA-dependent protein kinase (PKR), and inducible nitric oxide synthetase (20,21). The antiproliferative effect of IFN-β is complex and not well understood. Prolongation of the cell cycle and depletion of essential metabolites may underlie the antiproliferative effect in tumor cells and perhaps in lymphocytes (22,23). Type 1 IFNs inhibit DNA binding of the positive transcription factor E2F, resulting in reduced c-myc expression and prolongation of the cell cycle. IFN-β also may affect cell growth through PKR-mediated eIF2a phosphorylation and subsequent inhibition of mRNA translation (24). The immunomodulatory effect of IFN-β is multifaceted. Similar to other IFNs, IFN-β enhances the expression of HLA class I molecules (25). This may contribute to the antiviral effect of IFNs by rendering infected cells more susceptible to lysis by cytotoxic T-cells (26). In contrast to IFN-γ, which upregulates HLA class II, IFN-β inhibits class II molecules induced by IFN-γ in a variety of cell types (27–32) and subsequently inhibits antigen presentation (26). IFN-β also may effect Th cell function by inhibiting Th1 cytokine production, including IFN-γ, interleukin-12, and tumor necrosis factor (TNF) (33–35) and by promoting Th2 cytokine secretion such as interleukin (IL)–10 (36). An IFN-α/β inducible protein called ISG15 has been identified (37). This protein is secreted by lymphocytes and monocytes, induces IFN-γ in T-cells, enhances natural killer (NK) cell activity, and, hence, is believed to mediate some of the immunomodulatory effects of IFN-α/β. More recently, a novel gene designated NKLAM (NK lytic-associated molecule) was identified, whose expression is associated with NK cells' enhanced cytolytic activity in response to IFN-β (38). Using oligonucleotide microarrays assays, several IFN-stimulated and IFN-repressed genes have been identified (39). Understanding the function of these genes undoubtedly will enhance our understanding of the biologic and therapeutic effects of this molecule.

## MECHANISMS OF IFN-β THERAPEUTIC EFFECT IN MS

The present mechanism of action of IFN-β in MS is believed to occur at three levels: 1) the systemic immune system, 2) the blood–brain barrier, and 3) possibly in the CNS compartment. Although there is evidence that IFN-β has significant effects on the peripheral immune system and the blood–brain barrier in MS, there is very little evidence that the drug enters the CNS; therefore, its effect in the CNS compartment is speculative.

### T-Cell Activation

T-cell activation requires the interaction of at least three sets of molecules with their corresponding ligands on antigen-presenting cells. These include the trimolecular complex, adhesion molecules, and costimulation molecules (Figure 13.2). There is evidence that IFN-β1 can interfere with these three groups of molecules and downregulate T-cell activation. At the trimolecular complex level, there is strong evidence that IFN-β inhibits antigen presentation by peripheral blood mononuclear cells (PBMCs) and by other accessory cells (26). The mechanism for inhibition of antigen presentation is not completely understood, but, in addition to IFN-β effect on HLA, class II expression on antigen-presenting cells could involve an effect on antigen processing independent of the levels of class II or an inhibitory effect on differentiation of immunocompetent dendritic cells (40,41). In fact, one study found that IFN-β treatment in vivo may result in enhanced HLA class II expression on macrophages (40). This raises the possibility that IFN-β inhibition of antigen presentation may in fact be independent of its effect on class II molecules and involve an effect on antigen processing or perhaps on other molecules involved in T-cell activation.

Two classes of accessory molecules have been shown to be modulated by IFN-β treatment and con-

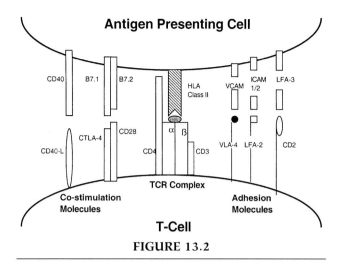

**FIGURE 13.2**

A schematic representation of the molecular interaction between T-cells and antigen-presenting cells. ICAM, intercellular cell adheshion molecule; LFA, leukocyte function antigen; TCR, T-cell receptor; VCAM, vascular cell adhesion molecule; VLA, very late activated antigen.

ceptually contribute to its therapeutic effect (42). These include the CD28–B7 and the CD40–CD40 ligand signaling pathways. The B7 molecule is expressed on a variety of antigen-presenting cells including macrophages, B-cells, and some T-cells. It consists of two forms: B7.1 (CD80) and B7.2 (CD86). Whereas B7.2 is constitutively expressed at low levels, B7.1 is inducible by inflammation. The ligand for B7.1 is CD28, which is expressed on T-cells and is responsible for T-cell activation. Another ligand on T-cells that binds to B7.2 is CTLA-4, which appears later in the course of T-cell activation and could be involved in inhibiting the inflammatory response. B7.1 and, to a lesser extent, B7.2 have been found to be overexpressed on the PBMCs in MS patients. Treatment with IFN-β inhibited B7.1 expression on lymphocytes and, to a lesser extent, B7.2. However, expression of these molecules was increased on monocytes in response to IFN-β treatment (42–44). How these changes in B7 molecules relate to the therapeutic effect of IFN-β in MS patients is not clear at the present time. IFN-β treatment in MS also targets a second group of accessory molecules, the CD40–CD40 ligand pathway. Interaction of CD40 on antigen-presenting cells with the CD40 ligand on T-cells leads to IL-12 secretion by the antigen-presenting cell, which in turn upregulates IL-12 receptors on T-cells. This consequently leads to increased IFN-γ secretion by T-cells (45). CD40 ligand expression was elevated on T-cells from MS patients, and this overexpression was normalized by treatment with IFN-β (46). In addition, several studies found an inhibitory effect of IFN-β on inducible IL-12 secretion by PBMCs. Two independent studies showed that IFN-β inhibits CD40-mediated IL-12 secretion by human antigen-presenting cells independent of the T-cell response (40,47). Therefore, inhibition of the CD40-mediated IL-12 pathway by IFN-β might have a positive therapeutic impact in MS because IL-12 and IFN-γ are deleterious cytokines in this disease. The third group of molecules involved in T-cell activation consists of the adhesion molecules. IFN-β does not seem to affect the level of expression of LFA-1 or ICAM-1 but might have a modest inhibitory effect on IFN-γ–induced VLA-4 on monocytes. However, increased level of soluble VCAM-1 as a result of IFN-β treatment has been reported in vivo and in vitro (48,49). This could block the VCAM–VLA-4 interaction and thus interfere with T-cell activation.

The finding that MS is associated with low mean NK cell activity and that this defect may be corrected by IFN-β has been challenged recently by the findings of Kastrukoff et al. (50) who demonstrated a positive relation between mean NK cell functional activity and the total number of active lesions on MRI in a serial study of relapsing-remitting MS patients. Further, they showed that high-dose IFN-β treatment can result in an inverse relation between mean NK cell functional activity and total number of active lesions on magnetic resonance imaging (MRI) over 2 years. The investigators concluded that patients with higher mean NK cell functional activity may be not only at greater risk for the development of active lesions but also more likely to respond to IFN-β.

IFN-β also may reduce T-cell activation by reducing T-cell IFN-γ receptor binding on lymphocytes (51). Moreover, IFN-β treatment may augment activation-induced T-cell death in MS (52). Consequently, pathogenically activated T-cells may be more susceptible to IFN-β driven cell death than nonactivated T-cells. However, this hypothesis has been challenged by Zipp et al. (53) who found that, although IFN-β moderately enhances the expression of the death receptor CD95 on human myelin basic protein (MBP)–specific T-cells, this treatment does not induce apoptosis.

## Induction of Cytokines Shift

It is now accepted that, in MS and experimental autoimmune encephalomyelitis (EAE), Th cells of the Th1 phenotype, which secrete inflammatory cytokines, play an important role in the pathogenesis of the inflammatory lesion. Conversely, Th2 cells, which secrete anti-inflammatory cytokines, are believed to participate in recovery and tissue repair. Cytokines that have been incriminated in the pathogenesis of MS include IFN-γ, IL-12, and TNF-α, whereas cytokines that have been associated with recovery include IL-4, IL-10, and TGF-β (54). Many studies have examined the effect of IFN-β on Th1

and Th2 cytokine messenger RNAs or protein secretion in PBMC in vitro and in vivo (55–69). The overwhelming finding is that IFN-β inhibits Th1 cytokines including IFN-γ, IL-12, and TNF, whereas IL-10 and TGF-β are enhanced. This suggests that the therapeutic effect of IFN-β could be the result of cytokine shifts in favor of a Th2 response. During the past few years, numerous studies examined the ex vivo cytokine changes associated with IFN-β treatment in MS patients. Those studies examined cytokine protein secretion, messenger RNA expression, and in some cases cytokine receptor changes. The results of some of these studies are summarized in Table 13.1. The in vivo findings seem to parallel the in vitro findings in the sense that Th1 cytokines are inhibited, whereas Th2 cytokines are enhanced by IFN-β treatment in MS patients. Of recent interest is the reciprocal relationship between IL-12 and IL-10 (70) and their role in response to IFN-β in MS patients (69). Recent studies in our laboratory indicated that IFN-β1b inhibits IL-12 production in PBMC and that this inhibition is mediated by IL-10 (69). IL-12 and IL-10 negatively regulate each other (70). A recent study in patients with MS associated a decrease in IL-10 and an increase in IL-12 p40 mRNA with disease activity in MS, whereas an increase in IL-10 correlated with recovery (71). Therefore, IFN-β efficacy in MS may be related to an inhibitory effect on IL-12, and patients who respond by inhibiting IL-12 and enhancing IL-10 production may be more likely to respond clinically to such treatment.

The observation that blocking antibodies to IFN-β, which are associated with a decline in clinical response, block the immunoregulatory effect of the drug, suggests

---

### TABLE 13.1
#### In Vivo Cytokine Modulation by IFN-β Treatment in Multiple Sclerosis

| MODULATION | CYTOKINE/RECEPTOR | REFERENCES |
|---|---|---|
| Inhibition (Th1 cytokines) | IFN-γ, IL-12 | 55–57, 69 |
| | TNF-α | 58–60 |
| Enhanced (Th2 cytokines) | IL-10 | 57,61,62 |
| | TGF-β | 63 |
| | TGF-β-R2 | 63 |
| | IL-1-RA | 64 |
| | TNFR1 and 2 | 64 |
| Unchanged | IL-1β, IL-6 | 67,68 |
| | IL-10 | |
| | TNF-α | |

IFN-γ, interferon-γ; IL, interleukin; R, receptor; TGF, transforming growth factor; Th, T-helper cell; TNF, tumor necrosis factor.

that cytokine shifts is an important therapeutic mechanism in MS (72).

It is worth pointing out that not all ex vivo studies agree on the cytokine changes associated with IFN-β treatment in MS (73–78). The apparent discrepancies in the results could be related to a number of factors including the clinical and genetic heterogeneities of the MS population studied, the methods used to examine cytokine expression, and variables related to the dose and kinetics of the different types of IFN-β administered.

## Effects of IFN-β on MBP-Reactive T-Cells

The therapeutic effect of IFN-β may be due in part to a direct effect on autoreactive T-cells. Studies have demonstrated that IFN-β-1b decreases the proliferation and precursor frequency of MBP-reactive T-cells in vitro. MBP-reactive T-cells exposed to IFN-β also manifest a reduction in TNF-α and IFN-γ secretion and an enhancement of IL-10 and IL-4 secretion, consistent with Th1 to Th2 shift induced by this drug (56,69–71,74,75). There is also some evidence, although controversial (53,77), that IFN-β enhances apoptosis of MBP-reactive T-cells (57) (Table 13.2).

## Effect of IFN-β on CD8⁺ T-Cells

IFN-β promoted the proliferation CD8⁺ T-cells, which could have therapeutic consequences for MS (78). First, a reduction in T-cell suppressor activity was associated with MS, and IFN-β treatment seemed to correct this defect (79). By enhancing the proliferation of CD8⁺ T-cells and, therefore, the secretion of Th2 cytokines such as TGF-β, IFN-β may correct the suppressor T-cell defect and enhance immune suppression. By augmenting the proliferation of CD8⁺ T-cells, IFN-β also may enhance viral surveillance by cytotoxic T-cells, if MS were to be caused by a viral infection. The latter also could be enhanced by the upregulation of class I molecule expression induced by IFN-β on a variety of target cells (80).

## Effect of IFN-β at the BBB

IFN-β has a dramatic effect in reducing gadolinium-enhanced MRI lesions (81). Because gadolinium enhancement is a reflection of BBB leakiness, a therapeutic effect of IFN-β at the level of the BBB is possible. This effect may involve interference with T-cell adhesion and diapedesis across the BBB. Our studies indicated that IFN-β treatment of human umbilical vein endothelial cells (UVECs) does not inhibit the expression of the adhesion molecules ICAM-1, VCAM, or E-selectin, (82) nor does it affect the functional adhesion of phytohemagylutinin (PHA)-activated lymphoblasts to UVECs (83). On the contrary, IFN-β seems to enhance adhesion molecule expression induced by IFN-γ, TNF-α, or IL-1 on UVECs. It was also reported that soluble VCAM serum levels increase significantly in IFN-β–treated patients, and the levels correlated with the reduction in MRI disease activity (48). These observations suggest that IFN-β interferes with T-cell/BBB adhesion by enhancing the expression and release of soluble adhesion molecules, which in turn can bind T-cells and block their ability to adhere to the BBB (48–84). In addition, we and others (85) observed that IFN-β inhibits IFN-γ–induced VLA-4 (the ligand for VCAM) on monocytes, which could reduce T-cell/BBB adhesion. The effect of IFN-β on VLA-4 may be significant in view of the observations that expression of this adhesion molecule on T-cells correlates with encephalitogenecity (86), and its expression is increased on cerebrospinal fluid lymphocytes in MS (87). IFN-β also may interfere with T-cell/endothelial cell adhesion by inhibiting class II expression on endothelial cells, which can function as ligands for T-cells (88,89). Recent studies also indicated that IFN-β inhibits the matrix metalloproteinases involved in the digestion of the matrix membrane of the BBB and therefore could interfere with T-cell migration to the CNS (90–97). Collectively, these findings are consistent with the proposition that IFN-β inhibits the opening of the BBB in MS.

---

**TABLE 13.2**
*Effects on Myelin Basic Protein–reactive T-Cells*

Decreased proliferation and precursor frequency (69–71).
Enhanced IL-10 ± IL-4 secretion (69–71).
Decreased TNF-α and IFN-γ secretion (56,69,71).
Possible enhanced apoptosis (57).

---

IFN-γ, interferon-γ; IL, interleukin; TNF-α, tumor necrosis factor-α.

---

**TABLE 13.3**
*Possible Interferon-β Effects at the Blood–Brain Barrier*

---

- Increased soluble VCAM, blocks VCAM-1/VLA-4 binding
- Decreased VLA-4 on monocytes, decreased homing to the CNS
- Modest increase in ICAM-1 and E-selectin on endothelial cells of uncertain significance.
- Migration: inhibition of metalloproteinase-9.

---

CNS, central nervous system; ICAM, intercellular cell adheshion molecule; VCAM. vascular cell adhesion molecule; VLA, very late activated antigen.

## Potential IFN-β Effects
## in the CNS

The effects of IFN-β in the CNS are poorly understood. Changes in cerebrospinal fluid immune markers such as a reduction in white blood cell count and IFN-γ expression have been observed in IFN-β–treated MS patients (98). These observations suggest, but do not necessarily implicate, a central effect. Theoretically, IFN-β could inhibit T-cell activation in the CNS through an inhibitory effect on class II and costimulatory molecule expression on resident antigen-presenting cells and possibly on other molecules involved in antigen processing and presentation. The effect of IFN-β on IFN-γ–induced class II expression appears to depend on the cell type and the species. For example, IFN-β inhibits IFN-γ–induced class II (DR) on cultured human astrocytes and astrocytoma cell lines (99,29) and on mouse astrocytes (S Dhib-Jalbut, unpublished data). However, IFN-β effect on human fetal astrocytes class II (DR) expression has not been consistent (100), although it seems to inhibit the antigen-presenting capacity of this cell type (101). The relevance of IFN-β effects on astrocytes has been questioned based on the observations that astrocytes are not the predominant class II–expressing cell in the MS lesion and by the lack of their expression of the costimulatory molecule B7 (102). The effect of IFN-β on class II in microglia is also unclear. Although it has been reported to inhibit IFN-γ–induced class II in neonatal rodent microglia, (102) IFN-β has no effect on IFN-γ–upregulated class II (DR) expression on cultured adult human microglia (100). However, in a functional assay we found that IFN-β inhibits presentation of alloantigens, thus raising the possibility that IFN-β affects other HLA molecules or that it interferes with antigen processing or with molecules involved in the transport and loading of peptide antigens. Other potential therapeutic targets for IFN-β in the CNS could involve its ability to inhibit molecules involved in myelin damage including nitric oxide (103,104), proteases (105), and free radicals (106), produced in macrophages and microglia.

IFN-β has also increased astrocytic production of nerve growth factor, which has been reported to promote oligodendrocyte proliferation and processes extension (107). Therefore, IFN-β could have a role in repair and remyelination. However, this in vitro effect is IFN-β dose dependent, so its in vivo significance is unclear at the present time because it is unknown whether IFN-β achieves biologically active levels in the CNS.

### Acknowledgment

Supported by grants from the National Institutes of Neurological Disorders and Stroke (K-24 NS02082) and the Department of Veteran's Affairs.

## References

1. Isaacs A, Lindenman J. Virus interference. I. *Proc R Soc Lond (Biol)*. 1957; 147:258–267.
2. Siegal FP, Kadowaki N, Shodell M, et al. The nature of the principal type 1 interferon-producing cells in human blood. *Science* 1999; 284:1835–1837.
3. Fleischmann WR, Ramamurthy V, Stanton GJ, Baron S, Dianzani F. Interferon: Mode of action and clinical applications. In: Smith R (ed.), *Interferon Treatment of Neurologic Disorders*. New York: Marcel Decker, 1988; 1–42
4. De Maeyer E, De Maeyer-Guignard J. The interferon gene family. In: De Maeyer E, De Maeyer-Guignard J (eds.), *Interferons and Other Regulatory Cytokines*. New York: John Wiley & Sons, 1988; 5–38.
5. Lin L. Betaseron. *Dev Biol Stand*. 1998; 96:97–104.
6. Revel M, Kalinka P. *Glycosylated Interferon-Beta in Multiple Sclerosis: Clinical Research and Therapy*. London: Martin Dunitz Ltd; 1997; 243–254.
7. Billiau A. Interferon beta in the cytokine network: An anti-inflammatory pathway. *Mult Scler* 1995; 1:S2–S4.
8. Novick D, Cohen B, Rubinstein M. The human interferon alpha/beta receptor: characterization and molecular cloning. *Cell* 1994; 77:391–400.
9. Uze G, Lutfalla G, Gresser I. Genetic transfer of a functional human IFN alpha receptor into mouse cells; cloning and expression of its cDNA. *Cell* 1990; 60:225–234.
10. Runkel L, deDios C, Karpusas M, et al. Systematic mutational mapping of sites on human interferon-beta-1a that are important for receptor binding and functional activity. *Biochemistry* 2000; 39:2538–2551.
11. Pattyn E, Van Ostade X, Schauvliege L, et al. Dimerization of the interferon type I receptor IFN-αR2-2 is sufficient for induction of interferon effector genes but not for full antiviral activity. *J Biol Chem* 1999; 274:34838–34845.
12. Senda T, Shmazu T, Matsuda S, et al. Three dimensional crystal structure of recombinant murine interferon-β. *EMBO J* 1992; 11:3193–3201.
13. Piehler J, Schreiber G. Mutational and structural analysis of the binding interface between type I interferons and their receptor IFN-αr2. *J Mol Biol* 1999; 294:223–237.
14. Pfeffer LM, Donner DB. The down-regulation of Interferon-α receptors in human lymphoblastoid cells: Relation to cellular responsiveness to the anti-proliferative action of a-interferon. *Cancer Res* 1990; 50:2654–2657.
15. Muller M, Brisco J, Laxton C, et al. The protein tyrosine kinase JAK1 complements defects in interferon alpha/beta and gamma signal transduction. *Nature* 1993; 366:129–135.
16. Darnell J, Kerr IM, Stark GR. Jak-STAT pathways and transductional activation in response to IFNs and other extracellular signaling proteins. *Science* 1994; 264:1415–1421.
17. Shuai K, Ziemiecki A, Wilks AF, et al. Polypeptide signaling to the nucleus through tyrosine phosphorylation of Jak and Stat protein. *Nature* 1993; 366:580–583.
18. Grumbach IM, Fish EN, Uddin S, et al. Activation of the Jak-Stat pathway in cells that exhibit selective sensitivity to the antiviral effects of IFN-beta compared with IFN-alpha. *J Interferon Cytokine Res* 1999; 19(7):797–801.
19. Arnason BG, Reder AT. Interferons and multiple sclerosis. *Clin Neuropharmacol* 1994; 17:495–547.
20. Borden EC, Hawkins MJ, Sielaff KM, et al. Clinical and biological effects of recombinant interferon beta administered intravenously daily in phase I trial. *J Interferon Cytokine Res* 1988; 8:357–366.
21. Baron S, Tyring SK, Fleischmann WR Jr, et al. The interferons, mechanisms of action and clinical applications. *JAMA* 1991; 266:1375–1383.
22. Borden EC. Interferons: Pleotropic cellular modulators. *Clin Immunol Immunopathol* 1992; 62:518–524.
23. Shearer M, Taylor-Papadimitriou J. Regulation of cell growth by interferon. *Cancer Metastasis Rev* 1987; 6:199–221.
24. Noronha A, Toscas A, Jensen MA. Interferon beta augments sup-

pressor cell function in multiple sclerosis. *Ann Neurol* 1990; 27:207–210.

25. Spear GT, Paulnock DM, Jordan RL, et al. Enhancement of monocyte class I and II histocompatibility antigen expression in man by in vivo beta interferon. *Clin Exp Immunol* 1987; 69:107–115.

26. Jiang H, Milo R, Swoveland P, et al. Interferon beta-1b reduces interferon gamma–induced antigen-presenting capacity of human glial and B cells. *J Neuroimmunol* 1995; 61:17–25.

27. Ling PD, Warren MK, Vogel SN. Antagonistic effect of interferon-beta on the interferon-gamma–induced expression of 1a antigen in murine macrophages. *J Immunol* 1985; 135:1857–1863.

28. Joseph J, Knobler RL, D'Imperio C, Lubin FD. Down-regulation of interferon-gamma–induced class II expression on human glioma cells by recombinant interferon-beta-effects of dosage treatment schedule. *J Neuroimmunol* 1988; 20:39–44.

29. Ransohoff RM, Devajyothi C, Esters ML, et al. Interferon-beta specifically inhibits interferon-gamma induced class II major histocompatibility complex gene transcription in a human astrocytoma cell line. *J Neuroimmunol* 1991; 33:103–112.

30. Panitch HS, Folus JS, Johnson KP. Beta interferon prevents HLA class II antigen induction by gamma interferon in MS [abstract]. *Neurology* 1989; 39:172.

31. Noronha A, Toscas A, Jensen MA. IFN-beta down-regulates IFN-gamma production by activated T cells in MS [abstract]. *Neurology* 1991; 41:219.

32. Noronha A, Toscas A, Jensen MA. Contrasting effects of alpha, beta, and gamma interferons on nonspecific suppressor cell functions in multiple sclerosis. *Ann Neurol* 1992; 31:103–116.

33. Noronha A, Toscas A, Jensen MA. Interferon beta decreases T-cell activation and interferon gamma production in multiple sclerosis. *J Neuroimmunol* 1993; 46:145–154.

34. Panitch HS, Folus JS, Johnson KP. Recombinant beta interferon inhibits gamma interferon production in multiple sclerosis [abstract]. *Ann Neurol* 1987; 22:139.

35. Dayal AS, Jensen MA, Lledo A, Arnason BGW. Interferon-gamma–secreting cells in multiple sclerosis patients treated with interferon beta-1b. *Neurology* 1995; 45:2173–2177.

36. Rudick RA, Ransohoff RM, Peppler R, et al. Interferon beta induces interleukin-10 expression: Relevance to multiple sclerosis. *Ann Neurol* 1996; 40:618–627.

37. D'Cunha J, Knight JE, Haas AL, Truitt RL, Borden EC. Immunoregulatory properties of ISG15, an interferon-induced cytokine. *Proc Natl Acad Sci USA* 1996; 93:211–215.

38. Kozlowski M, Schorey J, Portis T, Grigoriev V, Kornbluth J. NK lytic-associated molecule: A novel gene selectively expressed in cells with cytolytic function. *J Immunol* 1999; 163:1775–1785.

39. Der SD, Zhou A, Williams BR, Silverman RH. Identification of genes differentially regulated by interferon alpha, beta, or gamma using oligonucleotide arrays. *Proc Natl Acad Sci USA* 1998; 95:15623–15628.

40. Bartholome EJ, Willems F, Crusiaux A, et al. IFN-beta interferes with the differentiation of dendritic cells from peripheral blood mononuclear cells: Selective inhibition of CD40-dependent interleukin-12 secretion. *J Interferon Cytokine Res* 1999; 19:471–478.

41. McRae BL, Nagai T, Semnani RT, vanSeventer JM, van Seventer GA. Interferon-α and -β inhibit the in vitro differentiation of immunocompetent human dendritic cells from CD14+ precursors. *Blood* 2000; 96(1):210–217.

42. Genc K, Dona KL, Reder AT. Increased CD80-β cells in active multiple sclerosis and reversal by interferon beta-1b therapy. *J Clin Invest* 1997; 99:2664–2671.

43. Williams K, Ulvestad E, Antel JP. B7/BB-1 antigen expression on adult human microglia studied in vitro and in situ. *Eur J Immunol* 1994; 24:3031–3037.

44. Dangond F, Windhagen A, Groves CJ, Hafler DA. Constitutive expression of costimulatory molecules by human microglia and its relevance to CNS autoimmunity. *J Neuroimmunol* 1997; 76:132–138.

45. Balashov KE, Smith DR, Khoury SJ, et al. Increased interleukin 12 production in progressive multiple sclerosis: induction by activated CD4+ T-cells via CD40 ligand. *Proc Natl Acad Sci USA* 1997; 94:599–603.

46. Teleshova N, Bao W, Kivisakk P, et al. Elevated CD40 ligand expressing blood T-cell levels in multiple sclerosis are reversed by interferon-beta treatment. *Scand J Immunol* 2000; 51: 312–320.

47. McRae BL, Beilfuss BA, van Seventer GA. IFN-beta differentially regulates CD40-induced cytokine secretion by human dendritic cells. *J Immunol* 2000; 164:23–28.

48. Calabresi PA, Tranquill LR, Dambrosia JM, et al. Increases in soluble VCAM-1 correlate with a decrease in MRI lesions in multiple sclerosis treated with interferon beta-1b. *Ann Neurol* 1997; 41:669–674.

49. Kallman BA, Hummel V, Lindenlaub T, et al. Cytokine-induced modulation of cellular adhesion to human cerebral endothelial cells is mediated by soluble vascular cell adhesion molecule-1. *Brain* 2000; 123(4):687–697.

50. Kastrukoff LF, Morgan NG, Zecchini D, et al. Natural killer cells in relapsing-remitting MS: Effect of treatment with interferon beta-1B. *Neurology* 1999; 52:351–359.

51. Bongioanni P, Mosti S, Moscato G, et al. Decreases in T-cell tumor necrosis factor alpha binding with interferon beta treatment in patients with multiple sclerosis. *Arch Neurol* 1999; 56:71–78.

52. Kaser A, Deisenhammer F, Berger T, Tilg H. Interferon-beta 1b augments activation-induced T-cell death in multiple sclerosis patients. *Lancet* 1999; 353:1413–1414.

53. Zipp F, Beyer M, Gelderblom H, et al. No induction of apoptosis by IFN-beta in human antigen-specific T-cells. *Neurology* 2000; 54(2):485–487.

54. Martin R, McFarland HF. Immunological aspects of experimental allergic encephalomyelitis and multiple sclerosis. *Crit Rev Clin Lab Sci* 1995; 32:121–182.

55. Becher B, Giacomini PS, Pelletier D, et al. Interferon-gamma secretion by peripheral blood T-cell subsets in multiple sclerosis: Correlation with disease phase and interferon-beta therapy. *Ann Neurol* 1999; 45:247–250.

56. Bakhiet M, Ozenci V, Withagen C, et al. A new cell enzyme-linked immunosorbent assay demonstrates gamma interferon suppression by beta interferon in multiple sclerosis. *Clin Diagn Lab Immunol* 1999; 6:415–419.

57. Rep MH, Schrijver HM, van Lopik T, et al. Interferon (IFN)-beta treatment enhances CD95 and interleukin 10 expression but reduces interferon-gamma producing T-cells in MS patients. *J Neuroimmunol* 1999; 96:92–100.

58. Gayo A, Mozo L, Suarez A, et al. Interferon beta-1b treatment modulates TNFalpha and IFN-gamma spontaneous gene expression in MS. *Neurology* 1999; 52:1764–1770.

59. Bongioanni P, Lombardo F, Moscato G, Mosti S, Meucci G. T-cell interferon gamma receptor binding in interferon beta-1b-treated patients with multiple sclerosis. *Arch Neurol* 1999; 56:217–222.

60. Ossege LM, Sindern E, Voss B, Malin JP. Immunomodulatory effects of IFN-beta-1b on the mRNA-expression of TGFbeta-1 and TNFalpha in vitro. *Imunopharmacology* 1999; 43:39–46.

61. Ozenci V, Kouwenhoven M, Huang YM, et al. Multiple sclerosis: Levels of interleukin-10-secreting blood mononuclear cells are low in untreated patients but augmented during interferon-beta-1b treatment. *Scand J Immunol* 1999; 49:554–561.

62. Ozenci V, Kouwenhoven M, Huang Y, Kivisakk P, Link H. Multiple sclerosis is associated with an imbalance between tumour necrosis factor-alpha (TNF-alpha)- and IL-10–secreting blood cells that is corrected by interferon-beta (IFN-beta) treatment. *Clin Exp Immunol* 2000; 120:147–153.

63. Ossege LM, Sindern E, Patzold T, Malin JP. Immunomodulatory effects of interferon-beta-1b in vivo: Induction of the expression of transforming growth factor-beta1 and its receptor type II. *J Neuroimmunol* 1998; 91:73–81.

64. Perini P, Tiberio M, Sivieri S, et al. Interleukin-1 receptor antagonist, soluble tumor necrosis factor-alpha receptor type I and II, and soluble E-selectin serum levels in multiple sclerosis patients receiving weekly intramuscular injections of interferon-beta1a. *Eur Cytokine Netw* 2000; 11:81–86.

65. Duddy ME, Armstrong MA, Crockard AD, Hawkins SA. Changes in plasma cytokines induced by interferon-beta1a treatment in patients with multiple sclerosis. *J Neuroimmunol* 1999; 101:98–109.

66. Van Boxel-Dezaire AHH, van Trigt-Hoff CJ, Killestein J, et al. Contrasting responses to interferon b-1b treatment in relapsing-remitting multiple sclerosis: Does baseline interleukin-12p35 messenger RNA predict the efficacy of treatment? *Ann Neurol* 2000; 48:313–322.

67. Kozovska ME, Hong J, Zang YC, et al. Interferon beta induces T-helper 2 immune deviation in MS. *Neurology* 1999; 53:1692–1697.

68. Weber F, Janovskaja J, Polak T, Poser S, Rieckmann P. Effect of interferon beta on human myelin basic protein-specific T-cell lines: Comparison of IFN-beta-1a and IFN-beta-1b. *Neurology* 1999; 52:1069–1071.

69. Wang X, Chen M, Wandinger KP, Williams G, Dhib-Jalbut S. Interferon-beta inhibits IL-12 production in peripheral blood mononuclear cells in an IL-10 dependent mechanism: Relevance to interferon-1b therapeutic effects in multiple sclerosis. *J Immunology* 2000; 165:548–557.

70. Aste-Amezaga M, Ma X, Sartori A, Trinchieri G. Molecular mechanisms of the induction of IL-12 and its inhibition by IL-10. *J Immunol* 1998; 160:5936.

71. van Boxel-Dezaire AH, Hoff SC, van Oosten BW, et al. Decreased interleukin-10 and increased interleukin-12p40 mRNA are associated with disease activity and characterize different disease stages in multiple sclerosis. *Ann Neurol* 1999; 45:695.

72. Zang YCQ, Yang D, Hong J, et al. Immunoregulation and blocking antibodies induced by interferon beta treatment in MS. *Neurology* 2000; 55:397–404.

73. Ristori G, Montesperelli C, Gasperini C, et al. T-cell response to myelin basic protein before and after treatment with interferon beta in multiple sclerosis. *J Neuroimmunol* 1999; 99:91–96.

74. Matusevicius D, Kivisakk P, Navikas V, et al. Influence of IFN-beta1b (betaferon) on cytokine mRNA profiles in blood mononuclear cells and plasma levels of soluble VCAM-1 in multiple sclerosis. *Eur J Neurol* 1998; 5:265–275.

75. Khademi M, Wallstrom E, Andersson M, et al. Reduction of both pro- and anti-inflammatory cytokines after 6 months of interferon beta-1a treatment of multiple sclerosis. *J Neuroimmunol* 2000; 103:202–210.

76. Jansen M, Reinhard JF Jr. Interferon response heterogeneity: Activation of a pro-inflammatory response by interferon alpha and beta. A possible basis for diverse responses to interferon beta in MS. *J Leukoc Biol* 1999; 65:439–443.

77. Marrack P, Kappler J, Mitchell T. Type I interferons keep activated T-cells alive. *J Exp Med* 1999; 189(3):521–530.

78. Arnason BGW, Dayal A, Qu Z-X, et al. Mechanisms of action of beta interferon in multiple sclerosis. *Semin Immunopathol* 1996; 18:125–148.

79. Antel JP, Arnason BGW, Medof ME. Suppressor cell function in multiple sclerosis: Correlation with clinical disease activity. *Ann Neurol* 1979; 5:338–342.

80. Dhib-Jalbut S, Cowan EP. Direct Evidence that interferon-b mediates enhanced HLA-class I expression in measles virus-infected cells. *J of Immunol* 1993; 151:6248–6258.

81. Stone LA, Frank JA, Albert PS, et al. The effect of interferon-beta on blood-brain barrier disruption demonstrated by contrast-enhanced magnetic resonance imaging in relapsing-remitting multiple sclerosis. *Ann Neurol* 1995; 37:611–619.

82. Jiang H, Williams GJ, Dhib-Jalbut S. The effect of interferon beta-1b on cytokine-induced adhesion molecule expression. *Neurochem Int* 1997; 30:449–453.

83. Dhib-Jalbut S, Jiang H, Williams GJ. The effect of interferon beta-1b on lymphocyte-endothelial cell adhesion. *J Neuroimmunol* 1996; 71:215–222.

84. Kallmann BA, Hummel V, Lindenlaub T, et al. Cytokine-induced modulation of cellular adhesion to human cerebral endothelial cells is mediated by soluble vascular cell adhesion molecule-1. *Brain* 2000; 123:687–697.

85. Soilu-Hanninen M, Salmi A, Salonen R. Interferon-beta downregulates expresion of VLA-4 antigen and antagonizes interferon-gamma induced expression of HLA-DQ in human peripheral blood monocytes. *J Neuroimmunol* 1995; 60:99–106.

86. Baron JL, Mardi JA, Ruddle NH, et al. Surface expression of alpha 4 integrin by CD4 T-cells is required for their entry into brain parenchyma. *J Exp Med* 1993; 177:57–68.

87. Svenningsson A, Hansson G, Andersen O, et al. Adhesion molecule expression on cerebrospinal fluid T-lymphocytes in multiple sclerosis, aseptic meningitis, and normal controls. *Ann Neurol* 1993; 34:155–161.

88. Huynh HK, Oger J, Dorovini-Zis K. Interferon-β downregulates IFN-γ–induced class II MHC molecule expression and morphological changes in primary cultures of human brain microvessel endothelial cells. *J Neuroimmunol* 1995; 60:63–73.

89. Gelati M, Corsini E, Dufour A, et al. Immunological effects of in vivo interferon-beta1b treatment in ten patients with multiple sclerosis: A 1-year follow-up. *J Neurol* 1999; 246:569–573.

90. Stuve O, Dooley NP, Uhm JH, et al. Interferon beta-1b decreases the migration of T lymphocytes in vitro: effects on matrix metalloproteinase-9. *Ann Neurol* 1996; 40:853–863.

91. Leppart D, Waubant E, Burk MR, Oksenberg JR, Hauser SL. Interferon beta-1b inhibits gelatinase secretion and in vitro migration of human T-cells: A possible mechanism for treatment efficacy in multiple sclerosis. *Ann Neurol* 1996; 40:846–852.

92. Uhm JH, Dooley NP, Stuve O, et al. Migratory behavior of lymphocytes isolated from multiple sclerosis patients: Effects of interferon beta-1b therapy. *Ann Neurol* 1999; 46:319–324.

93. Corsini E, Gelati M, Dufour A, et al. Reduction of transendothelial migration of mononuclear cells in interferon-beta1b-treated multiple sclerosis patients. *Ann Neurol* 1999; 46:435.

94. Zou LP, Ma DH, Wei L, et al. IFN-beta suppresses experimental autoimmune neuritis in lewis rats by inhibiting the migration of inflammatory cells into peripheral nervous tissue. *J Neurosci Res* 1999; 56:123–130.

95. Trojano M, Avolio C, Liuzzi GM, et al. Changes of serum sICAM-1 and MP-9 induced by rIFN-beta-1b treatment in relapsing-remitting MS. *Neurology* 1999; 53:1402–1408.

96. Bever CT Jr, Rosenberg GA. Matrix metalloproteinases in multiple sclerosis: Targets of therapy or markers of injury? *Neurology* 1999; 53:1380–1381.

97. Lou J, Gasche Y, Zheng L, et al. Interferon-beta inhibits activated leukocyte migration through human brain microvascular endothelial cell monolayer. *Lab Invest* 1999; 79:1015–1025.

98. Rudick RA, Cookfair DL, Simonian NA, et al. Cerebrospinal fluid abnormalities in a phase III trial of Avonex (IFN-β-1a) for relapsing multiple sclerosis. The Multiple Sclerosis Collaborative Research Group. *J Neuroimmunol* 1999; 93:8–14.

99. Joseph J, Knobler RL, D'Imperio C, Lubin FD. Down-regulation of interferon-gamma-induced class II expression on human glioma cells by recombinant interferon-beta effects of dosage treatment schedule. *J Neuroimmunol* 1988, 20:39-44.

100. McLaurin J, Antel JP, Yong VW. Immune and non-immune actions of interferon-beta-1b on primary human neural cells. *Mult Scler* 1995; 1:10–19.

101. Jiang H, Milo R, Swoveland P, et al. Interferon beta-1b reduces interferon gamma-induced antigen-presenting capacity of human glial and B cells. *J Neuroimmunol* 1995; 61:17–25.

102. Hall GL, Compston A, Scolding NJ. Beta-interferon and multiple sclerosis. *Trends Neurosci* 1997; 20:63–67.

103. Deguchi M, Sakuta H, Uno K, Inaba K, Muramatsu S. Exogenous and endogenous type I interferons inhibit interferon-gamma–induced nitric oxide production and nitric oxide synthase expression in murine peritoneal macrophages. *J Interferon Cytokine Res* 1995; 15(11):977–984.

104. Guthikonda P, Baker J, Mattson DH. Interferon-beta-1-b (IFN-β) decreases induced nitric oxide (NO) production by a human astrocytoma cell line. *J Neuroimmunol* 1998; 82(2):133–139.

105. Garotta G, Talmadge KW, Pink JR, Dewald B, Baggiolini M. Functional antagonism between type I and type II interferons on human macrophages. *Biochem Biophys Res Commun* 1986; 140(3):948–954.

106. Ciera M, Bever CT. Gamma inteferon (gamma-IFN) induced increases in macrophage cathepsin B activity are blocked by alpha and beta IFN (type-I-IFN) [abstract]. *FASEB J*, 4:A339.

107. Boutros T, Croze E, Yong VW. Interferon-beta is a potent promoter of nerve growth factor production by astrocytes. *J Neurochem* 1997; 69(3):939–946.

# IV

# PATHOLOGY

# 14 The Pathology of Multiple Sclerosis and Its Variants

*Robert M. Herndon, M.D.*

D iseases of myelin comprise a variety of illnesses with varied etiology. They range from clearly infectious diseases such as progressive multifocal leucoencephalopathy to hereditary metabolic disorders such as adrenoleucodystrophy and metachromatic leucodystrophy to a group of disorders of unknown etiology (Table 14.1). Whether multiple sclerosis (MS) and its variants comprise a single disease with a highly varied course or a group of syndromes of diverse etiology remains controversial, although recent evidence suggests that it actually involves at least four different pathologic variants (1). Numerous clinical demyelinating disorders may be part of the MS spectrum or may represent different diseases with similar clinical and pathologic features. For years, many clinicians have felt that primary progressive MS and Devic syndrome (neuromyelitis optica) were distinct from relapsing remitting and secondary progressive MS. Balo concentric sclerosis was felt to be a different disease, but recent evidence has suggested that it is a variant of relapsing remitting MS. Whether the Marburg variant and acute disseminated encephalomyelitis (ADEM) are part of the MS spectrum or represent different disease entities remains a matter of debate. Recent immunopathologic studies are beginning to clarify these issues, but, ultimately, clarification of the relationship of the variants to each other

will have to await determination of the etiology of these conditions.

Recent developments in immunopathology have suggested that MS is several different diseases with a common clinical presentation (1). These immunopathologically different disorders are likely to have different etiologies. Guillian-Barre syndrome has been shown to have several variants caused by different agents including *Campylobacter jejuni*, cytomegalovirus, Epstein-Barr virus, *Mycoplasma pneumonia*, swine flu vaccine, and probably several others (2–4). Typical relapsing remitting MS now appears to have several variants, and these are likely to have different etiologies. The inflammatory demyelination in different cases has immunologic features that are sufficiently different from each other to suggest that this is really a group of diseases (1).

These demyelinating disorders appear to have central myelin and the cells that form central myelin, the oligodendrocytes, as the target of attack. MS usually does not affect peripheral myelin, although there are cases of a disease clinically and pathologically indistinguishable from MS in which there is also peripheral demyelination in a pattern indistinguishable from chronic inflammatory demyelinating polyneuropathy (5–7). Because there is good evidence that molecular mimicry is involved in Guillian-Barre syndrome (3), molecular mimicry of a shared epitope could cause this rare combination of cen-

**TABLE 14.1**
*Demyelinating Diseases*

Demyelination due to infectious agents (see Chapter 9)
    Progressive multifocal leucoencephalopathy
    Subacute sclerosing panencephalitis
Metabolic disorders of myelin
    Metachromatic leucodystrophy
    Globoid cell leucodystrophy
    Pelizaeus-Merzbacher disease
Peroxisomal disorders affecting myelin
    Generalized peroxisomal disorders
        Cerebrohepatorenal (Zellweger) syndrome
        Infantile Refsum disease (phytanic acid storage)
        Neonatal adrenoleucodystrophy
        Hyperpipecolic acidemia
    Single peroxisomal enzyme deficiencies with widespread pathology
        Thiolase deficiency
        Acyl-CoA oxidase deficiency
        Rhizomelic chondrodysplasia
    Single peroxisomal enzyme deficiencies with more restricted pathology
        Adrenoleukodystrophy complex
Diseases of unknown etiology
Multiple sclerosis
    Relapsing remitting/secondary progressive multiple sclerosis
    Marburg variant
    Neuromyelitis optica (Devic disease)
    Primary progressive multiple sclerosis
Acute disseminated encephalomyelitis
Fibrinoid leucodystrophy (Alexander disease)

tral and peripheral demyelination and lends further credence to the idea that it is an autoimmune disease. The increased risk of MS in first-order relatives of MS patients, the higher concordance rate in identical versus fraternal twins, and the overrepresentation of certain HLA types (8) point to significant genetic risk factors, although it is clear that no single gene is responsible for genetic susceptibility.

## ETIOLOGY

The etiology of MS remains unknown. The most widely accepted hypothesis is that it is an autoimmune disease induced by a virus or other infectious agent. The possibility of it being a primary infectious process with or without an associated autoimmune reaction has not been entirely ruled out despite repeated failure to identify a causative agent. Over the past four decades, there have been a number of reports of viruslike particles in brain tissue from MS patients (9). At least 14 different viruses have

been isolated from the brains of MS patients, yet none has been shown to be etiologically related (10). Cook listed 22 agents suspected of being related to MS for which substantial evidence of a causative role has not thus far appeared (11). The demonstration of viral nucleic acid by polymerase chain reaction in MS brain and cerebrospinal fluid (CSF) (12,13) has created some interest, but it has never been possible to clearly demonstrate a connection between any of these agents and the disease process. No agent has been found in 100 percent of active plaques. The demonstration of herpes viruses, in particular herpes I, II, and VI, in a significant proportion of MS plaques over the past decade (12,13), evidence that the anti-herpes drug acyclovir will reduce the number of attacks of MS (14), and, more recently, evidence for chlamydial infection (15) have renewed interest in infectious hypotheses. Because herpes viruses are activated by other infections and viral infections are known to precipitate some MS attacks, reactivation of herpes viruses may be related to some attacks or may be significant aggravating factor even if not causative. Only time will tell if any of these agents plays a role in disease causation. The report of a patient with MS developing acute optic neuritis two months after an allogenic bone marrow transplant for chronic myelogenous leukemia suggests that it is not purely an autoimmune disease (16). The possible role of infectious agents in MS is discussed in more detail in Chapters 7 and 8. Part of the problem in determining the role of infectious agents in MS may be multiple causation, as occurs in Guillian-Barre syndrome, in which several different agents can induce acute autoimmune neuropathies that are difficult to differentiate clinically (2).

Extensive effort has gone into the attempt to understand the role of the immune system in MS. Much of this effort has been directed toward understanding the immunology of experimental autoimmune encephalomyelitis (EAE), which is the most extensively studied animal model of the disease (see Chapter 6). This work has taught us an enormous amount regarding immunology in general and immunology as it applies to the human nervous system. Unfortunately, attempts to apply to MS what has been learned about EAE have rarely been successful. Numerous treatments that work well in EAE have failed completely when tried in MS, making it clear that MS is not simply EAE. However, there is good evidence that autoimmunity is involved in the disease, and immunomodulating agents such as the β interferons and glatiramer acetate and immunosuppressant drugs such as cyclophosphamide, methotrexate, and mitoxantrone can slow the disease process. With the development of a more detailed understanding of immunology and the ability to directly assess various immunologic components in situ, it is possible to begin to define the immune reaction in the acute plaque of MS and to begin to understand the nature of the immune reaction in MS, as discussed below.

## CLINICAL SPECTRUM OF HUMAN INFLAMMATORY DEMYELINATING DISEASES

The entities described here have at different times been considered distinct diseases and, largely because of overlap syndromes, been considered part of the MS spectrum. Recent advances in pathology are clarifying the relationships, but definitive answers to the relationship of these diseases remain to be established.

### Relapsing Remitting Multiple Sclerosis

This is the classic MS clinical pattern marked by exacerbations, with a variable amount of improvement between attacks

### Secondary Progressive Multiple Sclerosis

About 80 percent of relapsing remitting MS cases go on to develop a secondary progressive disease pattern, with a slowly progressive ascending paralysis from a few to 20 or so years after onset. This represents a later stage of relapsing remitting disease rather than a separate variant, although not all relapsing remitting MS goes on to develop secondary progression.

### Primary Progressive Multiple Sclerosis

This disease pattern has a later onset, usually after age 40 years, and begins with an insidious progression of disability affecting primarily the spinal cord without exacerbations or remissions. Unlike exacerbating remitting disease, in which two-thirds of the cases are female, primary progressive MS is only slightly more common in females with a ratio of about 1.3:1 (17). Magnetic resonance imaging (MRI) of the brain is sometimes normal in these cases, and MRI of the spinal cord may show only cord atrophy.

### Devic Syndrome (Neuromyelitis Optica)

Devic syndrome is an acute disorder in which optic neuritis and transverse myelitis occur within a short time of each other, with little or no involvement of other parts of the central nervous system (CNS) (18). It has generally been considered a monophasic disease without relapses after the initial episodes; however, numerous cases that begin with optic neuritis and transverse myelitis proceed to develop a relapsing remitting course similar to typical relapsing remitting MS, but with more severe residua from attacks and a more necrotic pathology. MRI in these cases shows no lesions within the brain itself but generally shows evidence of cord inflammation usually extending over three or more segments. Whether this is a variant of MS or a distinct disease remains controversial. It may

be a distinct disease entity, or the course and intensity differences may relate more to the genetic makeup of the host than to the etiology.

### Marburg Disease (Acute Multiple Sclerosis)

This acute, fulminant demyelinating disorder was first described by Otto Marburg in 1906 (19). It is a severe, unrelentingly progressive demyelinating disease that typically leads to death within a few months to a year.

### Balo Concentric Sclerosis

This has been thought to be an aggressive variant usually leading to death in weeks to months. It is marked by large plaques of demyelination with concentric bands of preserved or regenerated myelin. These bands can sometimes be seen on MRI. There is now good evidence that some cases with Balo-like lesions on MRI improve and have a course typical of relapsing remitting MS. It may be that the Balo type lesion is a feature of some early MS with very active remyelination, features that disappear as the disease progresses so that the concentric lesions are observed only pathologically in individuals who die soon after the onset of the disease.

### Acute Disseminated Encephalomyelitis

This is usually a monophasic demyelinating disorder that typically follows a viral infection. It appears to be closely analogous to EAE. The most severe cases are seen after measles infection, smallpox vaccination, or rabies vaccine. It is marked by the rapid, sometime sudden, onset of confusion, fever, and depressed consciousness, often with seizures and multiple focal neurologic signs such as ataxia, paraplegia, or cranial nerve signs. It can be fatal within days to weeks, although survivors often recover remarkably well over a period of many months.

## PATHOLOGY OF RELAPSING REMITTING MULTIPLE SCLEROSIS

The pathology of typical relapsing remitting MS consists of lesions (plaques) disseminated in location and varying in age, as would be expected from the clinical features. In addition, there is a second demyelinating process consisting of the demyelination of individual fibers or small groups of fibers that is best seen in the spinal cord. Plaques can be found wherever there is central myelin. They are present in white and gray matter, but the gray matter lesions are much less obvious and generally do not appear on MRI, possibly because of the relatively small amount of myelin present and a less intense inflammatory reaction. The lesions occur in different parts of the nervous system and are in different stages of activity or maturity. Lesions range from acute plaques with active inflammatory infiltrates and macrophages loaded with lipid and myelin degeneration products, through various degrees of lesser activity to plaques that are active only at their margin, to chronic, inactive demyelinated shrunken glial scars. Although plaques can appear anywhere there is central myelin, there is a predilection for the periventricular white matter, optic nerves, spinal cord, and juxtacortical areas.

Areas of white matter outside the plaques are not normal. They show biochemical abnormalities that some feel can be explained on the basis of Wallerian degeneration (18) and gliosis, whereas others believe that they represent an important aspect of the pathology, particularly in secondary progressive MS. (20). This appears to occur concurrently with plaque formation and consists of patchy demyelination in one or a few fibers with minimal inflammation. This is best seen in the spinal cord.

Recent reports by Lucchinetti et al. (1) and Lassman et al. (21) have dramatically altered our view of the pathology of MS. They described four different patterns of demyelination in active MS lesions based on a variety of modern staining and labeling techniques, suggesting that MS is a group of diseases with similar clinical and pathologic features rather than a single entity. Three of these patterns are seen in exacerbating remitting MS, and the fourth has been seen only in primary progressive MS. These recent observations already have had a major impact on our thinking regarding etiology and pathogenesis. It seems likely that the different patterns relate, at least in part, to different etiologies and may provide the basis for associating particular agents with particular disease patterns. They also explain some of the discrepancies found in the description of various investigators. The first two patterns appear to be autoimmune reactions against myelin, whereas the third and fourth patterns more closely resemble a disease primarily of oligodendrocytes. Pattern four appears to be associated exclusively with primary progressive MS, although it is likely that some cases that appear clinically to be primary progressive will have one of the other pathologies, because many cases of relapsing remitting MS are essentially silent clinically, and some apparently primary progressive cases are likely actually secondary progressive (22). The pathology of the fourth group is discussed below. The patterns can be summarized as follows.

## Pattern 1: Active Demyelination Associated with T-Lymphocyte and Macrophage-Dominated Inflammation without Significant Amounts of Antibody or Complement Deposition

Plaques were perivenular in location, and loss of all types of myelin protein appeared to occur simultaneously. There

was some diffuse immunoglobulin G (IgG) staining throughout the lesion. Staining for complement components was negative. This pattern comprised about 12 percent of the reported cases.

## Pattern 2: Active Perivenular Demyelination Associated with T-Lymphocyte and Macrophage-Dominated Inflammation with Extensive Antibody Deposition in the Tissue and in Astrocyte Cytoplasm

Complement C9 neoantigen was deposited at sites of active demyelination, indicating that the antibody plays a role in the demyelinating process. Plaque borders were well defined, and lymphocytic perivascular cuffs were frequent. Loss of all types of myelin protein appeared to occur simultaneously. There was heavy staining of myelin degradation products in the macrophages. In older, inactive plaques, there was variable loss of oligodendrocytes at the plaque borders, with reappearance of oligodendrocytes in the plaque centers. A high incidence of shadow plaques was seen in these cases, indicating that some remyelination is common. This was the most common pattern, comprising 53 percent of the reported cases. The formation of clathrin coated pits (caveolae) seen on electron microscopy reported by Prineas and Connell is consistent with a role for antibody in the demyelination; thus, these two cases were most likely type II (Figure 14.1) (23).

## Pattern 3: Active Demyelination with an Infiltrate of T Lymphocytes and Activated Macrophages and Microglia

No IgG deposition, possible preservation of a rim of myelin around venules, and the plaque borders were ill defined. With this lesion pattern, there was preferential loss of myelin-associated glycoprotein (MAG) relative to other myelin proteins such as MBP and proteolipid protein (PLP) as originally described by Itoyama et al. (24). A concentric (Balo type) pattern was seen in some of these cases. This pattern comprised about 30 percent of the cases.

Forty-three of the lesions examined by Lucchinetti and others were biopsies of initial clinical lesions. Thirty-three of these patients developed clinically definite MS in the follow-up period, including individuals with each of the first three disease patterns. Multiple lesions were examined from most of the cases, and the pattern was the same in all of the lesions from a given patient (1). Conversion of one pattern to another would seem possible, but, except for conversion of pattern 1 to pattern 2 with the development of an antibody reaction, conversion between types seemed a priori unlikely.

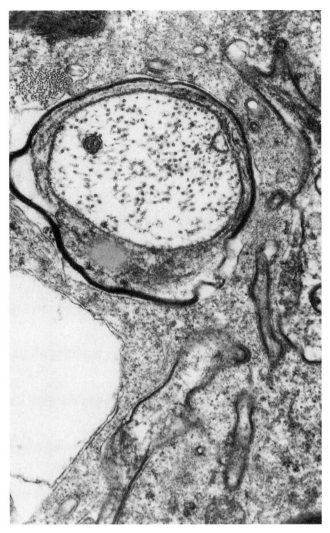

**FIGURE 14.1**

Electron micrograph showing a clathrin-coated pit on the surface of a macrophage (lower right center) and a remyelinating axon. Original magnification, 39000X. Reprinted from: *Neurology* 1978;28:S68–S75 (Figure 9), with permission.

## THE ACUTE PLAQUE

According to Prineas (25), most MS plaques appear to begin with margination and diapedesis of lymphocytes and macrophages forming perivascular cuffs about capillaries and venules. This is followed by diffuse parenchymal infiltration by inflammatory cells, edema, macrophage activity with stripping of myelin from axons, astrocytic hyperplasia, and the appearance of increased numbers of lipid-laden macrophages and demyelinated axons. Prineas also described a marked increase in the number of plasma cells in some cases, which would be consistent with a type 2 case. In contrast, Lumsden described plaques in which myelin frag-

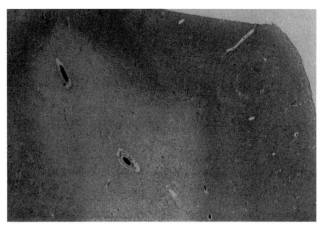

**FIGURE 14.2**

Hematoxylin and eosin stain of subacute multiple sclerosis plaque in the subcortical white matter, with a few perivascular inflammatory cells. At the top, the plaque extends into the cortical gray matter. The plaque edge stains more heavily with hematoxylin due to the concentration of inflammatory cells.

mentation preceded the appearance of macrophages. This would seem to correspond to a type 4 case of Lucchinetti et al. In type 2 cases, as plaques enlarge and coalesce, the initial perivenular distribution of the lesions becomes less apparent. The inflammatory reaction in the plaques usually is less pronounced in gray matter, probably because of the smaller amount of myelin in these areas and the correspondingly fewer macrophages needed to remove cellular debris.

Acute plaques begin in a perivenular location (25,26), and are marked by perivascular cuffs (Figure 14.2 and 14.3) of inflammatory cells including lym-

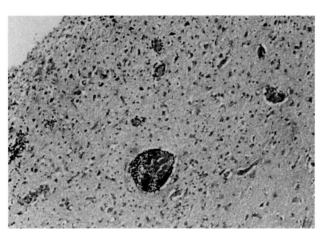

**FIGURE 14.3**

Perivascular cuff of lymphocytes and inflammatory infiltrate in an acute plaque. Hematoxylin and eosin stain.

phocytes, activated macrophages, microglia, and occasionally plasma cells. Polymorphonuclear leukocytes and eosinophils are rare except in Devic syndrome, in which they are much more common. Myelin breakdown occurs with stripping of myelin from the axons by macrophages, and many of the macrophages are filled with myelin debris and neutral lipid. Extracellular myelin debris is rarely, if ever, seen, but some of the myelin breakdown is extracellular, because recognizable myelin fragments are frequently seen on electron microscopy of CSF sediment taken at the time of an acute attack (27,28).

## CHRONIC ACTIVE AND INACTIVE PLAQUES

As plaques mature, the lipid-laden macrophages and microglia exit the central plaque area, which becomes hypocellular (Figure 14.4). Gliosis gradually increases, followed by gradual shrinkage of the plaque. The plaque margin may remain active with continuing or recurring activity, or the plaque margin may gradually lose inflammatory cells and become inactive. Plaque reactivation can commonly be seen on MRI during acute attacks, in which a known plaque shows ring enhancement thus indicating active inflammation with breakdown of the blood-brain barrier. The pathologic correlate of this recurring activity is a plaque with a gliotic, sparsely cellular center and a band of lipid-filled macrophages and lymphocytes at the plaque margin.

Considerable axonal interruption even in new acute plaques. Axonal interruption is marked by axonal ovoids that are easily demonstrated with special stains and confocal microscopy. Over time, these interrupted axons undergo retrograde degeneration and the ovoids disappear. Axonal damage is demonstrated on MR spectroscopy by loss of N-acetyl aspartate (NAA), an axonal marker (29). Trapp and colleagues reported an average of about 11,000 axonal ovoids/mm$^3$ in acute plaques, indicating that significant axonal loss begins early in the disease process (30,31). How much of the NAA loss is due to axonal interruption and how much is due to loss in axonal diameter and impairment of axonal transport remains to be determined. Demyelinated axons initially become irregular in diameter but in later stages appear to have a uniformly reduced diameter (Figure 14.4). They may lose as much as 50 percent or more of their diameter, which would reduce the axoplasmic volume by 75 percent, so that, even if the concentration in the axons remained the same, the amount would be markedly decreased. At the same time, axon transport is seriously impaired, which also could reduce the amount of NAA out of proportion to the actual axonal loss and might well decrease the concentration distal to the site of demyelination (see Chapter 16).

Wallerian degeneration due to axonal destruction in acute plaques can be extensive enough to be detected by MRI (32) (see Chapter 15). Additional axonal destruction occurs when older plaques are reactivated with demyelination at the plaque margins. The fact that sparing of axons is relative and not absolute has been known since the time of Charcot, but the extent of the damage to the axons has been only recently quantified. Cerebral atrophy and atrophy of the corpus callosum, which is commonly seen in advanced disease, is probably due to a combination of myelin and axonal loss and shrinkage due to scarring.

Most investigators now believe that axonal loss accounts for most of the chronic, irreversible disability in MS. Cumulative axonal loss in long pathways such as the pyramidal tracts and the dorsal columns of the spinal cord, where there may be several plaques along their course, is often very substantial. This in part accounts for the pallor that is frequently seen in these tracts at autopsy. It is important to recognize that axonal loss is an important factor in MS and that experimental efforts to improve conduction in surviving fibers will not affect those symptoms due to axonal loss, even though they may produce dramatic improvement in symptoms that are due to conduction failure in surviving axons.

Immunocytochemical studies of inflammatory cytokines indicate that most of the lymphocytes at the plaque margins are T-cells. CD4$^+$ T-cells (helper/inducer) are seen in the plaque margin and extend beyond the margin into periplaque white matter. CD8$^+$ T-cells (suppressor/cytotoxic) are fewer in number and more confined to the plaque margin. Occasional B cells and a few plasma cells may be seen. Macrophages may be seen

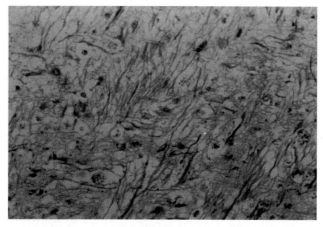

**FIGURE 14.4**

Inactive plaque center, with the axon stain showing numerous demyelinated axons and very little inflammation. The axons have a relatively uniform diameter, unlike newly demyelinated axons, which are irregularly dilated.

throughout the plaque but are rarely seen beyond the plaque margin (33).

## GRAY MATTER PLAQUES

Although juxtacortical plaques extending into the adjacent gray matter have long been recognized, isolated cortical plaques are rarely mentioned in the literature. Nevertheless, they are an important part of the pathology of MS. The failure to detect these plaques arises from two factors: they are much less inflammatory than white matter plaques and cannot be detected with myelin staining techniques. The instructions after staining with luxol fast blue, the most commonly used current myelin stain, is to destain until the gray matter no longer shows any staining. Thus gray matter plaques do not stain for myelin and are difficult to see with myelin stains. Gray matter involvement is frequently reported when plaques at the gray–white junction extend into the cortex, but isolated gray matter plaques were rarely discussed or commented on until the recent report of Peterson et al. (34). They reported a careful analysis of gray matter plaques and classified them into three types: type 1 were contiguous with subcortical lesions and accounted for 34 percent of the cortical lesions; type 2 were small, usually perivascular lesions confined to the cortex, and constituting 16 percent of the lesions; and type 3 extended from the cortical surface to layer 3 or 4 of the cortex, constituting 50 percent of the lesions (34). These plaques are much less inflammatory than those in the white matter, with only one-thirteenth as many CD3$^+$ lymphocytes and one-sixth as many microglia and macrophages (34). They found activated microglia apposed to and ensheathing neuronal perikarya and apical dendrites. Apoptotic neurons were increased in the cortical plaques. Transected neurites were found with an average density of 4119/mm$^3$, which is about one-third the number found in white matter plaques. They were about one-fourth as frequent in chronic gray matter plaques and much less common in inactive lesions. These cortical lesions may account for many of the cognitive changes seen in MS.

In chronic active lesions, astrocytes in and about the plaque express class I and class II histocompatibility antigens, although expression of class II antigens was both more common, intense, and consistent than expression of class I antigens (33,35). Class I and class II positive astrocytes extended into the periplaque area, but astrocytes outside the plaque and peri-plaque areas are negative for both antigens. Astrocytes in the plaque margin and peri-plaque area often stain for interferon-γ and a bit less frequently for interferon-β (33). Astrocytes in the plaque center and in normal-appearing tissue away from the plaques were consistently negative except in patients dying with intercurrent infections in whom staining was more generalized.

Staining for the intercellular adhesion molecule 1 (ICAM-1) revealed diffuse staining of the plaque periphery, most intense at the plaque margin but extending well beyond the zone of inflammation. Staining also was seen in perivascular cuffs, which included diffuse and cellular staining. LFA-1 is a ligand for ICAM-1 and is present on essentially all of the hematogenous cells in the plaque and peri-plaque areas. LFA-3, with its ligand CD2, is more selective for T-cells than ICAM-1, but it has a very similar distribution to that of ICAM-1 in the plaque and peri-plaque areas (33).

Old inactive plaques generally have sharp margins without hypercellularity, a few widely scattered T-cells, and do not stain for adhesion molecules or interferon. They are marked by gliosis and stain heavily for glial fibrillary acidic protein. Inflammatory cells are scarce, and most cells in the plaque are astrocytes. A few nonmyelinating oligodendroglia may be seen near the plaque margins.

Immunocytochemical studies have shown the inflammatory cells in the actively demyelinating central area of acute plaques to be mainly Ia-positive cells. These are mostly activated microglia and macrophages with a few T-cells and antibody-producing plasma cells. The T cells in the acute plaque are a mixture of T4$^+$ (helper-inducer) and T8$^+$ (suppressor/cytotoxic) lymphocytes and are more numerous near the center of the plaque, diminishing in numbers peripherally. As the lesion enlarges, T cells become relatively more numerous peripherally, whereas macrophages take their place centrally. T4$^+$ (helper) cells invade the normal appearing white matter about the lesion, whereas T8$^+$ (suppressor) cells are confined largely to the plaque margins and perivascular cuffs. The plaque margins contain increased numbers of oligodendrocytes, astrocytes, and inflammatory cells (33–35). As the lesions become more mature, myelin remnants and macrophages progressively disappear from the central part of the plaque (Figure 14.4), which eventually becomes a gliotic scar. At the plaque margin, a hypercellular "glial wall" contains lymphocytes, oligodendrocytes, and a few macrophages and astrocytes. In many instances, the disease process appears to continue, with low-grade activity at the plaque margins, manifested by lipid-laden macrophages and lymphocytes, often accompanied by a few thin perivascular cuffs. In chronic-active MS, inflammatory cells are scattered in small numbers through much of the normal-appearing white matter. These include T4$^+$, T8$^+$, and Ia$^+$ cells (35,36).

Chronic inactive MS plaques usually have a sharply demarcated border with little, if any, hypercellularity. Occasional T4$^+$ and Ia$^+$ cells are scattered throughout the lesions. At the edges, a few T4$^+$, T8$^+$, and Ia$^+$ cells, including macrophages and B lymphocytes, may be seen, and these also occur in small numbers throughout the otherwise normal-appearing white matter.

## REMYELINATION

Plaquelike areas of very pale myelin staining are a frequent occurrence in many cases of MS. On examination, these areas have increased cellularity and abnormally thin myelin sheaths of relatively uniform thickness (Figure 14.1 and 14.5). Numerous studies in experimental animals have demonstrated the characteristics of regenerated myelin with thin sheaths (Figure 14.6) and short internodes (Figure 14.7). The thickness of the myelin about individual axons in these shadow plaques bears no relationship to fiber diameter as it does in normally myelinated areas. Some have regarded these shadow plaques as evidence of partial demyelination; however, it is now clear that most, if not all, represent areas of remyelination (37).

Until the late 1950s, it was accepted dogma that remyelination did not occur and that oligodendroglia, like neurons, were endstage cells incapable of regeneration. Since Bunge et al. (38) first unequivocally demonstrated central remyelination in the cat in 1958, remyelination has been shown to occur in the CNS in essentially every species tested, including tadpole, mouse, rat, guinea pig, rabbit, cat, and dog (39). The characteristics of the shadow plaque are essentially identical to those of remyelinated areas in experimental animals: an increased number of oligodendrocytes that, contrary to traditional views, have been demonstrated to be capable of proliferation (40–42), thin myelin sheaths of relatively uniform thickness, and short internodes. The alternative possibility that shadow plaques arise from partial demyelination seems unlikely because partial demyelination has been convincingly demonstrated only during the acute phase of the demyelinating process or where the

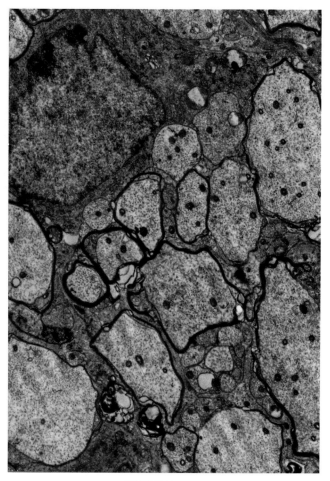

**FIGURE 14.6**

Electron micrograph of remyelination 28 days after mouse hepatitis virus inoculation. The newly regenerated myelin sheaths are very thin, and the myelin thickness bears no relationship to axon diameter. An oligodendrocyte can be seen at upper left. Original magnification, 5800X. Herndon RM and Weiner LP, unpublished observations.

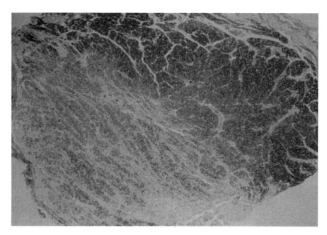

**FIGURE 14.5**

Luxol fast blue stain of a shadow plaque in optic nerve. Note the myelin pallor at lower left compared with the deeper staining of the undemyelinated area at upper right.

myelin is under mechanical pressure. In addition, these thin myelin sheaths, particularly those at plaque margins, have been shown to have short internodes (37). There is abundant evidence for remyelination in experimental animals and humans, and the appearance of shadow plaques and short internodes indicates that these are indeed remylinated fibers.

Regeneration of central myelin in some cases is accompanied by Schwann cell invasion of the CNS; consequently, the peripheral myelin can be seen within a demyelinated or remyelinated area (43). Schwann cells occur in small numbers in normal spinal cord, but it is uncertain whether they come from peripheral nerves innervating CNS blood vessels or occur independent of blood vessels. In pathologic conditions, most of the Schwann cell remyelination within CNS occurs near root

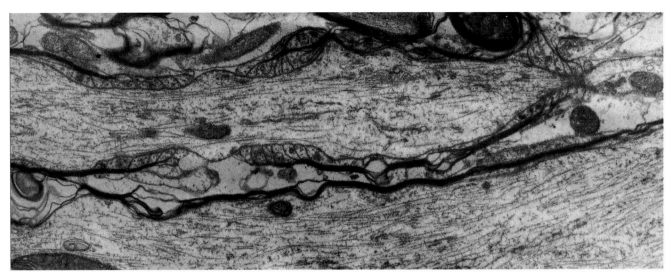

**FIGURE 14.7**

Remyelinated axon 28 days after mouse hepatitis virus inoculation. Two nodes are seen only 6 μm apart. Original magnification, 19000X. Herndon RM and Weiner LP, unpublished observations.

entry or exit zones. Breaches in the glial limitans caused by the demyelinating process allow Schwann cells in the nerve roots or autonomic nerves accompanying cerebral blood vessels to migrate into the central white matter, where they retain their capability to form myelin.

With progression of the pathologic process, recurrent demyelination at the plaque margins causes slow enlargement of the plaques. Although remyelination appears to be a regular event in early MS, it clearly becomes less common and less effective as the disease progresses, so that, at autopsy in patients with long standing disease, evidence of remyelination may be quite limited. Over time, demyelination of newly remyelinated areas may result in scarring, so that further remyelination cannot occur and the plaque becomes a hypocellular glial scar. Shadow plaques are thus more likely to be seen in autopsies of younger patients with continued active remitting disease (37), and much less common in older patients with inactive disease or chronically active, indolent disease progression. In most cases, the end result is a nervous system riddled with chronically scarred, inactive plaques and a considerable amount of Wallerian degeneration resulting in the pallor of long tracts in myelin-stained preparations.

## SECONDARY PROGRESSIVE MULTIPLE SCLEROSIS

Secondary progressive MS is usually marked by a slowly ascending paralysis or, much more rarely, progressive ataxia. It commonly occurs in patients in their 40s or early 50s who have had MS for a number of years. The pathologic substrate for this appears to be a progressive loss of axons in the spinal cord with cord atrophy. Examination of the cord, in addition to chronic inactive or occasionally active plaques, shows demyelination and/or degeneration of multiple individual fibers. Careful examination of the cord shows widely scattered individual fiber demyelination with a few scattered macrophages along the sheaths (20). This could result from an inadequate supply of transported materials with a resulting inability of the axon to adequately signal the myelin-forming oligodendrocytes. Certainly such scattered fiber demyelination could be a part of a dying axonopathy and thus the substrate for the slowly progressive ascending paralysis of secondary progressive MS (44) (Chapter 16).

What mechanisms could be invoked for such a process? It might be a problem in axonal transport, with retrograde degeneration, or axonal interruption secondary to scarring with Wallerian degeneration. The former seems more likely. Extensive studies in animals have shown that fast and slow axonal transport are markedly slowed by demyelination. Such axonal damage upstream would lead to an inadequate supply of the structural materials needed to maintain energy metabolism and axonal structure. These conditions, particularly if the axons metabolic resources are stretched due to induced sprouting of the distal axon to take over synapses vacated by death of other axons, could lead to a dying back axonopathy. Clinically this would result initially in death of the longest axons with gradual progression to shorter and shorter axons. The second major possibility is that they are undergoing Wallerian degeneration secondary to glial scar formation, with death of axons occurring in plaques as the extensive astrocytic scarring causes shrinkage of the plaques, thus compressing and choking off the axons. Either scenario could lead to an ascending paralysis, although one would expect that the second would cause a more scattered, less clearly ascending picture.

## PRIMARY PROGRESSIVE MULTIPLE SCLEROSIS

In the studies of Lucchinetti et al., all of the cases of primary progressive MS had pattern 4 (1). Inflammation was dominated by T lymphocytes, and macrophages, IgG, and complement deposition were absent. Death of oligodendrocytes ocurred in peri-plaque white matter adjacent to areas of demyelination. The dying oligodendrocytes demonstrated DNA fragmentation without features of apoptosis. Staining for the various myelin proteins showed an essentially simultaneous loss in staining for each of the proteins. Thus, it appears to be an oligodendrogliopathy.

Primary progressive MS constitutes about 10 percent of MS cases and is equally common in men and women. This pattern was the least common in the series of Lucchinetti et al., comprising 4 percent of the cases studied, and was the only one associated with a particular clinical disease pattern. Its association with primary progressive MS strongly supports the frequently expressed view that true primary progressive MS is a disease distinct from relapsing remitting and secondary progressive MS. Some cases that clinically appear as primary progressive disease undoubtedly will have the pathology of secondary progressive disease because relapsing remitting cases can be asymptomatic or nearly so (22) and thus may present clinically only when they move into the secondary progressive phase. Such cases show the pathology of secondary progressive disease even though clinical attacks were never observed. This will tend to confuse the clinical distinction between the disease types but is explained by the fact that a person can have multiple demyelinating events without symptoms in relapsing remitting MS, so that secondary progressive disease can masquerade clinically as primary progressive disease.

## ACUTE MULTIPLE SCLEROSIS (MARBURG DISEASE)

Acute MS is fortunately rather rare. It is marked by the rapid onset and almost continual progression of demyelination. It can begin in the hemispheres or the brainstem, and typical cases display on MRI multiple high signal areas that increase in size and become confluent. Many patients die within a few weeks to several months. Many of those who survive go on to have a typical relapsing remitting course.

Pathologically, it is marked by intense and widespread inflammation with T lymphocytes, large numbers of lipid-laden macrophages, and a scattering of B lymphocytes (18,19). The lipid-laden macrophages stain intensely for neutral lipid with oil red-O but show little staining with most myelin stains. Essentially, total demyelination occurs within the lesions, although beginning remyelination can be seen. Extensive IgG and complement product is deposited in the lesions, which pathologically resemble type 2 lesions of Lucchinetti et al. There is no evidence of death of oligodendroglia in the area surrounding the plaques. In semithin sections, partly digested bits of myelin are seen in macrophages. The demyelinated axons are irregularly constricted and dilated, unlike those in more chronic plaques, which have a more uniform diameter. Perivascular lymphocytic cuffs may be present but often are sparse.

Oligodendrocytes are usually considerably reduced in the acute lesions, although larger numbers may appear in somewhat older lesions (19), indicating that oligodendrocyte regeneration occurs in humans as it does in experimental animals.

## ACUTE DISSEMINATED ENCEPHALOMYELITIS

ADEM has a host of names, including perivenous encephalomyelitis, encephalitis periaxalis diffusa, acute hemorrhagic encephalomyelitis, postinfectious encephalomyelitis, and postvaccinal encephalomyelitis. Of the demyelinating diseases, this appears to correspond most closely to EAE. It is an acute diffuse inflammatory demyelinating disorder that often occurs 1 to 3 weeks after a viral infection or immunization. Its severity and intensity vary, but it usually runs a monophasic course, with a very small percentage later developing into a relapsing remitting disease. In those who survive the acute episode, slow improvement usually occurs over many months, often with remarkably good recovery and little residua. Most fatal cases follow smallpox vaccination or measles infection. The hemorrhagic form has been considered to represent a different entity by some (18), although some have considered it to be a more severe form of ADEM (45) because, in addition to the perivenous hemorrhages, perivenous inflammation and demyelination are regularly observed.

The gross pathology is marked by swelling and congestion, often with evidence of uncal and foraminal herniation. The fresh brain may show numerous petechia or simply appear swollen. Microscopically, it is marked by extensive perivenous inflammation and demyelination. The venules are surrounded by prominent cuffs of lymphocytes and macrophages. Often, long strips of perivenous demyelination occur, giving the tissue a reticulate appearance. In some cases, there is spread of macrophages and lymphocytes into the parenchyma. The macrophages may be laden with neutral lipid even rather early in the disease process.

In the hemorrhagic cases, in addition to the perivascular cuffs, there is edema and necrosis of blood vessels with fibrin deposition and numerous ring or ball hemorrhages. In these cases, there are usually numerous neutrophils in the infiltrate, and there may be areas of frank necrosis of tissue. Attempts to recover virus in these cases or to demonstrate by antibody staining or in situ hybridization have usually failed. Overall, the pathologic picture is essentially identical to EAE as seen in experimental animals (45).

## NEUROMYELITIS OPTICA (DEVIC DISEASE)

The place of neuromyelitis optica in the MS spectrum has long been in dispute. It has been said to be a monophasic disease, with optic neuritis and transverse myelitis occurring within a few weeks to a month or two of each other, without recurrences. However, it is clear that over half the cases that fit these criteria initially go on to develop relapses and remissions. Wingerchuk and coworkers reviewed 71 patients with neuromyelitis optica (46). Of these, 23 had a monophasic course and the other 48 had a relapsing remitting course. In the cases of monophasic illness, they noted that the initial optic neuritis and transverse myelitis occur quite close together, with a median of 5 days between the two events, whereas the median was 166 days for the relapsing cases. The relapsing cases had a poor prognosis with poor recovery between attacks. They frequently developed respiratory failure secondary to cervical cord disease.

Clinically Devic syndrome differs from typical MS in its clinical pattern and in the relatively poor recovery usually seen after the attacks. It also differs in its distribution in the population, being more common in Asians and Africans than in Caucasians. In Japan, the Devic pattern makes up about 7 percent of reported cases (47).

In the acute stages there is necrosis of the cord, usually extending over three or more segments. The cord is usually swollen and soft in the affected area. There may be additional demyelinating lesions in other cord segments but the brain itself is not involved. The CSF has a variable pleocytosis, often with 50 to 100 or more cells. These are predominantly lymphocytes with a variable number of monocytes and neutrophil leucocytes and occasionally a few eosinophil leucocytes. There may be extensive perivascular cuffs containing macrophages and granulocytes, including eosinophils and CD3$^+$ lymphocytes (48). The inflammation and necrosis are marked by extensive macrophage infiltration with lymphocytes and often polymorphonuclear leucocytes. Extensive deposition of IgG and C9 neoantigen is a marker for complement deposition in areas of myelin necrosis. Extensive oligodendrocyte destruction occurs, and all the myelin proteins disappear at about the same time. Thus the pathology resembles a more severe, necrotic pattern similar to the type 2 of Lucchinetti et al. It differs in that much of the IgG and complement deposition is on and around blood vessels in the Devic's cases (48).

In the late stages, cavitation and necrosis of gray and white matter occurs in the cord, and most of the length of the cord is affected. There is extensive scarring with marked hyalinization and thickening of blood vessels and perivascular fibrosis (49). Numerous macrophages are present in necrotic areas. In the optic nerves, similar necrosis and thickening and hyalinization of blood vessels is not seen, but demyelination typically includes the entire optic chiasm.

Axonal destruction in the lesions is much greater than that usually seen in MS. The destructiveness of the lesions is emphasized by the clinical findings, with relatively poor recovery from the lesions. For example, complete blindness is extremely rare in exacerbating remitting MS but common in neuromyelitis optica. Similarly, permanent paraplegia or quadriplegia is rare after a single attack of relapsing remitting MS but fairly common in Devic disease.

## STRUCTURES RESEMBLING INFECTIOUS AGENTS IN MS TISSUES

Despite a number of reports of "viruslike particles" seen by electron microscopy of MS biopsy and postmortem material (9,50,51), credible morphologic evidence for the presence of true virions has not been reported. Dense bodies surrounded by a membrane have been seen intracellularly, mainly in macrophages, in proximity to actively demyelinating areas. These are of variable size, do not closely resemble any particular virus or class of viruses, and are generally regarded as myelin breakdown products. Many other investigators, beginning with Prineas in 1972 (9), have reported "paramyxoviruslike" tubules in the nuclei of inflammatory cells in MS plaques. These consist of strands of 18- to 20-nm intranuclear filaments or tubules. In size and appearance, they resemble the nucleocapsid of paramyxoviruses. They have been seen in a variety of conditions including normal tissues fixed under acidic conditions (R.M. Herndon, unpublished observations) and appear to be chromatin strands, which have an altered appearance due to the metabolic state of the cell or conditions of tissue fixation (52).

With newer techniques of polymerase chain reaction, representational difference analysis, in situ hybridization, and immunocytochemical techniques, viruses are frequently found in MS plaques. The effort to tie viruses found in brain to the disease process has failed thus far. The viruses of greatest interest are the herpes viruses. These viruses are found latent in nervous tissue, are activated by other viral infections, just as new attacks of MS frequently follow viral infection, and might activate an inflammatory process in the nervous system resulting in a new attack of MS. Challoner et al. (12) reported the detection of herpes type 6 in MS brain using polymerase chain reaction and representational difference analysis followed by localization in plaques using immunocytochemistry. Subsequently, Sanders et al. (13) detected several herpes viruses in brain tissue (Table 14.2). Although several were more common in MS brains and more common in MS plaques, the differences did not reach statistical significance. Many of these viruses are carried in macrophages, so they would be more likely to appear in sites with large numbers of macrophages, such as MS plaques. Nothing in this work indicated an etiologic relationship to MS, but the presence of latent viruses, which are easily activated in plaques, suggests that they could contribute to the pathology.

## CHLAMYDIA PNEUMONIAE

The presence of *Chlamydia pneumonia* in the CSF of individuals with MS has been demonstrated by polymerase chain reaction and culture (15,53) and is discussed in detail in Chapter 10. *Chlamydia* has not been reported pathologically in MS tissue thus far, but structures resembling microorganisms compatible with *C. pneumonia* have been seen in the CSF sediment in MS cases (R.M. Herndon, unpublished observations). Whether this will prove to be related to the disease or yet another incidental occurrence remains to be determined.

### TABLE 14.2
*Herpes Viruses in Brain Tissue*

| VIRUS PLAQUE | MS BRAIN PLAQUE | ACTIVE BRAIN | INACTIVE | CONTROL |
|---|---|---|---|---|
| Herpes simplex | 37% | 41% | 20% | 28% |
| Herpes 6 | 57% | 32% | 17% | 43% |
| Varicella zoster virus | 43% | 14% | 10% | 32% |
| Epstein-Barr virus | 27% | 5% | 10% | 38% |
| Cytomegalovirus | 16% | 9% | 10% | 22% |

Adapted from: *J Neurovirol* 1996; 2:249–258.

## CONCLUSION

MS is an inflammatory demyelinating disorder or, more likely, a group of disorders of unknown but most likely autoimmune or infectious origin. Current pathologic evidence suggests that MS may have more than one etiology and that primary progressive MS is a separate disease. Much of the permanent disability in MS results from axonal destruction, which falls most heavily on very long pathways such as the pyramidal tract supplying the legs and the dorsal columns carrying sensory information from the legs. These long pathways take multiple hits over the years, with increasing axonal destruction leading to the loss of lower extremity function so common in advanced MS. Other aspects of the disease, such as incoordination and imbalance are caused by delayed and degraded information resulting from slowed conduction of proprioceptive information and the inability to monitor, on line, motor processes due to conduction delays and signal dispersion occurring as the signals pass through demyelinated areas, as discussed further in the chapter on pathophysiology. Every attack, even subclinical ones, causes some permanent damage, and it is the accumulation of damage from repeated demyelinating episodes that accounts for most of the long-term disability. It is this progressive accumulation of damage that provides the best rationale for early use of disease-altering therapies.

## References

1. Lucchinetti C, Bruck W, Parisi J, et al. Heterogeneity of multiple sclerosis lesions:implications for the pathogenesis of demyelination. *Ann Neurol* 2000; 47:707–717.
2. Hughes, RA, Hadden RD, Gregson NA, Smith KJ. Pathogenesis of Guillain-Barre syndrome. *J Neuroimmunol* 1999; 100:74–97.
3. Ho TW, McKhann GM, Griffin JW. Human autoimmune neuropathies. *Annu Rev Neurosci* 1998; 21:187–226.
4. Schonberger LB, Bregman DJ, Sullivan-Bolyai JZ, et al. Guillian-Barre syndrome following vaccination in the National Influenza Immunization Program, United States 1976–1977. *Am J Epidemiol* 1979; 110:105–123.
5. Mendell JR, Kolkin S, Kissel JT, et al. Evidence for central nervous system demyelination in chronic inflammatory demyelinating polyradiculoneuropathy. *Neurology* 1987; 37:1291–1294.
6. Ormerod IE, Waddy HM, Kermode AG, Murray NM, Thomas PK. Involvement of the central nervous system in chronic inflammatory demyelinating polyneuropathy: a clinical, electrophysiological and magnetic resonance imaging study. *J Neurol Neurosurg Psychiatry.* 199053:789–793.
7. Stojkovic T, de Seze J, Hurtevent JF, et al. Visual evoked potentials study in chronic idiopathic inflammatory demyelinating polyneuropathy. *Clin Neurophysiol* 2000111:2285–2291.
8. Compston A. The genetics of multiple sclerosis. *J Neurovirol* 2000; (suppl 2):S5–S9.
9. Prineas J. Paramyxovirus-like particles associated with acute demyelination in chronic relapsing multiple sclerosis. *Science* 1972; 178:760–763.
10. Johnson RT. The virology of demyelinating diseases. *Ann Neurol* 1994; 36:S54–S60.
11. Cook SD. Evidence for a viral etiology of multiple sclerosis. In: Cook SD (ed.), *Handbook of Multiple Sclerosis*. New York: Marcel Dekker; 2001.

12. Challoner PB, Smith KT, Parker JD, et al. Plaque-associated expression of human herpesvirus 6 in multiple sclerosis. *Proc Nat Acad Sci USA* 1995; 92:7440–7444.

13. Sanders VJ, Felisan S, Waddell A, Tourtellotte WW. Detection of herpesvirdae in postmortem multiple sclerosis brain tissue and controls by polymerase chain reaction. *J Neurovirol* 1996; 2:249–258.

14. Lycke J, Svennerholm B, Hjelmquist E, et al. Acyclovir treatment of relapsing-remitting multiple sclerosis. A randomized, placebo-controlled, double blind study. *J Neurol* 1996; 243:214–224.

15. Sriram S, Stratton CW, Yao S, et al. Chlamydia pneumoniae infection of the central nervous system in multiple sclerosis. *Ann Neurol* 1999; 46:6–14.

16. Jeffrey DR, Alshami E. Allogenic bone marrow transplantation in multiple sclerosis. *Neurology* 1998; 50(suppl 4):A147.

17. Cottrell DA, Kremenchutzky M, Rice GP, et al. The natural history of multiple sclerosis: a geographically based study. 5. The clincal features and natural history of primary progressive multiple sclerosis. *Brain* 1999; 122:625–639.

18. Prineas JW, McDonald WI. Demyelinating diseases. In: Graham DI, Lantos PL (eds.), *Greenfields Neuropathology*. 6th ed. 813–896.

19. Marburg O. Die sogenannte "akute multiple Sklerose" Jahrb. *Psychiat Neurol* (Leizig) 1906; 27:213–311.

20. Adams CWM. The general pathology of multiple sclerosisi: morphological and chemical aspect of the lesions. In: Hallpike JF, Adams CWM, Tourtellotte WW (eds.), *Multiple Sclerosis*. Baltimore: Williams & Wilkins; 1983; 203–240.

21. Lassman H, Raine CS, Antel J, Prineas JW. Immunopathology of multiple sclerosis: Report on an international meeting held at the Institute of Neurology of the University of Vienna. *J Neuroimmunol* 1998; 86:213–217.

22. Gilbert JJ, Sadler M. Unsuspected multiple sclerosis. *Arch Neurol* 1983; 40:533–536.

23. Prineas JW, Connell F. The fine structure of chronically active multiple sclerosis plaques. *Neurology* 1978; 28:S68–S75.

24. Itoyama Y, Sternberger NH, Webster HD, et al. Immunocytochemical observations on the distribution of myelin-associated glycoprotein and myelin basic protein in multiple sclerosis lesions. *Ann Neurol* 1980; 7:167–177.

25. Prineas JW. Pathology of the early lesions of multiple sclerosis. *Hum Pathol* 1975; 6:531–535.

26. Dow RS, Berglund G. Vascular pattern of lesions of multiple sclerosis. *Arch Neurol Psychiat* 1942; 47:1–18.

27. Herndon RM, Johnson MA. A method for the electron microscopic study of cerebrospinal fluid sediment. *J Neuropathol Exp Neurol* 1970; 29:320–330.

28. Herndon RM, Kasckow J. Electron microscopic studies of cerebrospinal fluid sediment in demyelinating disease. *Ann Neurol* 1978; 4:515–523.

29. Stefano N de, Narayanan S, Francis GS, et al. Evidence of axonal damage in the early stages of multiple sclerosis and its relevance to disability. *Arch Neurol* 2001; 58:65–70.

30. Trapp BD, Peterson J, Ransohoff RM, et al. Axonal transection in the lesions of multiple sclerosis. *N Engl J Med* 1998; 338:278–285.

31. Trapp BD, Bo L, Mork S, Chang A. Pathogenesis of tissue injury in MS lesions. *J Neuroimmunol* 1999; 98:49–56.

32. Simon JH, Kinkel RP, Jacobs L, et al. A Wallerian degeneration pattern in patients at risk of MS. *Neurology* 2000; 54:1155–1160.

33. Traugott U. On the role of astrocytes for lesion pathogenesis. In: Herndon RM, Seil FJ, (eds.), *Multiple Sclerosis: Current Status of Research and Treatment*. New York: Demos, 1994; 13–31.

34. Peterson JW, Bö L, Mörk S, Chang A, Trapp BD. Transected neurites, apoptotic neurons, and reduced inflammation in cortical multiple sclerosis lesions. *Ann Neurol* 2001; 50:389–400.

35. Traugott U, Reinherz EL, Raine CS. Multiple sclerosis: Distribution of T-cells, T-cell subsets and Ia positive macrophages in lesions of different ages. *J Neuroimmunol* 1983; 4:201–221.

36. Traugott U, Raine CS. Further lymphocyte characterization in the central nervous system in multiple sclerosis. *Ann NY Acad Sci* 1984; 436:163.

37. Prineas JW, Connell F. Remyelination in multiple sclerosis. *Ann Neurol* 1979; 5:22–31.

38. Bunge MB, Bunge RP, Ris H. Ultrastructural study of remyelination in an experimental lesion in adult cat spinal cord. *J Biophys Biochem Cytol* 1961; 10: 67–94.

39. Hommes OR. Remyelination in human CNS lesions. *Prog Brain Res* 1980; 53:39–63.

40. Herndon RM, Price DL, Weiner LP. Regeneration of oligodendroglia during recovery from demyelinating disease. *Science* 1977; 195:693–694.

41. Arenella L, Herndon RM. Mature oligodendrocytes: Division following experimental demyelination in adult animals. *Arch Neurol* 1984; 41:1162–1165.

42. Ludwin SK. Proliferation of mature oligodendrocytes after trauma to the central nervous system. *Nature* 1984; 308:274–276.

43. Itoyama Y, Webster H deF, Richardson EP, Trapp BD. Schwann cell remyelination of demyelinated axons in spinal cord multiple sclerosis lesions. *Ann Neurol* 1983; 14:339–346.

44. Herndon RM. Why secondary progressive multiple sclerosis is a relentlessly progressive illness? *Arch Neurol* 2002; 59:301–304.

45. Hart MN, Earle KM. Haemorrhagic and perivenous encephalitis: A clinico-pathological review of 38 cases. *J Neurol Neurosurg Psychiatry* 1975; 38:585–591.

46. Wingerchuk DM, Hogancamp WF, O'Brien PC, Weinshenker BG. The clinical course of neuromyelitis optica (Devic syndrome). *Neurology* 1999; 53:1107–1114.

47. Kuroiwa Y, Igata A, Itahara K, Koshijima S, Tusbaki T. Nationwide survey of multiple sclerosis in Japan. Clinical analysis of 1,084 cases. *Neurology* 1975; 25:845–851.

48. Lucchinetti CF, Mandler RN, McGovern D, et al. A role for humeral mechanisms in the pathogenesis of Devic's neuromyelitis optica. *Brain* 2002; 125:1450–1461.

49. Mandler RN, Davis LE, Jeffery DR, Kornfeld M. Devic neuromyelitis optica: a clinicopathological study of 8 patients. *Ann Neurol* 1993; 34:162–168.

50. Raine CS, Powers JM, Suzuki K. Acute multiple sclerosis—confirmation of "paramyxovirus-like" tubules. *Arch Neurol* 1974; 30:39–46.

51. Field EJ, Cowshall S, Narang HK, Bell TM. Viruses in multiple sclerosis? *Lancet* 1972; ii:280–281.

52. Raine CS, Schaumberg HH, Snyder DK, Suzuki K. Intranuclear "Paramyxovirus-like" material in multiple sclerosis, adrenoleukodystrophy and Kuf's disease. *J Neurol Sci* 1975; 25:29–41.

53. Sriram S, Stratton CW, Yao S-Y, et al. Chlamydia pneumoniae infection of the central nervous system in multiple sclerosis. *Ann Neurol* 1999; 46:6–14.

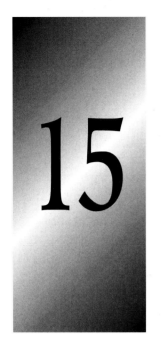

# 15

# Pathology of Multiple Sclerosis as Revealed by In Vivo Magnetic Resonance–Based Approaches

*Jack H. Simon M.D., Ph.D.*

Magnetic resonance imaging (MRI) and spectroscopy methods have contributed enormously to our understanding of multiple sclerosis (MS), including its early diagnosis, prognostic information, the natural history, and the effect of therapeutic intervention (1). I summarize our current understanding of the pathology of MS from the perspective of conventional and advanced MR-based methodologies, including concepts of the focal MS lesion, the global pathology of MS, and the potential relationships between focal and global injury as seen in the brain and spinal cord.

## NATURAL HISTORY OF THE MS LESION BASED ON MRI

Although possibly an oversimplification, the evolution of MS pathology generally follows a characteristic course that is conveniently viewed from the perspective of the isolated acute lesion, developing de novo from normal tissue, into a chronic lesion. From the beginning, temporally related but spatially distant effects may be initially subtle but become more apparent as disease progresses in time.

## The Earliest MS Lesion—Before Those Visualized by Conventional MRI

Until recently, the initial event in the evolution of the MS lesion was that detected by MR imaging as a contrast enhancing lesion that was typically also hyperintense on T2-weighted images (T2-hyperintense); Figure 15.1. Several studies now suggest that there are MR-detectable changes in brain tissue that precede the conventionally visualized MR lesion. Goodkin et al. (2) described newly enhancing lesions arising from what appeared to be normal-appearing white matter (NAWM), yet quantitative T2-relaxation, T1-intensity, and magnetization transfer measures indicated pre-existing white matter abnormality when using the contralateral homologous NAWM regions as control. Werring et al. (3) described a similar finding based on water diffusion measures. They found a steady, moderate increase in the average diffusion coefficient in the prelesion NAWM. Filippi et al. (4) and Pike et al. (5) also described a pre-existing reduction in the mean magnetization transfer ratio (MTR) in NAWM that subsequently developed focal enhancing lesions.

Although this finding of prelesion pathology appears to be consistent across most, although not all series (6), the time course for these changes is more controversial, ranging from intervals of months to years. The significance of these findings is also not known. For example,

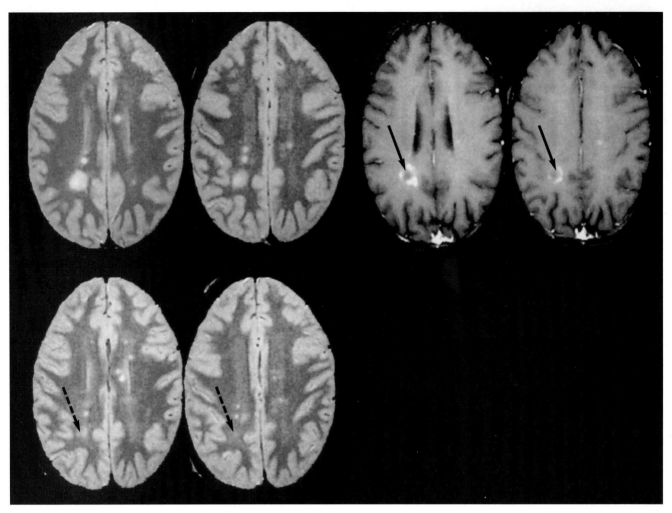

**FIGURE 15.1**

Multiple sclerosis lesions. **Top:** Acute enhancing lesion and the T2-hyperintense counterpart. The enhancing lesion (arrow) is a marker for the inflammatory stage. The T2-hyperintense lesion is nonspecific with regard to pathology. In the acute stages, the T2 hyperintensity results from inflammation, demyelination, and water space dysruption including reversible edema. Some acute lesions are hypointense on T1-weighted images, primarily due to edema fluid. **Bottom:** After several weeks, the T2-hyperintense lesion volume shrinks, leaving a stable residual lesion, the T2 footprint (dashed arrow), which is also nonspecific regarding pathology.

do these represent the true point at which pathology is initiated, well before major disruption of the blood–brain barrier as determined by gadolinium enhancement, or might these represent areas of prior injury more likely to be subsequent sites of essentially unrelated additional acute events?

### The Early Inflammatory MS Lesion

The first conventional imaging sign of an acute MS lesion is the focal enhancing lesion (Figure 15.1). These lesions meet a threshold of a sufficiently disturbed blood–brain barrier such that they are readily visible on standard postcontrast enhanced T1-weighted MR

images. We typically describe enhancing lesions as present when lesions more than a few millimeters in diameter appear. However, it should be recognized that smaller (e.g., 1–2 mm in diameter) areas of pathologic enhancement could exist, but by standard visual criteria would not be reliably separated from vascular enhancement or "noise" in an image. Normally, the clinically approved MR contrast agents that are ionic or non-ionic gadolinium chelates in the range of 600 to 1000 daltons are effectively confined to the intravascular space in the brain and spinal cord by the tight junctions of the endothelial cells making up the blood–brain barrier (BBB) (7). The inflammatory and immune events central to MS, primarily or secondarily, are thought to

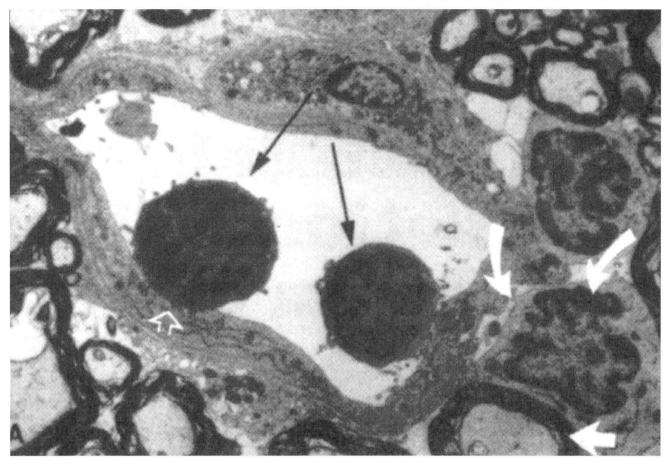

**FIGURE 15.2**

Lymphocyte migration through the blood–brain barrier in experimental demyelination. Lymphocytes attached to the endothelial surface of the postcapillary venule in experimental demyelination (adaptively transferred experimental allergic encephalomyelitis). Electron micrograph shows mouse spinal cord after sensitization to emulsion of mouse spinal cord and Freund adjuvant. Two intraluminal lymphocytes (long arrows) are attached to the postcapillary endothelium (short open arrow). Lymphocytes have migrated through the endothelium (curved arrows) and abut myelinated nerve fibers (short closed arrow). A similar process occurs to allow gadolinium-chelate entry through the blood–brain barrier, which occurs simultaneous to these cellular events and serves as a convenient marker for the inflammatory events early in the demyelination process. Reprinted with permission from *Magn Reson Imaging* 1999;17:731–737.

disrupt the endothelial tight junctions, making gadolinium enhancement (leakage into the interstitial spaces) a convenient marker for many of the early events in the inflammatory–demyelination cascade of events (8–10). The association between enhancing lesions and the acute inflammatory stage of individual MS lesions is based on few correlative MRI autopsy or MRI biopsy studies in humans. Nevertheless, this has become a well-accepted principle (11–13). Further support for the inflammatory lesion–lesion enhancement association was provided by studies of experimental allergic encephalomyelitis (EAE), where a good temporal–spatial correlation had been established (14–17) (Figure 15.2). More exquisite probes of the BBB in MS have been proposed, based on magnetically tagged or gadolinium-tagged lymphocytes

and macrophages, but these approaches are not as practical in human MS. More sensitive methodologies are likely to be revealing because there is immunohistochemical evidence for leakage of serum proteins across the BBB in old plaques (18), that are not detected by standard enhanced MRI methods. Dynamic contrast enhanced MRI is a potential MRI approach for detection of leakage of gadolinium chelates through a defective BBB (19–20), but this approach has not shown practical application to date. However, by factoring in the influence of BBB leakage, it becomes feasible to determine the regional cerebral blood volume (rCBV) by MRI. By this approach, (21) we learned that acute MS lesions have an increased rCBV compared to NAWM, presumably related to cerebral vasodilation.

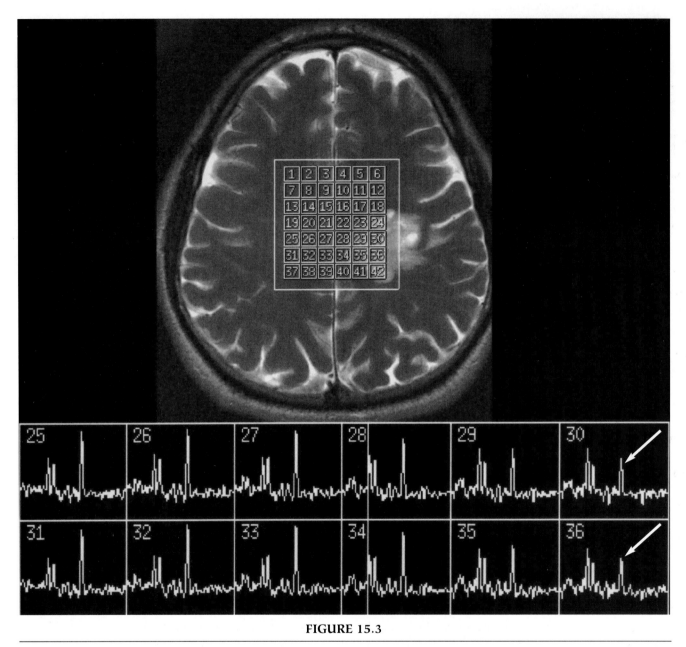

**FIGURE 15.3**

Reduced NAA by proton magnetic resonance spectroscopy in a large, acute demyelinating lesion. Multivoxel spectroscopy shows reduced area under the NAA peak (arrow) within a focal lesion, as compared with adjacent voxels.

Once gadolinium enhancement is observed in the acute MS lesion, it remains visible for about 2 to 8 weeks in most cases (22,23), but enhancement can last from less than 1 week (23) to as long as 16 weeks. Enhancing lesions tend to start out as small homogeneous areas, some of which progress to ringlike enhancement after about 4 weeks (24).

In contrast to relapsing and secondary progressive MS, the acute lesions of primary progressive MS appear to be less intensely inflammatory based on their histopathology and the reduced numbers of enhancing lesions observed by MRI (25,26). Despite this quantitative difference, primary progressive MS shows typical conventional imaging features as compared with relapsing MS (27).

There is now good evidence from biopsy and autopsy series that the acute, inflammatory MS lesion is accompanied by an impressive degree of axonal injury, including full transection within the lesion and along its borders (28,29). The MR spectroscopy literature provides in vivo evidence supporting axonal injury in early MS lesions as well. For example, the concentration of N-

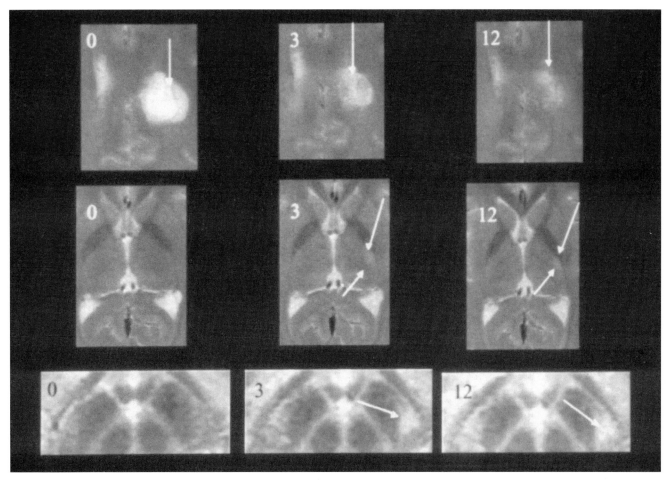

**FIGURE 15.4**

Wallerian degeneration pattern in the corticospinal tract, developing secondary to an acute multiple sclerosis–like lesion in a patient with a monosymptomatic clinical event and a positive magnetic resonance imaging. Such secondary degenerations are probably more common in multiple sclerosis than initially recognized but are difficult to detect in relapsing or more advanced stages of disease due to numerous, superimposed lesions. Reprinted from *J Neuroimmunol*, 1999;98:7–15.

acetylaspartate, a neuronal marker (30–32) is reduced in focal, acute MS-like lesions in patients with a clinically isolated syndrome and a positive MRI (33,34) (Figure 15. 3). Independent evidence from longitudinal studies of patients at risk for MS shows focal enhancing (i.e., inflammatory) lesions are also the precursor to neuronal tract injury, which may contribute to secondary abnormalities of the NAWM (35,36) (Figure 15.4).

### The Acute T2-hyperintense Lesion

The vast majority of acute, enhancing MS lesions are hyperintense on T2-weighted imaging, the T2-hyperintense area including and extending beyond the borders of the enhancing component of the lesion. The more peripheral areas of T2-hyperintensity most likely represent reversible, perilesional edema. Overall, the T2-hyperintense lesion is a relatively nonspecific manifestation of a

locally disturbed water environment and, as such, is nonspecific regarding pathology. In some cases, a rim of T2-hypointensity may be seen. This has been hypothesized to be from the zone of macrophage infiltration along the border of actively demyelinating lesions (11,37). Other regional differences have been described in acute MS lesions based on magnetization transfer or diffusion imaging methods evaluating the core or the periphery of individual lesions or based on the stage of lesion, which may relate in part to histologic variation (38–41).

### Lesion Regression Stages

After reaching a maximal T2-hyperintense lesion size over a period of about 4 to 8 weeks, the T2-hyperintensity (42,43) and the underlying gadolinium enhancing areas decrease over a period of weeks (44,45) (Figure 15.1). Visually, MR enhancement becomes completely non-

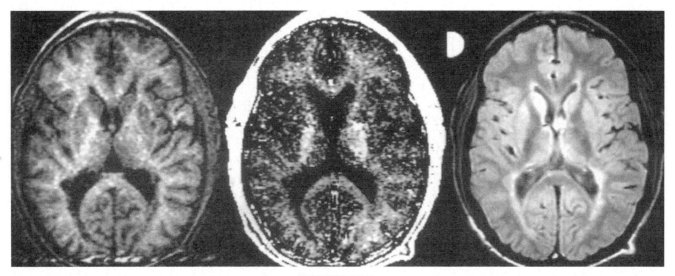

**FIGURE 15.5**

A magnetization transfer ratio (MTR) image (left), a myelin water map (center), and a proton density weighted image (right) from a patient with multiple sclerosis. The myelin water map is based on myelin water percentage at each voxel, determined by considering the multiexponential T2 relaxation decay curve. The MTR and myelin water percentages are uncorrelated in normal white and gray matter, but there is a small significant correlation in multiple sclerosis lesions. Reprinted with permission from *Magn Reson Med* 1998;40:763–758.

apparent during these late subacute stages of lesion evolution. Although this finding suggests that the BBB damage is returning to normal, the barrier is likely to continue to be partially damaged, as indicated by the leakage of serum protein observed in biopsied lesions, irrespective of activity, and as seen in long-standing MS plaques (11,18). After several months, the original MS lesion becomes a smaller residual area of focal T2-hyperintensity. This T2-hyperintense area is the "footprint" of the prior acute event. The footprint is typically about one-third to one-half the size of the initial lesion (42,43). After stabilizing, the vast majority of these lesions will not change over a period of many years, although reactivation, with lesion activity along the periphery or more centrally, does occur in a minority of lesions within a few years, probably analogous to the reactivation described in the pathology literature (46,47).

### The Chronic MS Lesion—T2 Footprints

The chronic MS lesion appears on T2-weighted images as a focal area of elevated signal intensity or as a confluent region of T2-hyperintensity. The ratio of volume of focal to volume of confluent lesion is proportional to the duration of disease in MS population studies. For example, in the earliest stages of disease, as in patients with a clinically isolated syndrome (CIS) and a positive MRI resembling demyelination (CIS+MRI), all the lesions are focal. In a fraction of relapsing MS patients, focal lesions remain the most common finding; many patients will have

regions of confluent lesions. This fraction increases in secondary progressive MS as the mean duration of disease also increases. Confluent lesions have two etiologies. They are in many cases the result of multiple, focal, adjacent lesions that then appear inseparable. More speculative is the hypothesis that confluence results from secondary degeneration around focal lesions or shrinkage of tissue around focal lesions.

Lesions that are hyperintense on T2-weighted images are described as nonspecific with regard to the underlying pathology, but there is some potential to use information from T2-weighted images to categorize these lesions. An early approach to classifying T2-hyperintense lesions was based on maps of the average T2-relaxation time determined from standard two or experimental four-echo spin-echo imaging because some lesion heterogeneity was expected based on known variations in T2 (and T1) relaxation times among lesions (48). A more refined approach to lesion characterization has been described based on the collection of MR data with large numbers of echoes (eg, 32) spanning very short, moderate, and long echo delay times (49–52). This allows more accurate measures of T2 relaxation and at the same time dissection of T2-relaxation curves into multiexponential T2-relaxation components (Figure 15.5). The shortest component may be related to myelin water, an intermediate component possibly related to extracellular water and cytoplasm; a long component may be related to cerebrospinal fluid (49–52). By analyzing the multiexponential decay, normal variations in water content and myelin

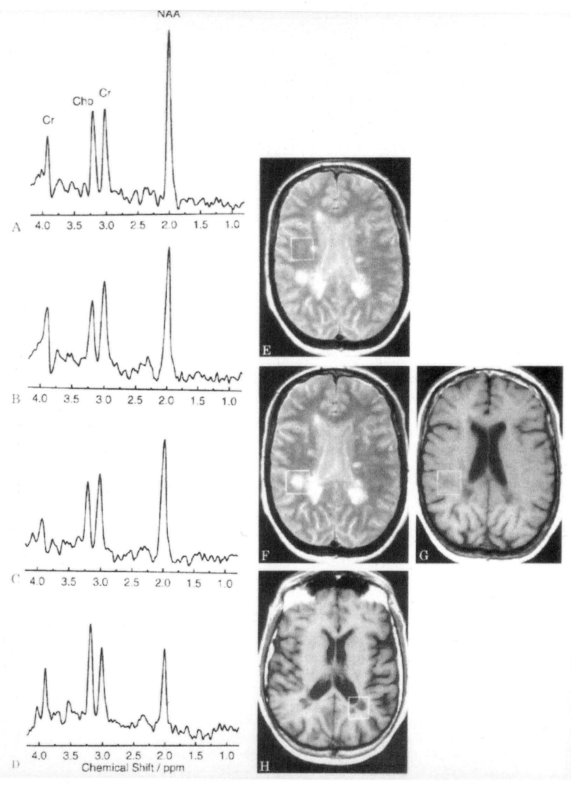

**FIGURE 15.6**

Major reduction in N-acetylaspartate in chronic T1-hypointense lesions, suggesting injury and loss of axons. Compared with the spectrum from normal white matter (NAWM) (**A**), there is a progressive reduction in NAA in NAWM (**B**), from a voxel in a mildly hypointense T1 lesion (**C**), and significant reduction in a typical T1-hypointense lesion (**D**). **E** shows NAWM in a patient with multiple sclerosis; **F** and **G** a T2-hyperintense, mildly T1-hypointense lesion; and H a severely hypointense lesion on T1-weighted image. Reprinted from Van Waldermeer MA, et al. *Ann Neurol* 1999;46:79–87.

water percentage can be seen in normal white and gray matters. Reductions in the moderately short T2-relaxation component have been proposed as a relatively specific marker of demyelination in humans (48–51) and animals (52). Supporting this are recent pathology–MRI correlative studies in MS showing that the moderately short T2 fraction is reduced in chronic MS lesions (50). Experimental evidence shows that, even though both the T2 relaxation measures and MTR assess myelin, they are not equivalent (Figure 15.5). Although the MTR measure may be sensitive to changes to myelin induced by inflammation, the short T2 component is a more specific indicator of myelin content in tissue (51–52).

## Chronic T1-hypointense Lesions

In contrast to the uniform appearance of lesions on standard T2-weighted imaging, T1-weighted images show that chronic MS lesions can be separated into two distinct groups. Most chronic T2-hyperintense lesions are isointense to NAWM (same signal intensity) on T1-weighted images. A smaller fraction of the chronic T2-hyperintense lesions are hypointense to NAWM (lower signal) on T1-weighted images (53–56) (Figure 15.6) Based on population studies, the fraction of hypo- to isointense lesion area on T1-weighted images increases with disease duration or disease stage. In CIS+MRI, most patients have no or a few T1-hypointense lesions. In relapsing MS, about 10 to 20 percent of the T2 lesion volume shows chronic T1-hypointensity (57). That fraction increases in secondary progressive MS.

Good evidence exists that the chronic T1-hypointense lesion fraction is white matter foci enriched for severe injury compared with lesions that are T1-isointense. By histopathologic–ex vivo MRI analyses of autopsy material, the T1-hypointense lesions are characterized primarily by their reduced axonal density, then by their greater matrix dysruption, and less so by their number of reactive astrocytes or their degree of demyelination (56). In vivo, the chronic T1-hypointense lesions have reduced MTRs (58), elevations in diffusion coefficient (41,59), and reduced fractional anisotropy (41). Compared with isointense T1 lesions, hypointense T1 lesions also show a reduction in NAA (55,60) (Figure 15.6). Chronic plaques that appear hypointense on T1-weighted images also show reduced rCBV (21).

## Assessing the Severity of Injury in the Chronic MS Lesion

Based on simple classification schemes using intensity on T1-weighted images or T2-relaxation data, acute and chronic MS lesions are not homogeneous with regard to the underlying pathology. Full characterization of lesions has been an unfulfilled promise. More sophisticated mul-

tivariable analyses are feasible in principle by using combined MR-based approaches (e.g., diffusion based measurements, MTR, T2 and T1 relaxation time measures, chemical characterization by MRS). This is particularly important as evidence mounts for discrete lesion patterns as observed in the recent pathology literature based on immunologic and neurobiologic markers (61), where four patterns of "MS" lesions have been described. Types 1 and 2 show close similarities to T-cell–mediated or T-cell plus antibody–mediated EAE, respectively. Types 3 and 4 are thought to suggest primary oligodendrocyte dystrophy. Whereas patterns of demyelination were heterogeneous in type between patients, they were homogeneous in type within individuals. Although extremely provocative, the relevance of these classifications to everyday MS is not known because there is almost certainly case selection bias in the unusual cases that come to biopsy or autopsy. In the future, a more complete characterization of the focal MS lesion in vivo might include a marker for remyelination (62), neuronal concentration N-acetylasparate (NAA), neuronal (axonal) architecture (diffusion), oligodendrocytes (MR spectroscopy), and specific cellular infiltration. Unfortunately, imaging of specifically tagged cells with iron particles or other markers remains a bench, not a bedside, approach to MS lesion characterization.

Another important area of interest is using a lesion's initial MR characteristics to predict its future: i.e., does it become an area of severe damage and does it remyelinate? The relationship between the area, location, or duration of contrast enhancement and subsequent outcome has been evaluated in several series, with variable conclusions (63). In one series (63) persistently enhancing lesions were more likely to result in T1 holes, but size, location, and configuration ultimately were unrelated to outcome.

## THE NORMAL APPEARING WHITE MATTER IN MS

Although a great deal of attention has been directed at focal MS lesions in the brain and spinal cord, initially by pathology and now by MRI, there is renewed interest in nonfocal or microscopic pathology—that appearing in the NAWN or, more comprehensively, the normal-appearing brain or spinal cord tissue. Abnormality of the NAWM may have several etiologies. Microscopic lesions may be contributory, as indicated in the pathology literature (64). Abnormal NAWM may result from neuronal tract degeneration. Some abnormalities are likely to be artifacts of contamination with focal lesions, the so-called partial volume errors.

The strongest MR evidence for microscopic involvement comes from the highest spatial resolution MR methods, those based on magnetization transfer experiments, with secondary support from lower, but modest resolution diffusion studies, and then from the low-resolution MRS studies. Changes in MTR occur independently of changes on T2-weighted images, and MTR is considered more sensitive than T2-weighted imaging in assessing NAWM in MS (65–71). In general, greater deviation from normal tissue values is seen in secondary progressive MS compared to relapsing MS, for primary progressive MS compared with normal, and for secondary progressive MS NAWM compared with primary progressive MS (69,71). Little is known about the specific pathologies reflected in changes in the MTR, and they are likely multiple. Animal demyelination model studies show that a low MTR correlates with myelin loss and axonal destruction (66). Edema elevates MTR (72). The MTR is an early indicator of Wallerian degeneration in visual tract degeneration after experimental section of the feline visual tract (66) and is more sensitive than conventional spin-echo imaging in that application.

After Christiansen et al. (73) first reported results for water diffusion in MS, subsequent studies have confirmed abnormal diffusion values in focal MS lesions (41,59,74–76), and abnormal diffusion or anisotropy values in the NAWM compared with white matter in normal controls (41,59,74,77–78). Werring et al. (74) and Bammer et al. (41) reported elevated water diffusion values based on the diffusion tensor. Reduced fractional isotropy has also been reported (41,74), although not in all white matter regions (41) (Figure 15.7).

Abnormally low NAA levels have been found in the NAWM in relapsing and progressive MS. Fu et al. (79) found that, although focal lesions in both groups show similarly decreased NAA, the NAA levels in the NAWM were lower for the secondary progressive group. Overall, the reduced NAA in the NAWM accounted for most of the decrease in NAA in the brains in relapsing MS patients followed longitudinally. Although it is commonly accepted that decreases in NAA:creatine ratios determined by MR spectroscopy are the result of reductions in the NAA fraction, in some cases this interpretation has been challenged. Rooney et al. (80) also found a reduced NAA:creatine ratio in the NAWM in relapsing and progressive MS, but evaluation of the absolute concentrations indicated that the ratio reduction was due primarily to increases in the creatine + phosphocreatine resonances. They speculated that the pathologic NAWM harbored increased glial cells, as reflected in the elevated creatine content.

Few studies have addressed the NAWM in earliest MS, as in patients presenting with clinically isolated syndrome and a positive MRI. Mixed results for abnormality have been reported (81,82).

## NEURONAL TRACT DEGENERATION IN MS

Axonal injury including transection occurs within early inflammatory MS lesions and along their periphery

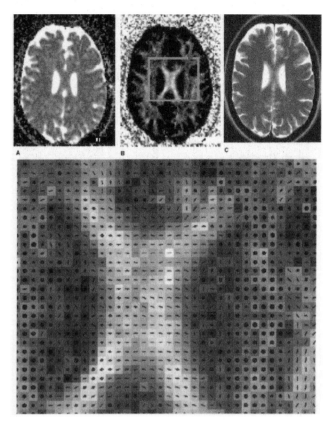

**FIGURE 15.7**

Water diffusion measures in multiple sclerosis (MS). Water diffusion can be measured in vivo by several magnetic resonance (MR) methods. The diffusion tensor approach involves a relatively rigorous data acquisition that allows analyses of diffusion independent of the orientation of the brain to the magnetic gradients in the MR instrument. After acquiring the information for the diffusion tensor, several kinds of data can be displayed. **A.** The mean diffusivity is displayed in a patient with early MS. Arrow indicates focal lesion with increased diffusivity. **B.** This image shows the fractional anisotropy map, with high signal indicative of strongly oriented axons, such as in the corpus callosum (central X-shaped structure). The MS lesion shows decreased anisotropy. **C.** This image shows the corresponding T2-weighted image. **D.** The fiber direction map from the corpus callosum is indicated by lines (through slice component) and circles (components perpendicular to slice).

(28,29) therefore it is likely that these injuries are causally related to more distant axonal degeneration as well. Neural tract degeneration, distant from focal MS lesions, although until recently thought to be rare in MS, has been hypothesized to account for tissue loss in the upper spinal cord in MS, as seen by MRI (83), and may be an important factor in cerebral tissue loss (35,84,85).

The evidence for tract degeneration in MS is largely circumstantial or indirect, but recent studies have provided good evidence that this type of injury does occur

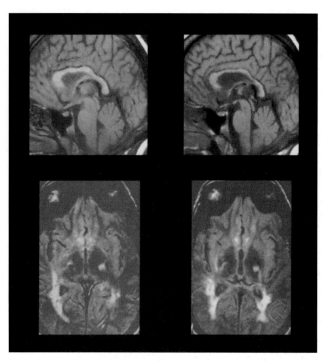

**FIGURE 15.8**

**Top.** Atrophy of the corpus callosum in multiple sclerosis, thought to be related to reduction in the number of axons. Atrophy of the corpus callosum over a 2-year interval in a patient with relapsing multiple sclerosis. **Bottom.** Atrophy resulting in enlarged third ventricle on T2-weighted image. Reprinted from *J Neuroimmunol* 1999;98:7–15.

and occurs in the earliest stages of disease. Evangelou et al (86) detected axonal loss in the NAWM of the corpus callosum in eight postmortem brains from MS patients compared with controls. This confirmed previous reports of volume loss in the corpus callosum in MS in vivo (87) (Figure 15.8) and extended these findings by showing a 53% reduction in axonal number, which was proportionate to reduction in cross-sectional area (86). Ganter et al. (88) found substantial reductions in nerve fiber density in the spinal cord (lateral columns, corticospinal tracts) in patients lacking focal plaques in those regions. De Stefano et al. (89) found abnormally low NAA:creatine ratios in homologous voxels in the contralateral hemisphere 1 month after focal demyelinating lesion development. Similarly, Werring et al. (3) found contralateral abnormalities based on diffusion measures.

My colleagues and I found two indications of tract degeneration temporally and spatially related to acute lesions in the earliest stages of MS (35,36). Changes in the corticospinal tract (Figure 15.4) resembles that seen for Wallerian degeneration in stroke (35). The second pattern suggesting tract degeneration after focal lesions resulted in T2-hyperintenity extending across the corpus callosum over months to years (36). Abnormalities extending

across the callosum may have some relation to findings of decreased NAA and increased transcallosal diffusion coefficient, as discussed above (3,89). Bammer et al. (41) speculated that the abnormally low fractional anisotropy in their studies of otherwise NAWM indicate fiber tract changes remote from MS lesions rather than from diffuse astrocytic hyperplasia and perivascular infiltration. NAA is also decreased along the visual pathways in MS (90). Enlargement of the third ventricle, striking already at the time of the relapsing stages of MS, occurs, presumably related to volume loss in the adjacent tissues. Because few focal lesions are seen in the thalamus by imaging or pathology, the working assumption is that this atrophy may be related to tract degeneration in the thalamus, although there may be an additional contribution from focal lesions or tract degeneration in the internal capsule fibers lateral to the thalamus (85,91).

## MORE DIFFUSE AND GLOBAL EFFECTS OF INJURY—CNS ATROPHY

Although atrophy of the central nervous system (CNS) in MS is well known from the pathology, and primarily autopsy literature (92,93), atrophy was thought until very recently to be a late or rare event in MS (93,94). The recent neuroimaging literature, however, shows that atrophy is not rare; it is initiated in the early stages of disease, and may progress at a surprisingly rapid pace (85,95–97). CNS atrophy in MS can be focal, affecting the central white matter and resulting in ventricular expansion, or global, resulting in a reduced spinal cord area or brain volume. In many cases, in the later stages of disease, focal and global atrophy is seen. Although there is very little direct pathology–MRI correlative data, CNS atrophy in MS is thought to be the result of variable contributions including loss of myelin and axonal loss or thinning (83,98,99). Myelin, of course, represents an important volume fraction of the normal white matter, and microscopy routinely confirms considerable myelin loss in MS lesions (11). The etiology of focal atrophy is believed to be related to focal pathology—likely demyelination, axonal injury, and matrix disruption. The etiology of global atrophy is more speculative but likely is the result of numerous focal lesions, distant degeneration, and possibly other unknown diffuse effects (e.g., "humoral" factors).

Although inflammatory lesions are associated with axonal injury (28,29) and demyelination, large studies have failed to show strong relationships between inflammatory activity and subsequent atrophy. This may be because we use relatively crude methods to evaluate inflammation (enhancing lesion counts), or because atrophy to date has been evaluated over relatively short intervals. However, several, but not all, (85,95,100,101) stud-

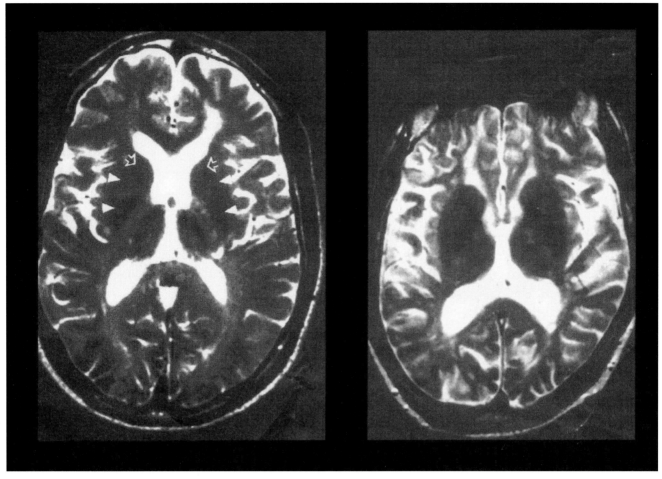

**FIGURE 15.9**

T2-shortened (black-T2) areas in the basal ganglia in multiple sclerosis. The pathologic accumulation of ferritin iron in the basal ganglia in MS has been hypothesized to be the result of interrupted iron transport in neuronal degeneration. Reprinted from Balishi with permission. *Neuoreport* 2000;11:15–21.

ies have detected at least some relationship between inflammation (enhancing lesions) and atrophy. One interesting study of humanized antileukocyte (CD52) monoclonal antibody (Campath 1H) in secondary progressive MS showed progression of brain atrophy and clinical disability despite early and effective suppression of inflammation based on enhancing lesions (102). However, atrophy during the study correlated with the extent of cerebral inflammation (enhancement) in the pretreatment phase, suggesting the possibility of linkage between enhancing (inflammatory) lesions and atrophy, although somewhat temporally dissociated. In the trial of interferon-β1a (Avonex®) in relapsing MS, a reduction in the rate of atrophy was seen in the second year (95). One can hypothesize that delayed slowing of atrophy by effective therapy is explained if atrophy, even after effective therapy, is already set in motion before treatment by prior inflammatory events, which play out over several months to a

year. That time course is in fact seen for atrophy subsequent to Wallerian degeneration in the CNS after stroke and is the time course of the Wallerian degeneration pattern in patients in the earliest stages of MS (35,36).

## OTHER SIGNS OF NEURONAL DEGENERATION—T2-SHORTENED (BLACK-T2) AREAS

Specific regions of the normal brain show decreased signal (T2 shortening) on T2-weighted imaging. There is a good correlation between these areas and iron accumulation, with the iron as ferritin (ferric) iron, as suggested by Perls-stained autopsy material. The principal early iron-containing regions in the brain include the globus pallidus, dentate nucleus, substantia nigra pars reticularis, red nucleus, and, with normal aging, the putamen.

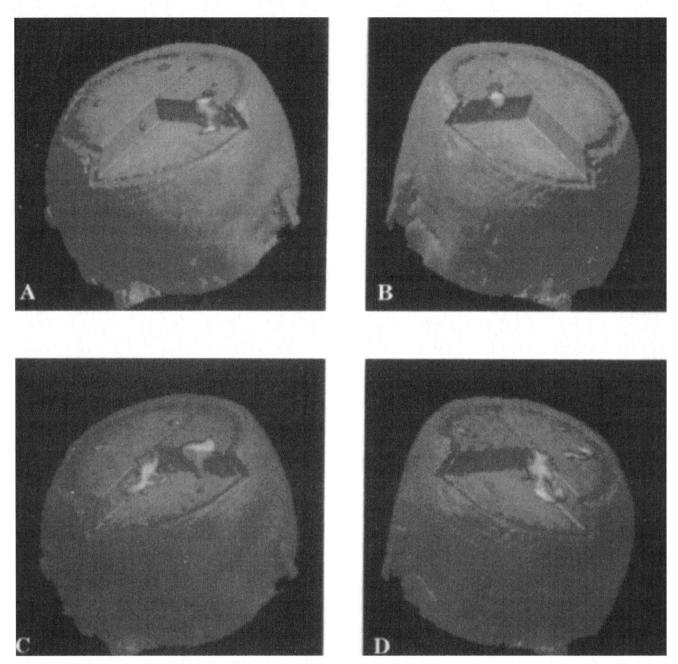

**FIGURE 15.10**

Abnormal cortical activation pattern by functional magnetic resonance imaging in multiple sclerosis. Activation due to finger tapping in a normal control subject (**A.** right hand; **B.** left hand) and a patient with multiple sclerosis (**C.** right hand; **D.** left hand). Activation in the contralateral sensorimotor cortex and supplementary motor cortex. The patient shows increased activation in the ipsilateral sensorimotor cortex and the supplementary motor area, hypothesized to be related to cortical reorganization or unmasking of latent pathways. Reprinted from Lee with permission. *Ann Neurol* 2000;47:606–613.

Pathologic iron accumulation has been described in MS in most (103–105) but not all, series(106). Abnormal degrees of T2-shortening, independent of age have been described in the thalamus, putamen, and caudate, followed in frequency by the Rolandic cortex (103) (Figure 15.9).These regions of T2 shortening seem to be related to longer disease duration and advanced neurologic disability (103,105). Although the basis for abnormal iron accumulation is not known, one theory is that axonal damage may induce an impaired transport of iron, thus resulting in an accumulation of ferritin in the thalamus and putamen.

## PLASTICITY AND RECOVERY

Functional MRI (fMRI) is likely to become an important method to evaluate neuronal systems in MS. Several early studies associated motor impairment in MS with fMRI activation over greater cortical regions (107–110), including recruitment of contralateral and ipsilateral supplementary motor cortex (108,109). These findings have been interpreted as suggesting that cortical reorganization or use of latent pathways may be mechanisms that contribute to functional recovery (108,109). In one study, unilateral optic neuritis was associated with a reduction in the area of activation in the primary visual cortex and a decreased activation for the unaffected eye (111).

## CONCLUSION

In vivo MR analyses using the wide range of methodologies that are currently available provide a great opportunity to determine the pathology of MS in vivo, by complementing and extending what can be learned from direct pathologic examination. Although MR-based methods are always limited by the inherently low signal to noise in the procedure, the virtually unlimited variety of pulse sequences in nuclear magnetic resonance (NMR) and the improved means to evaluate those data have already greatly extended our understanding of MS, from its early to late stages. Future innovations, particularly in high-field, high-resolution imaging approaches (112), MR spectroscopy (113), and molecular tagging approaches (114) will no doubt accelerate our understanding of the underlying pathology, its classification in individuals and patient groups, in predicting good and poor pathologic outcomes, and in monitoring therapeutic intervention.

## References

1. Simon JH. In: Burks JS, Johnson KP (eds.), *Multiple Sclerosis. Diagnosis, Medical Management, and Rehabilitation.* Magnetic resonance imaging in the diagnosis of multiple sclerosis, elucidation of disease, course, and determining prognosis. Demos Medical Publishers. New York. 2000; 99–126.
2. Goodkin DE, Rooney WD, Sloan R, et al. A serial study of new MS lesions and the white matter from which they arise. *Neurology* 1998; 51(6):1689–1697.
3. Werring DJ, Brassat D, Droogan AG, et al. The pathogenesis of lesions and normal-appearing white matter changes in multiple sclerosis: a serial diffusion MRI study. *Brain* 2000; 123(pt 8):1667–1676.
4. Filippi M, Rocca MA, Martino G, Horsfield MA, Comi G. Magnetization transfer changes in the normal appearing white matter precede the appearance of enhancing lesions in patients with multiple sclerosis. *Ann Neurol* 1998; 43(6):809–814.
5. Pike GB, De Stefano N, Narayanan S, et al. Multiple sclerosis: magnetization transfer MR imaging of white matter before lesion appearance on T2-weighted images. *Radiology* 2000; 215(3):824–830.
6. Silver NC, Lai M, Symms MR, et al. Serial magnetization transfer imaging to characterize the early evolution of new MS lesions. *Neurology* 1998; 51(3):758–764.
7. Hirano A, Kawanami T, Llena JF. Electron microscopy of the blood–brain barrier in disease. *Microsc Res Tech* 1994; 27:543–556.
8. Calabresi PA, Tranquill LR, Dambrosia JM, et al. Increase in soluble VCAM-1 correlate with a decrease in MRI lesions in multiple sclerosis treated with interferon β-1b. *Ann Neurol* 1997; 41:669–674.
9. Giovannoni G, Lai M, Thorpe J, et al. Longitudinal study of soluble adhesion molecules in multiple sclerosis: Correlation with gadolinium enhanced magnetic resonance imaging. *Neurology* 1997; 48:1557–1565.
10. Trojano M, Avoilio C, Simone IL, et al. Soluble intercellular adhesion molecule-1 in serum and cerebrospinal fluid of clinically active relapsing-remitting multiple sclerosis. *Neurology* 1996; 47:1535–1541.
11. Bruck W, Bitsch A, Kolenda H, et al. Inflammatory central nervous system demyelination: Correlation of magnetic resonance imaging findings with lesion pathology. *Ann Neurol* 1997; 42:783–793.
12. Katz D, Taubenberger JK, Cannella B, et al. Correlation between magnetic resonance imaging findings and lesion development in chronic, active multiple sclerosis. *Ann Neurol* 1993; 34:661–669.
13. Nesbit GM, Forbes GS, Scheithauer BW, et al. Multiple sclerosis: Histopathologic and and/or CT correlation in 37 cases at biopsy and three cases at autopsy. *Radiology* 1991; 180(2):467–474.
14. Hawkins CP, Munro PMG, Mackenzie F, et al. Duration and selectivity of blood-brain barrier breakdown in chronic relapsing experimental allergic encephalomyelitis studied by gadolinium-DTPA and protein markers. *Brain* 1990; 113:365–378.
15. Karlik SJ, Munoz D, St Louis J, Strejan G. Correlation between MRI and clinico-pathological manifestations in Lewis rats protected from experimental allergic encephalomyelitis by acylated synthetic peptide of myelin basic protein. *Magn Reson Imaging.* 1999; 17(5):731–737.
16. Namer IJ, Steibel J, Piddlesden SJ, et al. Magnetic resonance imaging of antibody-mediated demyelinating experimental allergic encephalomyelitis. *J Neuroimmun* 1994; 54:41–50.
17. Seeldrayers PA, Syha J, Morrisey SP, et al. Magnetic resonance imaging investigation of blood-brain barrier damage in adoptive transfer experimental autoimmune encephalomyelitis. *J Neuroimmun* 1993; 46:199–206.
18. Kwon EE, Prineas JW. Blood–brain barrier abnormalities in long-standing multiple sclerosis lesions. An immunohistochemical study. *J Neuropathol Exp Neurol* 1994; 53(6):625–636.
19. Larsson HB, Tofts PS. Measurement of blood-brain barrier permeability using dynamic Gd-DTPA scanning—a comparison of methods. *Magn Reson Med* 1992; 24(1):174–176.
20. Tofts PS, Kermode AG. Measurement of the blood-brain barrier permeability and leakage space using dynamic MR imaging. 1. Fundamental concepts. *Magn Reson Med* 1991; 17(2):357–367.
21. Haselhorst R, Kappos L, Bilecen D, et al. Dynamic susceptibility contrast MR imaging of plaque development in multiple sclerosis: application of an extended blood-brain barrier leakage correction. *J Magn Reson Imaging* 2000; 11(5):495–505.
22. Harris JO, Frank JA, Patronas N, et al. Serial gadolinium-enhanced magnetic resonance imaging scans in patients with early, relapsing-remitting multiple sclerosis: Implications for clinical trials and natural history. *Ann Neurol* 1991; 29:548–555.
23. Lai HM, Hodgson T, Gawne-Cain M, et al. A preliminary study into the sensitivity of disease activity detection by serial weekly magnetic resonance imaging in multiple sclerosis. *J Neurol Neurosurg Psychiatry* 1996; 60:339–341.
24. Guttmann CRG, Ahn SS, Hsu L, et al. The evolution of multiple sclerosis lesions on serial MR. *AJNR* 1995; 16:1481–1491.
25. Silver NC, Good CD, Barker GJ, et al. Sensitivity of contrast enhanced MRI in multiple sclerosis. Effects of gadolinium dose, magnetization transfer contrast and delayed imaging. *Brain* 1997; 120:1149–1161.
26. Thompson AJ, Polman CH, Miller DH, et al. Primary progressive multiple sclerosis. *Brain* 1997; 120:1085–1096.
27. Kremenchutzky M, Lee D, Rice GP, Ebers GC. Diagnostic brain MRI findings in primary progressive multiple sclerosis. *Mult Scler* 2000; 6(2):81–85.

28. Ferguson B, Matyszak MK, Esiri MM, Perry VH. Axonal damage in acute multiple sclerosis lesions. *Brain* 1997; 120:393–399.
29. Trapp BD, Peterson J, Pansohoff RM, et. al. Axonal transection in the lesions of multiple sclerosis. *N Engl J Med* 1998; 338:278–285.
30. Arnold DL. Magnetic resonance spectroscopy: imaging axonal damage in MS. *J Neuroimmunol* 1999; 98(1):2–6.
31. Miller BL. A review of chemical issues in 1H NMR spectroscopy: N-acetyl-L-aspartate, creatine and choline. *NMR Biomedicine* 1991; 4:47–52.
32. Morissey SP. Magnetic resonance spectroscopy in experimental allergic encephalomyelitis. In: Filippi M, Arnold DL, Comi G. (eds.), *Magnetic Resonance Spectroscopy in Multiple Sclerosis*. Milan: Springer-Verlag 2001; (4):51–59.
33. Brex PA, Gomez-Anson B, Parker GJ, et al. Proton MR spectroscopy in clinically isolated syndromes suggestive of multiple sclerosis. *J Neurol Sci* 1999; 166(1):16–22.
34. De Stefano N, Narayanan S, Matthews PM, et al. In vivo evidence for axonal dysfunction remote from focal cerebral demyelination of the type seen in multiple sclerosis. *Brain* 1999; 122(pt 10):1933–1939.
35. Simon JH, Kinkel RP, Jacobs L, et al. A Wallerian degeneration pattern in patients at risk for MS. *Neurology* 2000; 54:1155–1160.
36. Simon JH, Jacobs L, Kinkel RP. Transcallosal bands: A sign of neuronal tract degeneration in early MS? *Neurology* 2001; 57:1888–1890.
37. Powell T, Sussman JG, Davies-Jones GAB. MR imaging in acute multiple sclerosis: ringlike appearance in plaques suggesting the presence of paramagnetic free radicals. *AJNR* 1992; 13:1544–1546.
38. Roychowdhury S, Maldjian JA, Grossman RI. Multiple sclerosis: comparison of trace apparent diffusion coefficients with MR enhancement pattern of lesions. *AJNR Am J Neuroradiol* 2000; 21(5):869–874.
39. Cercignani M, Iannucci G, Rocca MA, et al. Pathologic damage in MS assessed by diffusion-weighted and magnetization transfer MRI. *Neurology* 2000; 54(5):1139–1144.
40. Tievsky AL, Ptak T, Farkas J. Investigation of apparent diffusion coefficient and diffusion tensor anisotrophy in acute and chronic multiple sclerosis lesions. *AJNR* 1999; 20(8):1491–1499.
41. Bammer R, Augustin M, Strasser-Fuchs S, et al. Magnetic resonance diffusion tensor imaging for characterizing diffuse and focal white matter abnormalities in multiple sclerosis. *Magn Reson Med* 2000; 44(4):583–591.
42. Koopsmans RA, Li DKB, Oger JJF, et al. The lesion of multiple sclerosis: Imaging of acute and chronic stages. *Neurology* 1989; 39:959–963.
43. Wiebe S, Lee DH, Karlik SJ, et al. Serial cranial and spinal cord magnetic resonance imaging in multiple sclerosis. *Ann Neurol* 1992; 32:643–650.
44. Kermode AG, Tofts PS, Thompson AJ, et al. Heterogeneity of blood-brain barrier changes in multiple sclerosis: an MRI study with gadolinium-DTPA enhancement. *Neurology* 1990; 40(2):229–235.
45. Miller DH, Rudge P, Johnson G, et al. Serial gadolinium enhanced magnetic resonance imaging in multiple sclerosis. *Brain* 1988; 111:927–939.
46. Prineas JW, Barnard RO, Revesz T, et al. Multiple sclerosis. Pathology of recurrent lesions. *Brain* 1993; 116(pt 3):681–693.
47. Prineas JW, Barnard RO, Kwon EE, et al. Multiple sclerosis: remyelination of nascent lesions. *Ann Neurol* 1993; 33(2):137–151.
48. Larsson HBW, Frederiksen J, Kjaer L, et al. In Vivo determination of T1 and T2 in the brain of patients with severe but stable multiple sclerosis. *Magn Reson Med* 1988; 7:43–55.
49. MacKay A, Whittall K, Adler J, et al. In vivo visualization of myelin water in brain by magnetic resonance. *Magn Reson Med* 1994; 31(6):673–677.
50. Moore GR, Leung E, MacKay AL, et al. A pathology-MRI study of the short-T2 component in formalin-fixed multiple sclerosis brain. *Neurology* 2000; 55(10):1506–1510.
51. Vavasour IM, Whittall KP, MacKay AL, et al. W. A comparison between magnetization transfer ratios and myelin water percentages in normals and multiple sclerosis patients. *Magn Reson Med* 1998; 40(5):763–768.
52. Gareau PJ, Rutt BK, Karlik SJ, Mitchell JR. Magnetization transfer and multicomponent T2 relaxation measurements with

histopathologic correlation in an experimental model of MS. *J Magn Reson Imaging* 2000; 11(6):586–595.
53. Truyen L, van Waesberghe JH, van Walderveen MA, et al. Accumulation of hypointense lesions ("black holes") on T1 spin-echo MRI correlates with disease progression in multiple sclerosis. *Neurology* 1996; 47(6):1469–1476.
54. van Waesberghe JH, van Walderveen MA, Castelijns JA, et al. Patterns of lesion development in multiple sclerosis: Longitudinal observations with T1-weighted spin-echo and magnetization transfer MR. *AJNR* 1998; 19(4):675–683.
55. van Walderveen MA, Barkhof F, Pouwels PJ, et al. Neuronal damage in T1-hypointense multiple sclerosis lesions demonstrated in vivo using proton magnetic resonance spectroscopy. *Ann Neurol* 1999; 46(1):79–87.
56. van Walderveen MA, Kamphorst W, Scheltens P, et al. Histopathologic correlate of hypointense lesions on T1-weighted spin-echo MRI in multiple sclerosis. *Neurology* 1998; 50(5):1282–1288.
57. Simon JH, Lull J, Jacobs LD, et al. A longitudinal study of T1 hypointense lesions in relapsing MS: MSCRG trial of interferon beta-1a. Multiple Sclerosis Collaborative Research Group. *Neurology* 2000; 55(2):185–192.
58. Loevner LA, Grossman RI, Cohen JA, et al. Microscopic disease in normal-appearing white matter on conventional MR images in patients with multiple sclerosis: Assessment with magnetization-transfer measurements. *Radiology* 1995; 196(2):511–515.
59. Filippi M, Iannucci G, Cercignani M, et al. A quantitative study of water diffusion in multiple sclerosis lesions and normal-appearing white matter using echo-planar imaging. *Arch Neurol* 2000; 57(7):1017–1021.
60. Brex PA, Parker GJ, Leary SM, et al. Lesion heterogeneity in multiple sclerosis: a study of the relations between appearances on T1 weighted images, T1 relaxation times, and metabolite concentrations. *J Neurol Neurosurg Psychiatry* 2000; 68(5):627–632.
61. Lucchinetti C, Bruck W, Parisi J, et al. Heterogeneity of multiple sclerosis lesions: Implications for the pathogenesis of demyelination. *Ann Neurol* 2000; 47(6):707–717.
62. Deloire-Grassin MS, Brochet B, Quesson B, et al. In vivo evaluation of remyelination in rat brain by magnetization transfer imaging. *J Neurol Sci* 2000; 178(1):10–16.
63. Ciccarelli O, Giugni E, Paolillo A, et al. Magnetic resonance outcome of new enhancing lesions in patients with relapsing-remitting multiple sclerosis. *Eur J Neurol* 1999; 6(4):455–459.
64. Allen IV, McKeown SR. A histological, histochemical and biochemical study of the macroscopically normal white matter in multiple sclerosis. *J Neurol Sci* 1979; 41(1):81–91.
65. Grossman RI. Application of magnetization transfer imaging to multiple sclerosis. *Neurology* 1999; 53(suppl 3)S8–S11.
66. Lexa FJ, Grossman RI, Rosenquist AC. Dyke Award Paper. MR of Wallerian degeneration in the feline visual system: characterization by magnetization transfer rate with histopathologic correlation. *Am J Neurorad* 1994; 15(2):201–212.
67. Loevner LA, Grossman RI, Cohen JA, et al. Microscopic disease in normal-appearing white matter on conventional MR images in patients with multiple sclerosis: Assessment with magnetization-transfer measurements. *Radiology* 1995; 196(2):511–515.
68. van Buchem MA, McGowan JC, Kolson DL, Polansky M, Grossman RI. Quantitative volumetric magnetization transfer analysis in multiple sclerosis: estimation of macroscopic and microscopic disease burden. *Magn Reson Med* 1996; 36(4):632–636.
69. Tortorella C, Viti B, Bozzali M, et al. A magnetization transfer histogram study of normal-appearing brain tissue in MS. *Neurology* 2000; 54(1):186–193.
70. Richert ND, Frank JA. Magnetization transfer imaging to monitor clinical trials in multiple sclerosis. *Neurology* 1999; 53(suppl 3):S29S32.
71. Filippi M, Inglese M, Rovaris M, et al. Magnetization transfer imaging to monitor the evolution of MS: a 1-year follow-up study. *Neurology* 2000; 55(7):940–946.
72. Dousset V, Grossman RI, Ramer KN, et al. Experimental allergic encephalomyelitis and multiple sclerosis: lLsion characterization with magnetization transfer imaging. *Radiology* 1992; 182(2):483–491.
73. Christiansen P, Gideon P, Thomsen C, et al. Increased water self-

diffusion in chronic plaques and in apparently normal white matter in patients with multiple sclerosis. *Acta Neurol Scand* 1993; 87(3):195–199.

74. Werring DJ, Clark CA, Barker GJ, Thompson AJ, Miller DH. Diffusion tensor imaging of lesions and normal-appearing white matter in multiple sclerosis. *Neurology* 1999; 52(8):1626–1632.

75. Tievsky AL, Ptak T, Farkas J. Investigation of apparent diffusion coefficient and diffusion tensor anisotrophy in acute and chronic multiple sclerosis lesions. *AJNR* 1999; 20(8):1491–1499.

76. Cercignani M, Iannucci G, Rocca MA, et al. Pathologic damage in MS assessed by diffusion-weighted and magnetization transfer MRI. *Neurology* 2000; 54(5):1139–1144.

77. Horsfield MA, Lai M, Webb SL, et al. Apparent diffusion coefficients in benign and secondary progressive multiple sclerosis by nuclear magnetic resonance. *Magn Reson Med* 1996; 36(3):393–400.

78. Droogan AG, Clark CA, Werring DJ, et al. Comparison of multiple sclerosis clinical subgroups using navigated spin echo diffusion-weighted imaging. *Magn Reson Imaging* 1999; 17(5):653–661.

79. Fu L, Matthews PM, De Stefano N, et al. Imaging axonal damage of normal-appearing white matter in multiple sclerosis. *Brain* 1998; 121(pt 1):103–113.

80. Rooney WD, Goodkin DE, Schuff N, et al. 1H MRSI of normal appearing white matter in multiple sclerosis. *Mult Scler* 1997; 3(4):231–237.

81. Iannucci G, Tortorella C, Rovaris M, et al. Prognostic value of MR and magnetization transfer imaging findings in patients with clinically isolated syndromes suggestive of multiple sclerosis at presentation. *AJNR* 2000; 21(6):1034–1038.

82. Kaiser JS, Grossman RI, Polansky M, et al. Magnetization transfer histogram analysis of monosymptomatic episodes of neurologic dysfunction: preliminary findings. *AJNR* 2000; 21(6):1043–1047.

83. McDonald WI. Rachelle Fishman-Matthew Moore Lecture. The pathological and clinical dynamics of multiple sclerosis. *J Neuropathol Exp Neurol* 1994; 53(4):338–343.

84. Simon JH. Brain and spinal cord atrophy in multiple sclerosis. Neuroimaging Clinics of North America. Frank JA (ed.) *Advances in Multiple Sclerosis*. WB Saunders, Philadelphia. 2000, 10(4)753–769.

85. Simon JH, Jacobs LD, Campion A, et al. A longitudinal study of brain atrophy in relapsing multiple sclerosis. *Neurology* 1999; 53:139–148.

86. Evangelou N, Esiri MM, Smith S, Palace J, Matthews PM. Quantitative pathological evidence for axonal loss in normal appearing white matter in multiple sclerosis. *Ann Neurol* 2000; 47:391–395.

87. Simon JH, Schiffer RB, Rudick RA, Herndon RM. Quantitative determination of MS-induced corpus callosum atrophy in vivo using MR imaging. *AJNR* 1987; 8(4):599–604.

88. Ganter P, Prince C, Esiri MM. Spinal cord axonal loss in multiple sclerosis: A post-mortem study. *Neuropathol Appl Neurobiol* 1999; 25(6):459–467.

89. De Stefano N, Narayanan S, Matthews PM, et al. In vivo evidence for axonal dysfunction remote from focal cerebral demyelination of the type seen in multiple sclerosis. *Brain* 1999; 122(pt 10):1933–1939.

90. Heide AC, Kraft GH, Slimp JC, et al. Cerebral N-acetylaspartate is low in patients with multiple sclerosis and abnormal visual evoked potentials. *AJNR* 1998; 19(6):1047–1054.

91. Simon JH. From enhancing lesions to brain atrophy in relapsing MS. *J Neuroimmunol* 1999; 98(1):7–15.

92. Barnard RO, Triggs M. Corpus callosum in multiple sclerosis. *J Neurol Neurosurg Psychiatry* 1974; 37:1259–1264.

93. Lumsden CE. The neuropathology of multiple sclerosis. In: Vinken PJ, Bruyn GW (eds.), *Handbook of Clinical Neurology, vol 9. Multiple Sclerosis and Other Demyelinating Diseases.* Amsterdam: Elsevier; 1970; 217–309.

94. Adams RD, Kubik CS. The morbid anatomy of the demyelinative diseases. *AJM* 1952; 12: 510–546.

95. Rudick RA, Fisher E, Lee JC, et al. Use of the brain parenchymal fraction to measure whole brain atrophy in relapsing-remitting MS. Multiple Sclerosis Collaborative Research Group. *Neurology* 1999; 53(8):1698–1704.

96. Simon JH. Brain and Spinal cord atrophy as a surrogate measure of disease progression in multiple sclerosis. *CNS Drugs* 2001, 15:427–436.

97. Brex PA, Jenkins R, Fox NC, et al. Detection of ventricular enlargement in patients at the earliest clinical stage of MS. *Neurology* 2000; 54(8):1689–1691.

98. Prineas JW. The neuropathology of multiple sclerosis. In: Koetsier JC (ed.), *Handbook of Clinical Neurology: Vol 3. Demyelinating Diseases.* Amsterdam: Elsevier Science Publishers; 1985; (47):213–257.

99. Prineas JW, Connell F, Raine CS. The fine structure of chronically active multiple sclerosis plaques. *Neurology* 1978; 28:68–75.

100. Coles AJ, Wing MG, Molyneux P, et al. Monoclonal antibody treatment exposes three mechanisms underlying the clinical course of multiple sclerosis. *Ann Neurol* 1999; 46(3):296–304.

101. Kappos L, Moeri D, Radue EW, et al. Predictive value of gadolinium-enhanced magnetic resonance imaging for relapse rate and changes in disability or impairment in multiple sclerosis: a meta-analysis. Gadolinium MRI Meta-analysis Group. *Lancet* 1999; 353(9157):964–969.

102. Paolillo A, Coles AJ, Molyneux PD, et al. Quantitative MRI in patients with secondary progressive MS treated with monoclonal antibody Campath 1H. *Neurology* 1999; 53(4):751–757.

103. Bakshi R, Shaikh ZA, Janardhan V. MRI T2 shortening ('black T2') in multiple sclerosis: frequency, location, and clinical correlation. *Neuroreport* 2000; 11(1):15–21.

104. Drayer B, Burger P, Hurwitz B, Dawson D, Cain J. Reduced signal intensity on MR images of thalamus and putamen in multiple sclerosis: Increased iron content? *AJR* 1987; 149(2):357–363.

105. Nishii T, Hirata A, Masaki T, et al. (Reduced signal intensity of T2 weighted MR imaging of thalamus and putamen in multiple sclerosis in Japan). *Rinsho Shinkeigaku* 2000; 40(7):677–682.

106. Grimaud J, Millar J, Thorpe JW, et al. Signal intensity on MRI of basal ganglia in multiple sclerosis. *J Neurol Neurosurg Psychiatry* 1995; 59(3):306–308.

107. Yousry TA, Berry I, Filippi M. Functional magnetic resonance imaging in multiple sclerosis. *J Neurol Neurosurg Psychiatry* 1998; 64(suppl 1):S85–S87.

108. Lee M, Reddy H, Johansen-Berg H, et al. The motor cortex shows adaptive functional changes to brain injury from multiple sclerosis. *Ann Neurol* 2000; 47(5):606–613.

109. Reddy H, Narayanan S, Matthews PM, et al. Relating axonal injury to functional recovery in MS. *Neurology* 2000; 54(1):236–239.

110. Rombouts SA, Lazeron RH, Scheltens P, et al. Visual activation patterns in patients with optic neuritis: an fMRI pilot study. *Neurology* 1998; 50(6):1896–1899.

111. Gareau PJ, Gati JS, Menon RS, et al. Reduced visual evoked responses in multiple sclerosis patients with optic neuritis: Comparison of functional magnetic resonance imaging and visual evoked potentials. *Mult Scler* 1999; 5(3):161–164.

112. Keiper MD, Grossman RI, Hirsch JA, et al. MR identification of white matter abnormalities in multiple sclerosis: A comparison between 1.5 T and 4 T. *AJNR* 1998; 19(8):1489–1493.

113. Bartha R, Drost DJ, Menon RS, Williamson PC. Comparison of the quantification precision of human short echo time (1)H spectroscopy at 1.5 and 4.0 Tesla. *Magn Reson Med* 2000; 44(2):185–192.

114. Xu S, Jordan EK, Brocke S, et al. Study of relapsing remitting experimental allergic encephalomyelitis SJL mouse model using MION-46L enhanced in vivo MRI: early histopathological correlation. *J Neurosci Res* 1998; 52(5):549–558.

# 16 Mechanisms of Repair, Adaptation, and Recovery of Function in Multiple Sclerosis

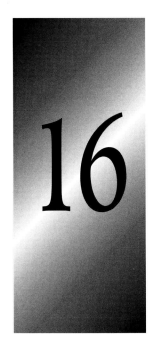

*Robert M. Herndon, M.D.*

Optic Neuritis...very rarely issues in complete blindness. This is peculiarly worthy of notice, especially if you remember that patches of sclerosis have been found, after death, occupying the whole thickness of the nerve trunks in the optic nerves, in cases, where during life, an enfeeblement of sight simply had been noted. This apparent disproportion between the symptoms and the lesion constitutes one of the most powerful arguments which can be invoked to show that the functional continuity of the nerve tubes is not absolutely interrupted...

Jean Martin Charcot, 1877 (1)

P atients with acute optic neuritis usually recover vision quite well and are left with minimal residual effects (2). Most patients with multiple sclerosis (MS) also recover from exacerbations early in the disease, sometimes without clinically detectable residua. Despite these examples of good functional recovery, the dogma in the 1950s was that oligodendrocytes, like neurons, could not reproduce, remyelination did not occur, and demyelinated fibers could not conduct. A little historic knowledge would have shown that the dogma regarding conduction by demyelinated fibers was incorrect (1). That remyelination does occur was first established by Bunge et al. who reported electron microscopic studies of remyelination in the cat spinal cord after bar-

botage induced demyelination in 1961 (3). Subsequently, remyelination has been demonstrated in a host of animals including humans (4). Studies demonstrating conduction in demyelinated fibers began in the peripheral nervous system in the early 1960s (5) and in the central nervous system (CNS) soon thereafter (6).

As MS progresses, the ability to recover from exacerbations decreases, and permanent irreversible disability accumulates. Recovery from exacerbations and adaptation to compensate for functional losses occurs over periods ranging from hours to months or even years. Multiple mechanisms contribute to functional improvement. The most important of these appear to be 1) resolution of the inflammatory response, 2) remyelination, 3) restoration of conduction in demyelinated fibers, 4) adaptation, and 5) neural plasticity. In this chapter I discuss known and postulated mechanisms of recovery, why the time course of recovery varies so widely, and why, ultimately, permanent, nonrecoverable disability accumulates.

## RESOLUTION OF THE INFLAMMATORY RESPONSE

The role of the inflammatory response itself in interfering with conduction, as opposed to the physical destruction and phagocytosis of myelin, has not been well characterized but is undoubtedly important. The local inflammation and edema are accompanied by release of numerous enzymes, chemokines, and cytokines into the extracellular space (see Chapters 11 and 12). Most of these enzymes are secreted by macrophages and are capable of damaging a variety of structures including myelin and axons. Enzymes released include a variety of proteases, lipases, neuraminidase, phosphatases, and glycosidases. Their actions are potentiated by complement (7). Phospholipase, in part by producing lysolecithins that have a powerful detergent effect, may be one of the most destructive to myelin. Phospholipase also interrupts conduction and alters or destroys sodium channels as measured by saxitoxin binding (8,9). Proteases alone appear to cause little damage to peripheral nodes of Ranvier, probably because the proteins are largely inaccessible to the enzymes; however, it is not known whether this holds for central nodes that, unlike peripheral nodes, are not covered by overlapping folds of myelin. In addition, in the presence of lipases, membrane proteins may become accessible to proteases that then cause further membrane damage. Damage from enzymes in the inflammatory milieu is not likely to be limited to ion channels on the axonal membrane but probably includes other functionally important surface structures.

Lipolytic enzymes in the inflammatory milieu such as phospholipase A2 can also damage the axonal membrane itself by creating lysolipids from the myelin lipids. These, through their detergent action, attack myelin and axonal membranes. Indeed, one model used to study demyelination in experimental animals is the focal injection of lysophosphatidyl choline (10), which is produced by the action of phospholipase on myelin lipids. Enzymes in the axonal membrane can inactivate lysolipids by re-acylating them, which provides some degree of protection, but when lysolipids are present in a high enough concentration, they may attack lipids in the axon and thus may contribute significantly to the axonal destruction that occurs acutely in the demyelinating lesions (11). In addition, the detergent effect of lysolipids released by the action of lipases contributes to the spread of myelin damage in the MS plaque. With resolution of the inflammation and disappearance of the inflammatory milieu, surviving axons that have retained their myelin can replace damaged ion channels essential to nerve conduction and regain the ability to conduct impulses. Demyelinated fibers need to undergo further changes before they can resume conduction, as detailed below. There is evidence that the nodal membrane is damaged by phospholipase and by lysolipids generated from myelin. Relatively little is known of the time course of replacement of damaged channels in the nodal region once the inflammatory response resolves. The process most likely occurs through slow transport. Partial replacement might occur rapidly by using channels already in the pipeline. However, generation of additional channels almost certainly occurs in the soma so that complete replacement may take time for the transport of additional channels from the soma. The process of replacement may be significantly impaired in axons, with additional demyelinated areas upstream from the new demyelinated region because transport is almost certain to be impaired.

## REMYELINATION

Our understanding of remyelination in the CNS began with the classic report on remyelination in cat spinal cord (3). Until that time, remyelination was thought not to occur in the CNS even though remyelination was well known in the peripheral nervous system. Since then, remyelination has been repeatedly demonstrated in a variety of experimental demyelinating conditions including experimental autoimmune encephalomyelitis (10,12,13), mouse hepatitis virus infection (14), Theilers virus infection (15), and in cuprizone (16), and lysolecithin-induced demyelination (17) in humans (18).

The characteristics of myelin generated during remyelination differ from those of normal myelin. Typically internodes are much shorter (Figure 16.1), the relationship between myelin thickness and fiber dimeter is lost, and fibers of widely different diameters have similar myelin thickness. With this information, it soon became clear that "shadow plaques" are not areas of partial demyelination but of remyelination. Subsequently, Prineas demonstrated that remyelination occurs regularly early in the course of relapsing-remitting MS but with decreasing frequency as the disease progresses, so there was little evidence of remyelination in advanced disease. In some cases, Wallerian degeneration in a tract will cause an area of pallor that superficially resembles a shadow plaque but is secondary to axon loss. Examination at high magnifications show that the myelin is of normal thickness but there are fewer than normal myelinated fibers.

Regeneration of oligodendrocytes (Figure 16.2) as part of the process of remyelination was demonstrated in experimental animals (14,16), and there is evidence of persistence and regeneration of oligodendrocytes in humans. The source of the newly generated oligodendrocytes involved in remyelination is most likely from undifferentiated glial precursor cells. That pre-existing mature oligodendrocytes can divide has been clearly demonstrated (19,20). Indeed, Ludwin (19) demonstrated division occurring in oligodendrocytes that had retained their attachment to myelin. In contrast, Blakemore produced evidence that the oligodendrocytes involved in remyelination are derived from undifferentiated glial precursor cells (21).

Little work has been done on conduction speed and safety in remyelinated central axons. In the periphery, remyelinated fibers can achieve 95 percent of their normal conduction rate. In the CNS, where the regenerated

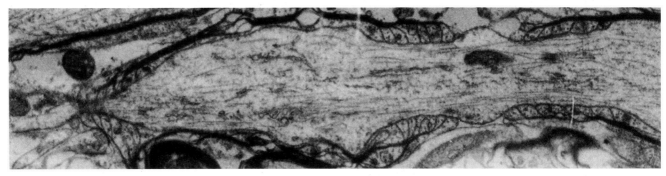

**FIGURE 16.1**

Electron micrograph of a remyelinated fiber. A node can be seen at the far left and another node can be seen right of center with adjacent paranodal loops. The fiber is from a mouse recovering from mouse hepatitis virus infection. The distance between the nodes is 6 μm. Magnification, 15000X. From Herndon RM, Weiner LP, unpublished data.

myelin remains thinner than normal, it is likely that conduction is slowed more than it is in the periphery, but I am unaware of any data on the speed or safety of conduction after remyelination over the full length of the previously demyelinated region. In any case, it is very clear that remyelination significantly improves conduction and plays an important role in recovery from acute attacks of MS.

## RESTORATION OF CONDUCTION IN DEMYELINATED FIBERS

The occurrence of conduction in demyelinated fibers was inferred by Charcot (1), but until the 1960s, little was known regarding how this occurred or what was necessary for restoration of conduction after demyelination. During the process of demyelination, conduction failure is probably invariable in the demyelinated fibers. Clinically silent lesions that have been demonstrated to occur in major motor and sensory pathways without causing clinically obvious deficits (21–23) probably occur when demyelination affects a minority of fibers in a pathway at any one time, leaving intact conduction in other fibers. Other lesions appear clinically silent because they occur in areas of the white matter that do not produce clinically eloquent deficits. The causes of conduction failure during demyelination are not completely understood but may include 1) damage to the nodal sodium channels (8,9),

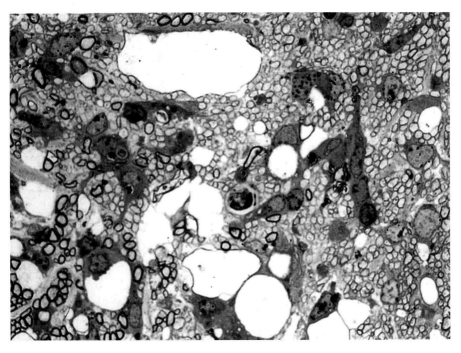

**FIGURE 16.2**

Autoradiograph of a regenerated oligodendrocytes and astrocytes labeled wih tritiated thymidine after mouse hepatitis virus infection. Thymidine in a dose of 6 ML/g was given every 12 hours from the 13th through the 19th day after intracerebral inoculation with mouse hepatitis virus. The mice were anesthetized and perfused with a glutaraldehyde/ paraformaldehyde fixative 28 days postinoculation. Note the uniformity of myelin thickness unrelated to fiber diameter and the silver grains overlying astrocytic and oligodendrocytic nuclei. Magnification, 400X. Herndon RM, Weiner, LP unpublished data. (X1200)

2) virtual absence of sodium channels from the internodal membrane (24–26), and 3) increased membrane capacitance (impedance mismatch) in the demyelinated region (25).

The internodal membrane normally contains very few sodium channels (24,27). Unmyelinated fibers in the rat sympathetic trunk have a sodium channel density of about $200/\mu m2$, close to the theoretical density needed for conduction based on computer simulation. If the sodium channels of a myelinated fiber were evenly distributed over the length of the fiber, the density would be much less than half that in most unmyelinated fibers and would be too few to support conduction (29). For continuous conduction to develop in a demyelinated axon, additional sodium channels must be inserted into the axonal membrane. When the axon is demyelinated, the sodium channels from the node remain clustered and do not spread out evenly over the axolemma (29). The sodium channels appear to be anchored at the node and remain clustered even after the myelin is gone. Thus insertion of new sodium channels is a prerequisite for the restoration of continuous conduction. The newly inserted sodium channels appear to be made in the soma, are transported down the axon by the slow transport system, and differ from those normally present at the nodes (29) but clearly are capable of supporting continuous conduction, albeit with a markedly decreased velocity and safety margin for conduction.

Increased membrane capacitance and the resulting increase in capacitative charge on the demyelinated axolemma results in an increase in the amount of current required to depolarize the membrane to threshold. The current, which must pass down the axon from the nearest node in the myelinated region, is normally insufficient to discharge the demyelinated membrane to threshold. This can be most easily understood if one regards the axolemma and myelin as the dielectric of a tubular capacitor, with the extracellular fluid and axoplasm serving as the plates (Figure 16.3). Because capacitance is inversely proportional to the distance between the two plates of a capacitor, the capacitance of a demyelinated fiber is many times that of a myelinated fiber, where numerous layers of myelin membrane separate the axoplasm and the extracellular space.

The current passing along the last myelinated segment to a demyelinated segment comes mainly from the last node, which may be as much as a millimeter away. This is normally insufficient to discharge the large capacitative charge on the demyelinated membrane and depolarize the demyelinated membrane to threshold (impedance mismatch). Thus, conduction fails at the junction of the myelinated and demyelinated segments even if the number of sodium channels in the demyelinated membrane has increased enough to support continuous conduction.

Conduction block due to impedance mismatch can be overcome in several ways. First, membrane capacitance can be decreased by increasing the distance between the two "plates" of the capacitor. This is accomplished by remyelination and is an effective and important mechanism in experimental animals and humans. In addition, the sodium current can be increased enough to discharge the additional capacitative charge on the demyelinated membrane. This is an important mechanism but depends on remyelination at the plaque margins.

Second, in preterminal axons, there is a need to increase the sodium current to depolarize the rather large unmyelinated membrane area of the terminal. This is accomplished by an anatomic arrangement where the last few internodes are much shorter than normal, allowing a summation of current from several adjacent nodes (30). Similarly, in demyelinated fibers, the sodium current can be increased by decreasing the distance between nodes just proximal to the area of demyelination. New myelin regenerated at the plaque margins has such short internodes. This allows summation of current from several nodes, which can discharge the added capacitance of the demyelinated membrane, thus triggering continuous conduction in the demyelinated segment.

Third, conduction can be improved by blocking potassium channels with compounds such as 4-aminopyridine. This slows the efflux of potassium, which tends to repolarize the membrane during conduction and improve the safety margin. This produces a noticeable symptomatic improvement (Davis). Unfortunately, the safety margin for 4-amino-pyridine is quite low; serious dose-dependent toxicity occurs, and as a result, although available from compounding pharmacies, it has not been commercialized.

Conduction that has been restored through a demyelinated segment is suboptimal (29). Experimental studies of demyelinated fibers show marked temperature sensitivity. This is thought to relate to the high Q10 in the sodium channels. Essentially all of the sodium channels in a node open during impulse conduction. The rate of closure is markedly increased by even a small increase in the temperature. As a result, the amount of sodium allowed to pass is reduced rapidly as temperature increases, and a rise in temperature of as little as 0.5°C above normal will cause conduction failure in some fibers (31). By the same token, cooling allows the channels to remain open longer, allowing more inward current and improving the safety margin for conduction.

The increased influx of sodium and efflux of potassium that occur as a result of the increased number of nodes and ion channels at the plaque margin and in the demyelinated segments is another important factor leading to rapid nerve fiber fatigue with conduction failure. Demyelinated fibers have a poor ability to conduct trains of impulses, in part due to an increased refractory period in the demyelinated segment. In addition, studies in experimentally demyelinated fibers have demonstrated a progressive reduction in longitudinal current amplitude

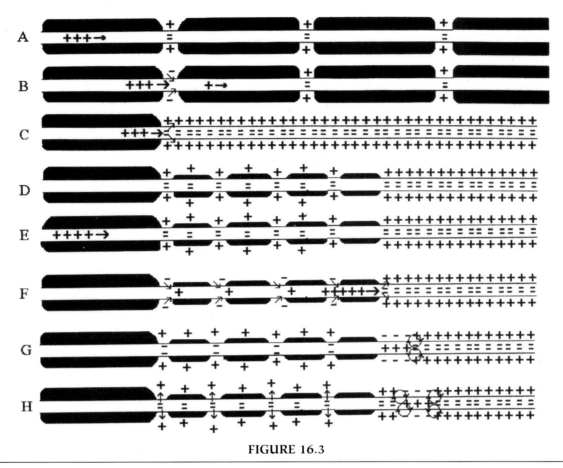

**FIGURE 16.3**

Cartoon of impulse conduction in myelinated, demyelinated, and partly remyelinated fibers. At rest, there is about a –70-mV positive charge across the membrane. **A.** A positive charge moves down the axon. **B.** This results in an initial outward current at the nodes, which opens sodium channels in the membrane resulting in an inward current (small arrows) with a reversal of the charge, and the positive current moves down toward the next node. **C.** Because the charge on the demyelinated membrane is much larger, the charge moving down the axon is insufficient to depolarize the membrane to threshold and conduction fails. **D.** Partial remyelination has occurred with abnormally short internodal segments and thin myelin. The charge on the partly remyelinated membrane is more than normal but less than on the totally demyelinated portion. **E.** An impulse moves down the normally myelinated portion of the nerve, which is sufficient to depolarize the nodes that, because they are very close together, depolarize almost simultaneously. The resulting summation of the current from several nodes is now sufficient to depolarize the initial portion of the demyelinated segment **F**, resulting in slow continuous conduction in the demyelinated segment **G**, with a wave of local depolarization followed by a wave of repolarization produced by potassium efflux **H**. For an excellent technical discussion of the effect of remyelination at the plaque margins on conduction, see Waxman et al. (25) and Waxman (30).

followed by conduction block that is attributed to an increase in intracellular sodium or an increase in extracellular potassium (25,31). The capacity of the sodium pump is soon overwhelmed by the increased sodium influx, leading to loss of the axon's membrane potential with conduction failure (nerve fiber fatigue). These and other features of demyelinated and partly remyelinated fibers explain some of the clinical features of motor fatigability and activity-related failure of neurologic function that are clinically prominent in MS.

Slowed conduction and conduction failure in demyelinated fibers has been well demonstrated in MS in the form of delays in and loss of evoked potentials. This has important clinical consequences. Delayed and degraded feedback from proprioceptors accounts for much of the imbalance and tremor in MS (33). In some patients this results in an inability to monitor arm or leg position concurrently with the movement, so that force cannot be adjusted to the demands of the task. This results in inaccurate movement and terminal tremor. The terminal tremor is often described as cerebellar but usually is due to problems related to delayed and degraded proprioceptive feedback. In addition, conduction failure due to nerve fiber fatigue, an increase in body temperature, or both accounts for many of the limitations in activity, such as walking, that MS patients experience.

## ADAPTATION

By adaptation I mean the substitution or modification of one function or functional system to compensate for another. This may be conscious or unconscious. In its most obvious form, this includes use of canes, walkers, and other equipment. In the mental sphere, it may take the form of notes, a diary, or other memory aids, but other important but much subtler and less well-known forms of adaptation exist.

The best known unconscious and essentially automatic adaptation in MS is substitution of vision for proprioception. Many with MS have impaired or delayed proprioceptive sensation from their feet and legs and cannot depend on proprioception for balance. These individuals routinely use vestibular and visual functions to compensate for the impaired or delayed proprioceptive sensation, usually without being aware of it (33). Such individuals have difficulty when they are out in the open, away from close visual references, and in the dark. For such individuals, a cane can provide another point of contact with the surface and augment proprioception. Similarly, when proprioception is impaired in the upper extremities, certain functions such as buttoning buttons or holding light objects becomes difficult. By watching their movements, they may be able to substitute vision for the inadequate proprioception.

Another form of adaptation is substituting consciously directed movements for what previously were automatic movements. This often happens with ambulation, for example. We normally are not particularly aware of the movement of our legs when we walk. With increasing motor deficits, conscious effort must be brought into play to get the legs to move where they should. Thus, conscious control is substituted to compensate for the deficit in an automatic behavior. Adaptation of this type has the benefit of partly restoring a function that has been lost, but it has a cost. That cost is in multitasking ability. It is a requirement for increased conscious attention to the activity and inability to attend to other activities because conscious effort must be directed to the activity in question. This is the reason some with MS complain that they cannot walk and talk at the same time.

## NEURAL PLASTICITY WITH RESTORATION OF FUNCTION

In the peripheral nervous system, partial denervation of a muscle is followed by sprouting of adjacent fibers that take over the vacated neuromuscular junctions. This results in recovery of motor strength and, electrophysiologically, in the development of polyphasic motor potentials. In the CNS, similar sprouting, with the formation of new synapses on vacated postsynaptic terminals is an established but less well-known phenomenon. Liu and Chambers (34) demonstrated extensive sprouting with formation of new contacts after spinal cord and nerve root lesions. After section of a dorsal root, fibers from adjacent dorsal roots sprouted, enlarged their territories, and took over the vacated synapses. Similar sprouting occurred after lesions in descending tracts and, in some cases, sprouting resulted in the extension of processes over quite long distances. Reinnervation of vacated synapses on anterior horn cells by sprouting dorsal root fibers is thought to be an important mechanism involved in the maintenance of extensor strength and the hyperreflexia seen after pyramidal tract damage. However, regrowth of fibers that have been interrupted in a plaque rarely occurs. Oligodendrocytes fail to support or possibly actively inhibit regrowth of disrupted axons (35), which in MS have been disrupted during the process of demyelination.

Sprouting probably also plays a role in cortical reorganization, although reinforcement of transmission through existing connections is thought to play an important role. That reinnervation can occur in central gray matter has been known for decades (36,37), but the extent of its role in cortical reorganization is unknown. There is very good evidence from positron emission tomography and functional magnetic resonance imaging data that cortical reorganization occurs with peripheral injury and that cortical resources can expand in response to central damage as in stroke or loss of peripheral structures (38,39). That the areas involved in information processing change and expand in response to damage from MS has been demonstrated using functional magnetic resonance imaging (40–42). This has other consequences. When extensive cortical areas are substituted to process information, these areas cannot simultaneously be processing other information efficiently. Thus, many previously automatic tasks require conscious attention, and multitasking becomes increasingly difficult. In addition, many with MS complain that visually busy environments are upsetting, so they avoid supermarkets, not because of difficulty getting about but because their visual processing is altered and less efficient and they have difficulty making sense of the visual cacophony surrounding them.

Another factor affecting function in MS is the inability to concentrate in the presence of distractions. It is important to recognize that ignoring distraction is an active process and involves processes that go back to the very first synapses in the pathway through which the information is arriving. The efficiency with which transmission of the distracting information can be shut down is impaired by the loss of fibers and impaired conduction in MS, thus leading to difficulty in shutting out unwanted stimuli. Restoration of conduction through demyelinated fibers likely plays a role in restoring the ability to concentrate and to deal with distractions; however, this situation is best dealt with by environmental adaptation, i.e., removing the distracting stimulus.

## FAILURE OF COMPENSATORY MECHANISMS

Despite relatively effective compensatory mechanisms, over time these mechanisms are overwhelmed and permanent deficits accumulate. Initially this is seen as a poorer recovery from acute attacks. Progressive loss of axons, which occurs with each attack, eventually reaches a point where the remaining axons can no longer carry the added load. Sprouting and remodeling of connections can no longer compensate. The disease then usually enters a secondary progressive phase that is most commonly manifested as a slowly ascending paralysis. Although the cause is not known, I hypothesized that it is a dying back axonopathy (43). In the CNS, when synaptic terminals are lost, sprouting occurs in adjacent terminals to replace the lost contacts (36,44). This puts an added metabolic burden on the axon terminals. The structural materials needed to enable sprouting come from the cell soma and are carried by the slow axonal transport system. Slow transport is impaired in areas of demyelination in the peripheral (45) and central (46) nervous systems. Thus, although there is likely to be an effective stimulus to sprout, the structural material needed to do so successfully is inadequate. In addition, because they presumably have sprouted previously as part of the compensatory process, the cells are already in metabolic overload. This occurs in postpolio syndrome, in which the added burden of disrupted transport is not present. It is marked by a dying back axonopathy with increasing paralysis (48). I postulated that secondary progressive MS is just such a dying back process and therefore is not amenable to alleviation by drugs, which are relatively effective in relapsing remitting MS (43).

## CONCLUSION

A variety of mechanisms is important in the recovery of function in MS. These include restoration of conduction after suppression of the inflammatory process and restoration of conduction in demyelinated fibers, sprouting of fibers to replace damaged or destroyed inputs to various structures, and cortical reorganization. These adaptive and reparative processes can restore function, but their ability to compensate is limited and has a cost that is most obvious in multitasking. With progressive damage, the ability to compensate is progressively overwhelmed. Permanent irreparable damage ensues with progressive disability and a conversion from a relapsing-remitting disease to a secondary progressive process.

## References

1. Charcot JM. *Lectures on Diseases of the Nervous System.* Sigerson G, trans. London: New Sydenham Society; 1877.
2. Beck RW, RW, Cleary PA. Optic Neuritis Study Group. Optic neuritis treatment trial: One-year follow-up results. *Arch Ophthalmol* 1993; 111:773–775.
3. Bunge MB, Bunge RP, Ris H. Ultrastructural study of remyelination in an experimental lesion in adult cat spinal cord. *J Biophys Biochem Cytol* 1961; 10:67–94.
4. Hommes OR. Remyelination in human CNS lesions. *Prog Brain Res* 1980; 53:39–63.
5. McDonald WI. The effects of experimental demyelination on conduction in peripheral nerve: a histological and electrophysiological study. II. Electrophysiological observations. *Brain* 1963; 86:501–524.
6. McDonald WI, Sears TA. The effects of experimental demyelination on conduction in the central nervous system. *Brain* 1970; 93:583–598.
7. Cammer W, Brosnan CF, Basile C, Bloom BR, Norton WT. Complement potentiates the degradation of myelin proteins by plasmin: Implications for a mechanism of inflammatory demyelination. *Brain Res* 1986; 364:91–101.
8. Kasckow J, Abood LG, Hoss W, Herndon RM. Mechanism of phospholipase A2-induced conduction block in bullfrog sciatic nerve II. Biochemistry. *Brain Res* 1986; 373:392–398.
9. Kasckow J, Abood LG, Hoss W, Herndon RM. Mechanism of phospholipase A2-induced conduction block in bullfrog sciatic nerve II. Biochemistry. *Brain Res* 1986; 373:392–398.
10. Blakemore WF, Eames RA, Smith KJ, McDonald WI. Remyelination in the spinal cord of the cat following intraspinal injection of lysolecithin. *J Neurol Sci* 1977; 33:31–43.
11. Trapp B, Peterson J, Ransohoff R, et al. Axonal transection in the lesions of multiple sclerosis. *N Engl J Med* 1998; 338:278–290.
12. Lampert PW. Demyelination and remyelination in experimental allergic encephalomyelitis. Further electron microscopic observations. *J Neuropath Exp Neurol* 1965; 24:371–385.
13. Prineas J, Raine CS, Wisniewski H. An ultrastructural study of experimental demyelination and remyelination. III. Chronic experimental allergic encephalomyelitis in the central nervous system. *Lab Invest* 1969; 21:472–483.
14. Herndon RM, Price DL, Weiner LP. Regeneration of oligodendroglia during recovery from demyelinating disease. *Science* 1977; 195:693–694.
15. Theiler's virus
16. Ludwin SK. An autoradiographic study of cellular proliferation in remyelination of the central nervous system. *Am J Pathol* 1979; 95:683–696.
17. Blakemore WF, Eames RA, Smith KJ, McDonald WI. Remyelination in the spinal cord of the cat following intraspinal injection of lysolecithin. *J Neurol Sci* 1977; 33:31–43.
18. Hommes OR. Remyelination in human CNS lesions. *Prog Brain Res* 1980; 129:269–278.
19. Ludwin SK. Proliferation of mature oligodendrocytes after trauma to the central nervous system. *Nature* 1984; 308:274–275.
20. Arenella L, Herndon RM. Mature oligodendrocytes: division following experimental demyelination in adult animals. *Arch Neurol* 1984; 41:1162–1165.
21. MacKay RP, Hirano S. Forms of benign multiple sclerosis: Report of two "clinically silent" cases discovered at autopsy. *Arch Neurol* 1967; 17:588–600.
22. Gilbert JJ, Sadler M. Unsuspected multiple sclerosis. *Arch Neurol* 1983; 40:533–536.
23. Herndon RM, Rudick RA. Multiple sclerosis: The spectrum of severity. *Arch Neurol* 1983; 50:531–532.
24. Ritchie JM, Rogart RB. The density of sodium channels in mammalian myelinated nerve fibers and the nature of the axonal mem-

brane under the myelin sheath. *Proc Natl Acad Sci USA* 1977; 74:211–215.

25. Waxman SG, Kocsis JD, Black JA. Pathophysiology of demyelinated axons. In: Waxman SG, Kocsis JD, Stys PK (eds.), *The Axon: Structure, Function and Pathophysiology.* New York: Oxford University Press; 1995; 438–461.

26. Ritchie JM. Sodium and potassium channels in regenerating and developing mammalian myelinated nerves. *Proc Royal Soc B* 1982; 215:273–287.

27. Querfurth HW, Armstrong R, Herndon RM. Sodium channels in normal and regenerated feline ventral spinal roots. *J Neurosci* 1987; 7:1705–1716.

28. Waxman SG. Voltage-gated ion channels in axons. Localization, function and development. In: Waxman SG, Kocsis JD, Stys PK (eds.), *The Axon: Structure, Function and Pathophysiology.* New York: Oxford University Press; 1995; 218–243.

29. Waxman SG. Clinicopathological correlations in multiple sclerosis and related disorders. In: Waxman SG, Ritchie JM, (eds.) *Demyelinating Diseases: Basic and Clinical Electrophysiology.* New York: Raven Press; 1981; 169–182.

30. Waxman SG. Conduction in myelinated, unmyelinated and demyelinated fibers. *Arch Neurol* 1977; 34:585.

31. Rasminsky M. The effects of temperature on conduction in demyelinated single nerve fibers. *Arch Neurol* 1973; 28:287–292.

32. Sears TA, Bostock H. Conduction failure in demyelination: is it inevitable? In: Waxman SG, Ritchie JM (eds.), *Demyelinating Diseases: Basic and Clinical Electrophysiology.* New York: Raven Press; 1981; 357–375.

33. Herndon RM, Horak F. Vertigo, imbalance and incoordination in multiple sclerosis. In: Johnson K, Burks J (eds.), *Multiple Sclerosis, Diagnosis and Management* New York: Demos Publications; 2000; 333–339.

34. Liu CN, Chambers W. Intraspinal sprouting of dorsal root axons; development of new collaterals and preterminals following partial denervation in the cat. *Arch Neurol Psychiat* 1958; 79:46–61.

35. Villegas-Perez MP, Vidal-Sanz M, Bray GM, Aguayo AJ. Influ-

ences of peripheral nerve grafts on the survival and regrowth of axotomized retinal ganglion cells. *J Neurosci* 1988; 8:265–280.

36. Cotman CW, Nadler J. Reactive synaptogenesis in the hippocampus. In: Cotman CW (ed.), *Neuronal Plasticity* New York: Raven Press; 1978; 227–271.

37. Raisman G. Neuronal plasticity in the septal nuclei of the adult rat. *Brain Res* 1969; 14:25–48.

38. Borsook D, Becerra L, Fishman S, et al. Acute plasticity in the human somatosensory cortex following amputation. *Neuroreport* 1998; 9:1013–1017.

39. Rossini PM, Caltagirone C, Castriota-Scanderbeg A, et al. Hand motor cortical area reorganiztion in stroke: A study with fMRI, MEG and TCS maps. *Neuroreport* 1998; 9:2141–2146.

40. Yousry TA, Berry I, Filippi M. Functional magnetic resonance imaging in multiple sclerosis. *J Neurol Neurosurg Psychiat* 1998; (suppl 1):S85–S87.

41. Lee M, Reddy H, Johansen-Berg H, et al. The motor cortex shows adaptive functional changes to brain injury in multiple sclerosis. *Ann Neurol* 2000; 47:606–613.

42. Reddy H, Narayanan S, Arnouteliss et al. Evidence for adaptive functional changes in the cerebral cortex with axonal injury from multiple sclerosis. *Brain* 2000; 123:2314–2320.

43. Herndon RM. Why is secondary progressive multiple sclerosis a relentless? Progressive illness? *Arch Neurol* 2002; 59:301–304.

44. Liu CN, Chambers W. Intraspinal sprouting of dorsal root axons; development of new collaterals and preterminals following partial denervation in the cat. *Arch Neurol Psychiat* 1958; 79:46–61.

45. de Waegh SM, Lee VM-Y, Brady ST. Local modulation of neurofilament phosphorylation, axonal caliber and slow axonal transport by myelinating Schwann cells. *Cell* 1992; 68:451–463.

46. Rao NA, Guy J, Sheffield PS. Effect of chronic demyelination on axonal transport in experimental allergic optic neuritis. *Invest Ophthalmol Visual Sci* 1981; 21:606–611.

47. Dalakas MC. Pathogenetic mechanisms of post-polio syndrome: morphological, electrophysiological, virological, and immunological correlations. *Ann NY Acad Sci* 1995; 753:167–185.

# Index

Note: Boldface numbers indicate illustrations; italic t indicates a table.